D0421773

DESIGN OF BIOMEDICAL DEVICES AND SYSTEMS

DESIGN OF BIOMEDICAL DEVICES AND SYSTEMS

Paul H. King
Vanderbilt University
Nashville, Tennessee, U.S.A.

Richard C. Fries
Datex–Ohmeda, Inc.
Madison, Wisconsin, U.S.A.

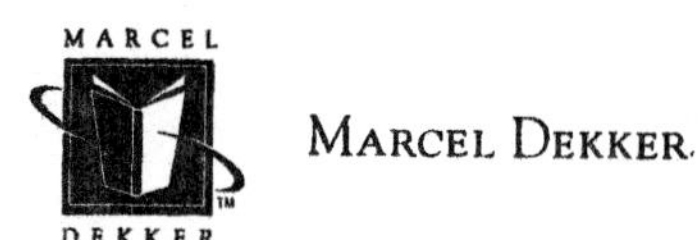

MARCEL DEKKER   NEW YORK

ISBN: 0-8247-0889-X

This book is printed on acid-free paper.

Headquarters
Marcel Dekker
270 Madison Avenue, New York, NY 10016
tel: 212-696-9000; fax: 212-685-4540

Eastern Hemisphere Distribution
Marcel Dekker AG
Hutgasse 4, Postfach 812, CH-4001 Basel, Switzerland
tel: 41-61-260-6300; fax: 41-61-260-6333

World Wide Web
http://www.dekker.com

The publisher offers discounts on this book when ordered in bulk quantities. For more information, write to Special Sales/Professional Marketing at the headquarters address above.

Current printing (last digit):
10 9 8 7 6 5 4

PRINTED IN THE UNITED STATES OF AMERICA

To

Sue

my wife and best friend

Paul H. King

To my wife

June

whose friendship, support, and love

make me whole

Richard C. Fries

Preface

This text is aimed generally at senior-bioengineering students who are in the formative stages of deciding what to do for a senior design project and who need to consider what the societal factors are that may or may not impact their project now or in the future. Portions of the text may be used in lower level classes, such as the sections on brainstorming and elementary idea generation techniques. Portions of the text may be used in early graduate level classes if one has had little exposure to the FDA and CE mark information. The text is meant to be fairly comprehensive, so that the needs of a variety of students working on a variety of topics (from databases to process analysis to device improvement) may have adequate information to begin a fairly comprehensive project.

Design of Biomedical Devices and Systems is the joint effort of two licensed engineers, one with over 30 years of experience as a reliability engineer in the biomedical device industry, and one with 30-plus years of teaching and research experience in teaching Biomedical Engineering, the latter 12 of them as sole instructor of a senior design course. The text is an intermingling of industrial experiences and earlier texts by the former (*Reliable Design of Medical Devices*) and class notes and class experiences by the latter.

The text opens with a general overview of the process and definition of design (Chapter 1). Next an outline of some fundamental idea generation, and design, decision and comparison tools is achieved, with a brief introduction to the process of inventive problem solving (Chapter 2). The use of Quality Function Deployment (QFD) diagrams is also introduced at this stage as a comparison tool.

Fundamental to successful design processes is the generation of a good design team, and the management thereof. Chapter 3 naturally sequences into the need for documentation techniques and requirements, and the use of databases in this endeavor. Reporting techniques for the student through those in industry are briefly covered in a discussion of posters, oral presentations, and progress reports.

Fundamental to a good design is correct and customer-driven product definition. Chapter 4 summarizes the product definition process, and reiterates and enlarges on the use of QFD in this process. Product documentation, record keeping, and levels of effort mandated by quality regulations and medical device regulations are reviewed in the following chapter.

Chapter 6 gives an overview of hardware and software design techniques that ensue from the earlier product specification tasks. Specifically addressed are means by which reliability goals may be achieved. Various models of the overall design process at this stage are reviewed, followed by a brief review of the use of a computerized design assist tool (innovation workbench) with a fairly significant design study, a brief synopsis of axiomatic design, and an outline of structured design (à la Pahl and Beitz.) The chapter concludes with an introduction to redesign and reverse engineering.

A brief overview of computer-aided design is given in Chapter 7, with an introduction to rapid prototyping.

Chapters 8 and 9 offer a good introduction to human factors issues and industrial design. Several of the techniques used to guard against human-caused errors are reviewed, as are techniques to increase usability. Workstation design and human expectations are also discussed, as are the methods used to test these in use.

Biomaterials and materials selection are the theme of Chapter 10, with heavy coverage of the various FDA (and some international) tests and test methods used for materials that may come into contact with users. Tests for toxicity, hemocompatabilty, irritation, reactivity, and sensitization are summarized.

Chapter 11 covers some safety topics not elsewhere dealt with in the text, specifically addressing safety as a component of the design process and one of several structured approaches to the consideration of safety in a design. One medical disaster is used as an example.

Prototyping and testing of samples is summarized in Chapter 12. Types of tests and considerations to determine mean-time-to-failure are given. This is a good introduction to the concept of reliability testing. This concept is then extended in Chapter 13, with overviews of quality control and improvement and a formal introduction to reliability and the possible outcome of its converse, liability. Not only are medical device errors discussed, but also errors by medical personnel are reviewed.

Chapter 14 reviews the FDA, both its history and the methods required to obtain clearance to market medical devices. Classification of medical devices and the related requirements are reviewed. Also included are the requirements for institutional review boards for human subject tests.

Good design will likely generate intellectual property; Chapter 15 gives a summary of protection of intellectual property via patents, copyrights, trademarks, and trade secrets.

Chapters 16 and 17 continue the theme of product testing and validation, and total system testing. Chapter 18 continues the discussion of regulations tracking, with an emphasis on European requirements for certification of medical devices. Chapter 19 covers manufacturing processes and how quality control issues continue at this phase of the design process and must be addressed. Chapter 20 covers liability issues that remain after the final users have put the device in use, and some of the safety issues that arise. Investigation of medical device accidents is also reviewed, as is investigation of traffic accidents.

Chapter 21 is a brief synopsis of professional issues that must be considered by the biomedical professional. Specifically, membership in professional societies, licensure, and professional ethics are discussed. Forensics and consulting are also briefly covered.

Chapter 22 covers a few miscellaneous issues not relevant to other chapters, such as learning from failure and designing for failure.

Chapter 23 is meant to be a resource chapter; nine different design case studies are reviewed. This material may be read as one or used in conjunction with earlier chapters as examples. .

Design in biomedical engineering and bioengineering is a moving target. This is an interesting and demanding field in terms of breadth and depth. Chapter 24 briefly captures some snapshots of "hot" design areas right now and in the near future.

ACKNOWLEDGMENTS

We are deeply indebted to many people for their encouragement, help, and constructive criticism in the preparation of this book.

We want to thank the students of BME 272 at Vanderbilt University for their review and constructive criticism of the draft of this book. Their input made this a better text.

Mostly, we thank our wives, Sue and June, who constantly encouraged us and who sacrificed much quality time together during the preparation of this book.

Paul H. King
Richard C. Fries

Contents

Chapter 1

Introduction to Biomedical Engineering Design

"Give a man a fish; you have fed him for today.
Teach a man to fish and you have fed him for a lifetime."
Author unknown

This text is designed to cover the design of Biomedical Engineering Devices and/or Systems. It is intended as a reference to guide thoughts and actions, by using prior experiences, classroom instruction, and otherwise, to the problem of designing something relevant to this field.

What is relevant to this field? Biomedical Engineering can be very broad in scope, dependent on interests and circumstances. Biomedical Engineers are expected to have some familiarity with Medical Devices, their design, their regulation, and use. They are further expected to consider safety aspects of the devices, and should consider the potential misuse of a device. Designers may be expected to involve themselves in the improvement of a process, such as the tending of patients in a hypertension clinic. They may get involved in biotechnology to manufacture products derived from mammalian cells, they may wind up in the manufacturing of implant devices for the treatment of diabetes. They may design a specialized brace for a single individual or design a medical device to be used by thousands of patients.

It is vital to understand the many meanings of the term design, and have some experience at problem solving using the design principles outlined in this text.

1.1 What Is Design?

It is useful to discuss design from two viewpoints this early in the text, first by discussing what it is **NOT**, then by discussing what it is and the many forms of it.

Design is **NOT** research, which may be defined as "a careful investigation or study, especially of a scholarly or scientific nature"[1] A design task may require research to accomplish a task, but it typically involves the integration of knowledge, rather than the generation of knowledge. Research may be done into the process of design and as such is sponsored by such groups as the NSF (see http://www.eng.nsf.gov/dmii/index.htm for the design, manufacturing and industrial innovation research division).

On the other hand, design is **NOT** craftsmanship. Designers are not nor should they be viewed as a craftsman. This work will involve brains and skills, not just skills.

Design as an action verb is to:

- To conceive, invent
- To formulate a plan for; devise
- To have as a goal or purpose; intend.[1]

Design work thus does not necessarily involve the manufacture of a physical device; it can be a plan or process, or a study to determine the same. Naturally, it can range from this level to the complete specification of a device and its manufacture.

Design as a noun (thing) incorporates the following:

- A drawing or sketch; especially a detailed plan for construction or manufacture.

- The purposeful arrangement of parts or details.
- The art or practice of making designs.
- An ornamental pattern.
- A plan or project.
- A reasoned purpose; intent.
- Often a secretive plot or scheme (Latin).[1]

Each of these terms has validity in the types of work that will be discussed in this text. Even the ornamental pattern qualifies as it is a product of the intellect, is therefore an invention, and may qualify as patentable intellectual property. How does a secretive plot qualify? Perhaps under the category of "trade secret," for example the recipe for the manufacture of Coca-Cola.

1.2 What Is the Thrust of this Text?

This text is aimed at introducing one to the application of design processes to a wide category of design problems in Biomedical Engineering. It is anticipated that the user of this text will be involved during the reading of this text in one or more design projects and/or exercises. It likely will best be used in parallel with some early design exercises, then referred to occasionally as a major design project is pursued. It is meant to be a part of the learning triad of hear/see/do, but not all of it.

The text also attempts to place the various steps in the design process in a logical order, typically that followed in engineering best practices for conducting and completing a design project. The process is generic and flexible, so that processes may be included or not, depending on the project.

1.3 What Might Be Designed?

A partial listing of senior level design projects follows:

Biomedical Devices:

- Modified patient brace for an individual
- Patient (or pet) tracking device
- Improved implantable EKG transmitter
- Improved safety warning system for an intensive care unit

- Improved patient monitoring for premature infants
- Development of a voice training system for patients with Parkinson's disease
- Development of a surgical tool for use in spina-bifida surgery
- Development of an adjustable tray for a spinal cord injured patient
- Modification of a riding mower for use by a paraplegic
- Development of a laser spot size measurement system

Biomedical Systems

- Improved patient record keeping system
- Revised and improved vaccine database system
- Comprehensive pain clinic data collection/billing system
- Development of a prostate cancer screening test
- Development of a skin disease database
- Development of a research ward database system
- Improved feeding apparatus for cystic fibrosis patients

Biomedical Processes

- A study of patient flow in an emergency room
- Improved patient communication in a breast cancer clinic
- A determination of clinic space and facility needs[2]

Note the keywords: improve, develop, revise, or study. Note also the keywords device, process, and system. Each of these terms will see major elaboration in the ensuing chapters. Design will on occasion involve invention, but seldom.

1.4 The Essentials of Design

A well-written newspaper article quickly answers the following questions:

- Who?
- What?
- Where?
- When?

- Why?
- How?

The process of design typically begins with such a listing, with the how portion being the major part of the endeavor. The most important part? The what section. If this section of the overall task is done well one will not need to backtrack and rework a design (normally). The first five steps are required for proper task clarification, the final term, unless specified, typically is the end result of the design task. Figure 1-1 is the generic design process in flowchart form.

If one properly defines the problem (ie understand the who/what/why/ when/where part) then one can hope for a tracing linearly to the solution evaluation section. If the solution is wrong, or if the problem definition is wrong, one will have to backtrack and rework the overall solution. There will be other rearrangements of this basic structure as the tasks of documentation, standards, testing, codes, trademarks and patents, etc are added. The most vital part of the design work will be to figure out what it is that one is asked to do.

Part of this problem will hopefully be minimized by prior educational experiences, which should have included medical nomenclature, some systems physiology, and medical instrumentation. If one is working with a non-engineer on your design project, some new communication skills may be needed. This will be especially true in dealing with most physician collaborators, who commonly go from diagnosis to treatment (or therapy) on a generally non-modifiable patient, while the designer is charged with the modification of a device or process.

1.5 How this Text Is Structured

This text will approach the process of design as generically as possible; the special constraints relevant to Biomedical Engineering will be added as necessary. Such constraints include, but are not limited to, the Food and Drug Administration (FDA) and its device classification and licensing rules, the Medical Device Directives (European), Clinical Trials issues, and others. As an introduction, the text will consider that most processes involve three main items, which are: information, material, and energy flows. Which term is stressed will largely determine the design process to follow. A cancer-screening

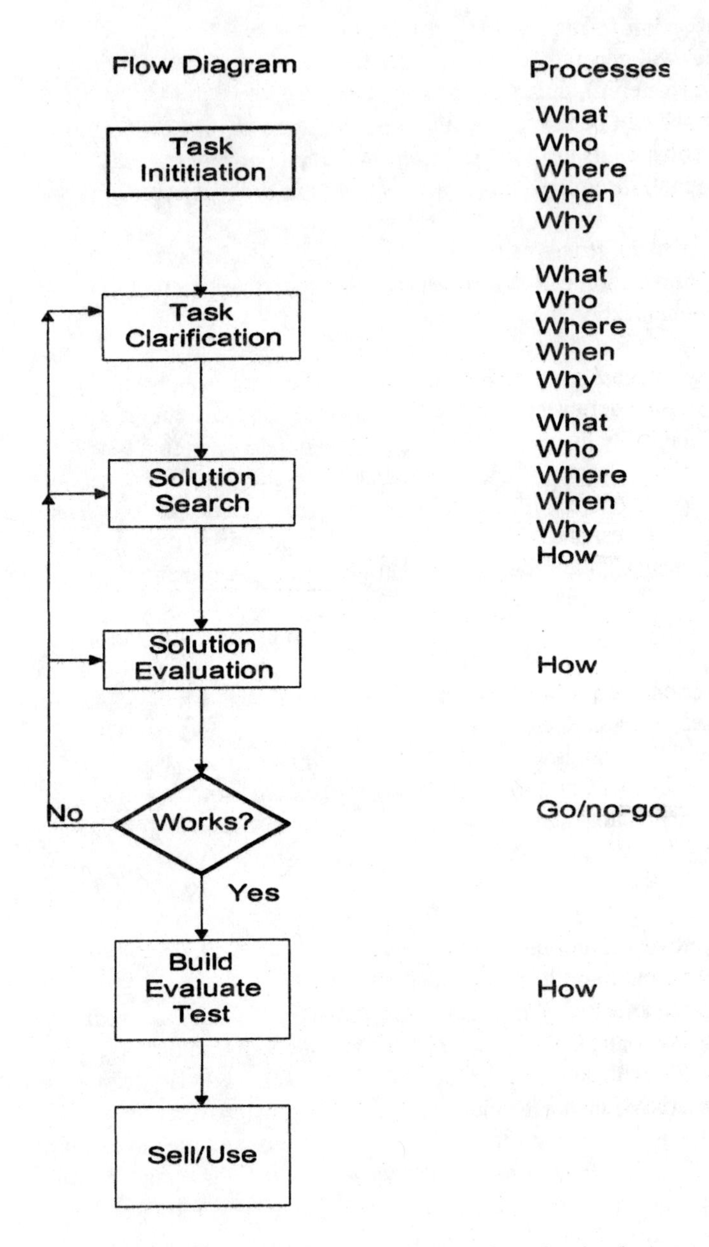

Figure 1-1 A generalized flow chart for the design process.

clinic is primarily an information gathering system, thus a flow chart approach (computer science) will generally be recommended. An enteral feeding unit is primarily a device (material), thus a more mechanical and/or electrical engineering approach will be used. A device to produce radiation for the treatment of cancer has as its primary function the delivery of energy; many engineering (and legal) disciplines are involved [Chapter 2].

The design team, structure, and reporting techniques are the framework upon which your information gathering, sharing and design activities rest. This teamwork and communication is essential [Chapter3].

The design process as an entity forms the basis for all remaining work in this text. The product definition phase and refinement of the who/what/where/when/why listings is mandatory for continuance and successful completion of a project [Chapter 4]. Expansion and justification of the project, as necessary, through development of a business plan, improved product specification and initial design specifications are next covered [Chapter 5]. Lastly, methods of design solution search techniques will be covered, from simple combinations of flowchart terms to structured and unstructured design methods [Chapter 6].

A series of chapters will cover design topics that will not be involved in all design processes, but should be familiar to designers and accessible should the occasion arise. These chapters include computer-aided design [7], human factors issues [8], industrial design [9], materials selection [10] and safety engineering [11], a mandatory issue. Further chapters include topics on prototyping, quality control, and product standards in the US and abroad [12,13,14].

A brief, but very important chapter will cover the issues of patenting, licensing, copyrights, and trade secrets [15]. Premarket testing issues, regulation tracking, and good manufacturing techniques comprise Chapters 16-19. Aftermarket issues involving liability, forensics, and professionalism are covered in Chapters 21 and 22, with some miscellaneous design issues covered in Chapter 22. Summarizing several design examples is the purpose of Chapter 23.

1.6 The Real Purpose of this Text

The real purpose of this text is to guide one in the tackling of a real-world design task relating to Biomedical Engineering. An ultimate goal is it is to prepare one for a career in design as advertised in the following web-based example advertisement (2000):

R&D Engineer
This position offers excellent growth opportunities for the highly motivated individual. Seeking engineer to assist our product development team in developing and testing proprietary medical device concepts. Candidate must be hands-on and able to work independently. Working knowledge of ISO and FDA requirements preferred. Principle responsibilities will include product design, testing, and analysis. Qualified candidate should have 1-3 years' experience with medical device company and BS in mechanical engineering, materials engineering, or biomedical engineering. Additional responsibilities may include animal testing, clinical evaluation, patent/literature searches, and support of ongoing development projects as required. Experience with biomaterials and mechanical design a plus."[3]

Homework Exercises

1. Often design projects are generated by persons concerned about improving the welfare of persons close to them (patients, family, friends). Think about your acquaintances and develop a design project definition. Be sure to detail the who/what/where/why/when specifics as much as is necessary.

2. An orthopedic physician has proposed that you study the effect of electrical stimulation on the healing rate of a bone fracture. Write this request up - briefly - as a research project. Rewrite this as a design project. Discuss the differences in the approaches.

3. You have done some form of design project in your personal life (device, plan of action, project, college choice, etc.). Briefly describe, for your instructor, your favorite project and any lessons learned from it.

4. This is a good time to look at your background in order to determine what areas you will be qualified to work in. Convey to your instructor the following information: Are you familiar with html use? FrontPage or the equivalent? VB or VBA use? Excel? Flowcharting? Access? PowerPoint? Web survey form generation? What are your special skills and interests? What professional experience have you had to date? What area are you most interested in for a design project?
5. The who/what/where/why/how/when construct is often used in newspaper writing. From your Sunday newspaper, extract one short news story and one obituary and analyze it for the above content. Turn in both articles and your commentary to the instructor.

References

[1]Microsoft Encarta, 1999.

[2]See http://vubme.vuse.vanderbilt.edu/King/bme272.htm for additional listings.

[3]Job opening listing Kensey Nash Corporation, Exton PA, May 2000. See http://www.kenseynash.com/ for current information.

Chapter 2

Fundamental Design Tools

"*Men have become the tools of their tools.*"
Henry David Thoreau

There are a series of design tools in current use that will be valuable in the design process as discussed in the remainder of this text. Some of these tools will be covered on an introductory level in this chapter. As design is in truth an information gathering and processing activity, these tools will reflect this process. Some of the tools involve interaction with humans, some with computer programs, some with physical devices. This text will cover solution search methodologies and function structure abstraction, including flowcharting techniques.

2.1 Brainstorming and Idea Generation Techniques

Without knowledge of idea generation techniques a designer may rely too heavily on prior knowledge or on making minor adjustments to a device or process that could be dramatically overhauled. Some of the more common idea generation techniques include brainstorming, Method 635, the Delphi method, and Synetics. There are variations on the themes as discussed below, and computer support and training tools exist for these and many other methods.

2.1.1 Brainstorming

A typical brainstorming group will consist of five to fifteen individuals generally chosen by the person who will be the discussion leader. The individuals should consist of the design team searching for a solution, and involve an additional mix of lay or other people who might be able to contribute due to their backgrounds. In a university environment, brainstorming teams consisting of several engineering students and two or three arts and science students are often much more effective than teams of just engineering students. The additional viewpoints are useful, as is the extra brainpower.

In preparation for the session, the leader should set a reasonable duration for the meeting (20-40 minutes) and stress that there will be no hierarchy and no criticism of any ideas presented. At the outset of the meeting, the leader should state or restate the problem to be solved and reiterate the rules for the meeting. The brainstorming discussion then begins, with the leader primarily trying to maintain a flow of information from single individuals, rather than having multiple people trying to talk at once. The leader may not lead the discussion, but may, during periods of long silence, suggest elaboration or expansion of earlier suggestions. All ideas are to be heard and posted, even the "ridiculous" ones, as they may in fact lead to a novel solution. No derogatory or dismissive comments are allowed. Someone, the leader or a designated secretary, should take minutes on the meeting. One suggested method is to write each idea on a post-it note for later reclassification.

At the end of the session, the group can evaluate, rank, and if desired classify all ideas. The rank ordering and evluation of the list then can become an agenda for the design team and its efforts. If the ideas are also classified, a design tool such as concept mapping can be used to categorize ideas and guide further work. Such a mapping for a brainstorming session on grades in a design course is illustrated in Figure 2.1 below. Note that the "ridiculous" ideas remain at this stage.

Brainstorming is generally useful in conditions when new ideas are needed and/or when a design group is deadlocked on methods to use in a design

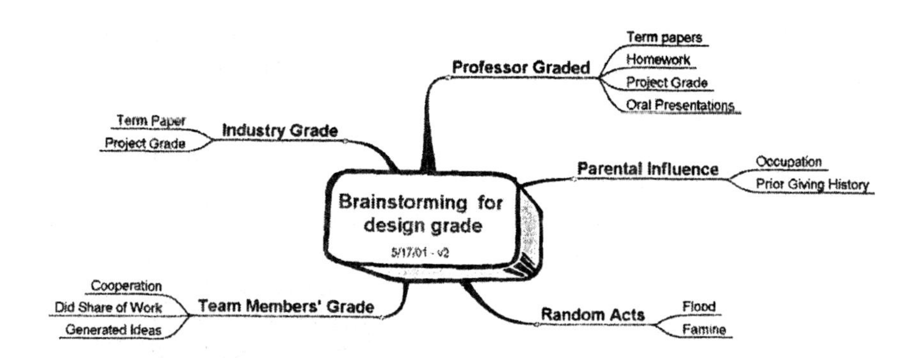

Figure 2.1 Concept map[1] for a brainstorming session on grade sources in a design course.

process. A drawback is that it relies on the abilities and backgrounds of the practitioners and on their willingness to speak up and give suggestions, even in areas outside of their competence.

2.1.2 Method 635

If shyness is a problem, or there is a problem getting people together, this method is ideal. Once again, a problem is presented in sufficient detail to specify what needs to be addressed, but without presenting a solution. Each of six individuals writes down three ideas for solution of the problem, typically on a large sheet of paper or tablet. At a preselected time these tablets are exchanged, each individual may now elaborate on the new ideas received or may generate three new ideas, or may simply relate the three original ideas (not preferred). Five exchanges take place such that no person gets back their original tablet and each of the six tablets holds as many as 18 ideas for problem solution.

This method is useful in that it is very systematic and can generate a large number of solutions if each individual has a modicum of originality and can build on other's ideas. It has a drawback in that each person works in isolation and thus the group synergy is missing.

2.1.3 Delphi method

This method is a polling process and can be valuable in both design processes and in situations where the future of a process is a subject of concern. The process typically consists of three steps. First, a series of suggested starting points for a design problem (or the future or a process) are generated by the process leader or by a panel of experts. These suggestions are regrouped and returned to the panelists, who are asked to add to the list. The resultant response list is then recollected and reordered, and the panel is asked to evaluate and comment on the reordered and expanded list.

An example of the use of this method might be to predict the future of the process of anesthesia during major surgery. Your preliminary letter to the chairs of anesthesiology at major medical centers might request a simple listing of key events in place now, and some suggested future modifications of these processes. Your next letter would list the several responses that you obtained and might ask for both a timetable and a list of additional comments. Your third round would ask for advice on the practicality of each of the predictions, and the necessity for related events to occur to make an event happen.

This method relies on the willingness of experts to respond to a questionnaire in a timely fashion. With most surveys running at a maximum of 30% return you will need strongly motivated individuals on your panel.

2.1.4 Synetics

Synetics is a term that describes a way of looking at analogies of terms relating to a problem as described. The process, briefly described, involves the following steps: First, the problem to be solved is presented to a small group. The group discusses the problem and the environment of the problem to the point that they are familiar with the problem and are able to articulate it. They then operate by looking at analogies and forcing relationships.[2]

An example of the use of this methodology might be looking at ways to close a defect in the heart, for example in the case of atrial septal defect. The problem is that there is a hole in the heart between the two atria, this hole needs to be closed by something that is small when introduced into the patient but large enough to cover and close the hole when deployed or opened. The key to this problem solution is to look at the key words in the last sentence: cover, close, open, small, large. These key terms should enable you to make a number of analogies regarding devices that do one or more of these things; the most obvious would be to make the analogy to an umbrella. Another could be to compare this with patching a tire on your car, thus a patch would be needed.

There are variations on this theme that can be used, such as by randomly picking words from a dictionary and trying to apply them to the problem solution (forcing a fit). This method is somewhat better than brainstorming, if the problem to be solved has an analogy and your group is willing to explore seemingly bizarre trains of thought.

2.1.5 Other methods

One interesting variation on brainstorming is a fairly structured approach proposed by Dr. Edward de Bono that utilizes "six thinking caps". During a meeting on problem solving the facilitator (blue hat) guides the conversations of others who wear white hats while gathering information, or red hats while expressing emotions, black hats while expressing caution, yellow hats while being enthusiastic, or green hats while being creative.[3] The objective of the hats is to allow persons to express feelings representative of the hats exclusively, rather than a combination of unstructured feelings as might be the case in a brainstorming situation. Changing hats allows one to "change gears" without "exposing" oneself.

2.2 Conventional Solution Searches

The above section discussed techniques that required the use of other live humans to begin a solution search. A far more vast supply of information exists in web-based and print literature, especially patent databases. Nature holds many examples of solutions to specific problems as plants and animals evolved to solve their own niche problems. Existing solutions and analogies should also be pursued.

2.2.1 Web-based and print literature

Several web based search engines exist, these include AltaVista, Direct Hit, Excite, Yahoo, Google, HotBot, Infoseek, Lycos, Northern Light, Web Crawler, and the like. Some services, such as Go Express Search spawn as many as eleven other search engines in an attempt to quickly search the web for requested information. Good services allow one to sort by relevance and to search using Boolean operators such that you can, for example search only for "Patent Ductus Arteriosis" AND "repair" in order to limit the amount of information that needs to be searched through.

Many libraries have computerized systems so that one can search, for example, titles for a specific term, such as electrocardiogram. As a prelude to this trip, it is useful to access Amazon.Com (www.amazon.com) on the web and use their search engine to find recent books that they stock. The search term "electrocardiogram" gave twelve hits in 2001 while the more generic term "design" gave 32,000 "hits."

Another excellent source for information is the U. S. Patent and Trademark site (www.uspto.gov) which allows one to search granted or pending patents in a period of time for key words. For example, the search term embolus searched for in the title of granted patents in the time period of 1996-2001 yielded four "hits". The site also lists other patent office sites, such as the Japanese site, some of which allow for similar patent key word searches.

Many trade magazines exist for product design and several are specific for medical product design. Some magazines (Medical Design Online and Medical Industry Today for example) send daily emails regarding work in the field, several maintain web sites that allow search functions for devices and products. (See http://vubme.vuse.vanderbilt.edu/King/design_education.htm for additional sources).

2.2.2 Solutions in nature and analogies

Many design problems may have been solved in nature and may be transferred to design problems at hand. For example, the motion and flexibility of a worm should be studied if one is to look at improved catheter designs. The Eiffel Tower design was said to be mimicry of how bones support weight. The Amazon website lists fourteen books on Biomimetics, several of which may apply depending on the problem at hand. The web site www.nature.com/nature has a search function that allows a search on such terms as biomimicry, one article, "Lifes' lessons in design"[4] is a standout example of design and biomimicry.

2.3 Function Analysis

Many design problems will involve the use of flowcharting tools to assist in understanding the processes under study in order to improve or modify them. Properly done, these flowcharts will assist in the analysis of delays, patient irritations, added costs, and the like. Several levels of analyses may be of use, from simple process charts, to fairly complicated combinations of signal, material, and information flows. Overall, the process of flowcharting can be an excellent communication tool.

2.3.1 Simple process charts

Process charts can be extremely simplistic and tell an unequivocal story. Figure 2.2 below details the process of putting a single bolt on a carburetor, one can almost image going through the process oneself.
The shapes used in the above diagram are fairly common, with many flow charting systems typically using circles or ellipses for processes, arrows for designation of flows, diamonds for storage, and "D"s for delays or wait states. The above example is an extremely short diagram, but is illustrative of ways to display this data and potentially to make use of it. An extensive diagramming of a system could allow one to ask the questions: Where can I get rid of delays? How is the transport of several parts to be facilitated to speed up this operation? How many operations are my workers being asked to do per minute? Why am I seeing carpal tunnel syndrome?

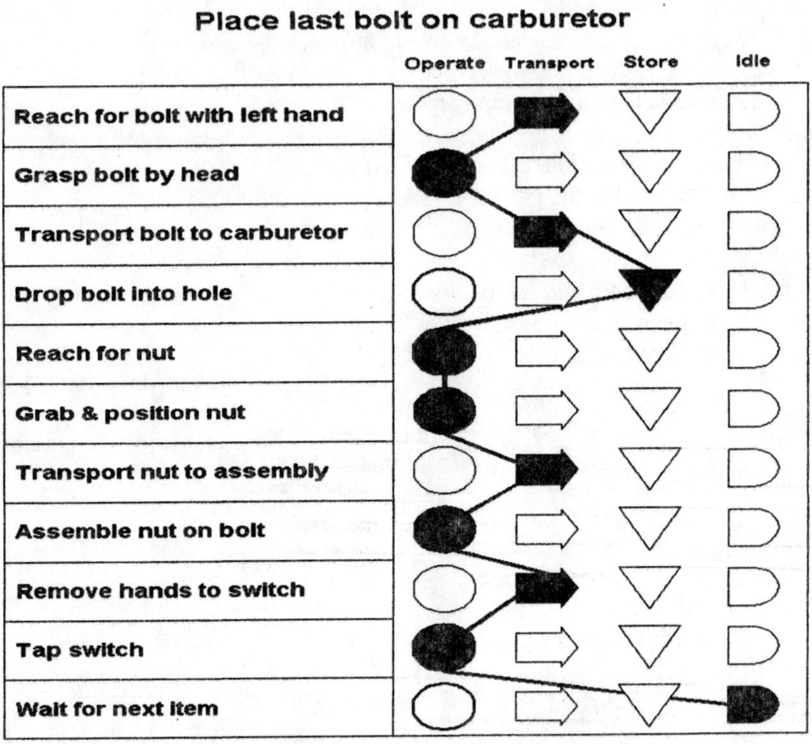

Place last bolt on carburetor

Operate Transport Store Idle

Reach for bolt with left hand
Grasp bolt by head
Transport bolt to carburetor
Drop bolt into hole
Reach for nut
Grab & position nut
Transport nut to assembly
Assemble nut on bolt
Remove hands to switch
Tap switch
Wait for next item

Figure 2.2 Process diagram for placing a single bolt on a system.

2.3.2 Clinic flow charts

Figure 2.3 below represents the path of a patient in a hypertension clinic. Note the linear nature of the path through the clinic and the emphasis on delays. This figure emphasizes the fact that this system is linear, that each event must be completed prior to the next beginning. From a patient point of view, this can be extremely frustrating, as the delay times accumulate. Overall waiting time for a patient is from 14 to 70 minutes for this process which involves only 8 minutes of interaction with professionals, 5 of that time with the physician. As the physician is the only one in charge of emptying rooms, he/she can be blamed for this waste of time.

2.3.3 Flowcharts with decision points

To speed up a clinic process, at least for some patients, ancillary personnel can be used in the patient care taking and advising process. Figure 2.4 demonstrates a modification of the above flow chart wherein a nurse or other medical practitioner can take the weight, pulse rate, medication listing and blood pressure data (if needed) and screen the patient to see if the patient needs to see the physician or can be seen by an RN or other healthcare worker for any update on medications or other matters. The diamond in the flowchart is a decision point, the y and n branches signify a yes or no branch condition.

This revision of the hypertension clinic allows three branching points, which on the average will allow for faster patient clinic visits by decreasing wait times via the use of ancillary personnel. Overall wait time has been reduced from 22-78 minutes to 7-20 minutes in this model. The physician time is utilized for "needy patients" rather than the entire clinic scheduled patient load. This can lead to improved clinic utilization if planned wisely, as many patients will be status quo and will not need a physician interaction. This model is analogous to well-run dentist offices where dental hygienists take care of the majority of patients' minor needs while the dentist takes care of the remainder.

Presented above has been some very rudimentary flowcharting information, the minimum necessary to understand some of the essentials needed for a starting analysis of clinic and other process analysis as a prelude to redesign of the process. Many other variations and embellishments on the above material are part of normal flowcharting programs, such as the use of color to identify particular paths, the use of additional annotation to indicate complaints about sections of the process, and the use of additional symbols specific to a number of other processes, such as design of databases, process diagrams for the food industry, etc. Some common variations for systems involving electromechanical devices involve the simultaneous overlay of material flows, information flows, and energy flows. Many commercial products have a wide variety of template patterns available for use. Two of the more commonly used commercial packages are Microsoft's Visio and Micrografx FlowCharter, a few

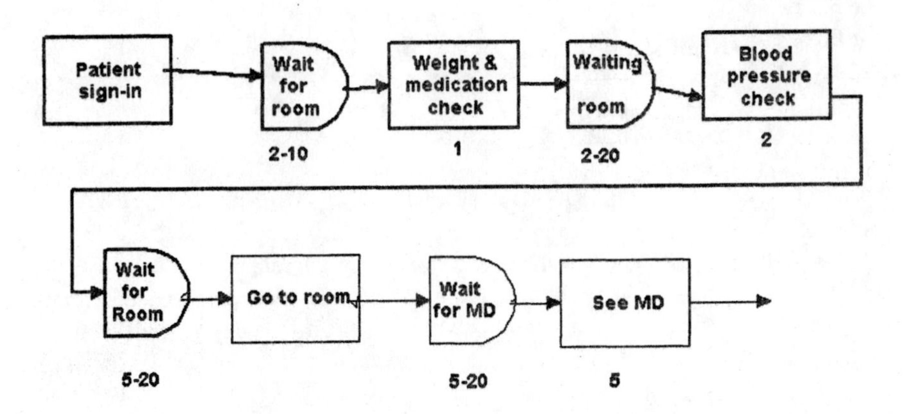

Figure 2.3 Blood pressure (hypertension) clinic flow chart. Numbers indicate length of delay or interaction time in minutes.

other programs are available on the web for free but most have a limited time trial associated with them. Software packages exist that emulate processes such as patient clinic visits such that variables such as the effect of the number of examination rooms or number of clinic staff may be varied and the effect of this on patient throughput estimated (High Performance Systems program Stella, for example).

2.4 Elementary Decision-Making Techniques

In Chapter 4 the need to define well the parameters involved in the design problem statement will be very strongly emphasized. Terms such as demand and wish will a part of the design analysis when design choices are being considered. Alternate terms involve objectives, quality, and function. The purpose of this section is to introduce some elementary concepts in the decision-making processes that may be selected in a solution search.

2.4.1 Selection chart

A selection chart that might be used in a design process is shown schematically in Figure 2.5 on the next page. The essence of the design chart is

Ideal Hypertension Clinic?

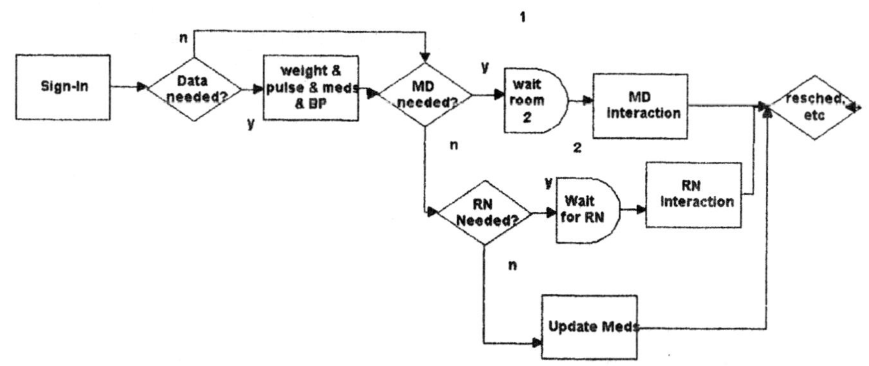

Figure 2.4 A faster hypertension clinic flowchart.

that design demands are listed vertically and concepts or design choices being considered to perform these demands are listed horizontally. If a design choice uncertain, a ? symbol. The final scoring with this simplistic chart simply asks the question – does this column (choice) meet all criteria? If not, the design choice is rejected. If there are only + and ? symbols, the particular choice will need to be investigated further.

As an example, consider the design decision for a proper writing implement for a grade school class in a damp environment. Figure 2.6 might be an example of a product selection matrix.

The above example is simplistic and is meant only as an example. The process can work very nicely if there are few choices and most are go-no go in nature. A drawback is that there are no "shades of gray" or partial solutions allowed, and, as will be seen in a later discussion on invention, conflicts yield only dismissal of the choice, rather than resolution of the conflict via an inventive problem solution.

2.4.2 Evaluation charts

The next level up in complexity to the above selection chart is an evaluation chart. This chart generally is used to assist in the ranking of various wishes, qualities, or other aspects of a proposed solution. Wishes or qualities are

	Choice Number			
Demand #	1	2	3	4
1	+	+	?	+
2	+	-	-	+
3	+	+	-	?
summary	go	no go	no go	recheck

Figure 2.5 A simplified design selection process diagram.

tabulated in a vertical column, each of these are assigned weights (importance) on an arbitrary scale, often ranging 1-10 for example. No zero values are assigned as this would dismiss this row as a valid choice. Each set of columns from this point on carry the value of the particular column's solution and the net weight of the product of the solution and the weighting given to that wish. The totals are then added for each proposed solution and the "winner" is normally the column with the highest total. A fabricated example for a Daddy Warbuck's transportation choices between New York City and Rome for vacation purposes is given in Figure 2.7.

In this example, the maximum possible score for a mode of transportation would be 100 (the total of the weights times the maximum weight of 5 each), thus the choice of an ocean liner meets 87% of the above persons wishes, versus the 59% figure for the commercial airliner. This method is subjective but is useful to help rank order a potentially large list of choices and wishes.

	Choice			
Demand #	Fountain Pen	Pencil	Chalk	Marker
Writes on paper	+	+	?	+
Won't stain hands	-	+	+	-
Damp paper tolerant	?	+	?	?
Summary	no go	go	recheck	no go

Figure 2.6 An example of a product selection matrix.

2.5 Objective Trees

The final minor evaluation process involves the generation of an objectives tree. This is a formulation that involves the assignment of priorities to a series of objectives and sub objectives such that a determination of the value of each of several sub-objectives is quantified in the designers' mind. At the first branching each sub-objective is given a weight such that the sum of all weights is one. At every successive branching the weights continue to sum to unity, but the overall weight of each branch is the product of all branchings prior. An example objectives tree to illustrate this process is given in Figure 2.8.

The objectives tree below is meant to be simple, but illustrative. In actual practice the tree may have many more branchings and levels of branching. The overall value of such diagrams is that they may give insight into overall priorities in a complicated situation. The drawback is that such trees are based upon the designers personal bias as to the value of each branch, which will be borne out by the values in the final column.

2.6 Introduction to Quality Function Deployment Diagrams

The process known as QFD or Quality Function Deployment[5] is a structured approach to assist in translating customer requirements into realistic goals and sometimes even manufacturing specifications, dependent on the level

		Commercial airline		Ocean Liner	
"wish"	weight	value	product	value	Product
High speed	3	5	15	2	6
Convenience	5	4	20	5	25
Comfort	5	3	15	5	25
Low cost	2	2	4	3	6
Food & Drink	5	1	5	5	25
Total			59		87

Figure 2.7 Transportation evaluation chart, maximum weight =5.

and complexity of the structures used. This section will give an overview of only the first level of the QFD process, that of building most of the first, and most valuable diagram, which is intended to relate the qualities that a customer wants to the functions that the device or process must perform. The deployment part of the process involves (generally) the manufacturing or other specification processes, this will be left for a later discussion. This process is in fact an extension of some of the material previously covered. A sample diagram will be used to introduce the topic (see Figure 2.9).

The QFD diagram below is similar to ones that would normally be used in product comparison and product planning exercises. The function of the device is normally plotted on the vertical axis of a grid that is used for the comparison of "your product" and the competitors. In this case, we might posit that the function of marriage is to enable a couple to have legally recognized sex, reproduction, and companionship. The qualities desired in thispartner are elaborated on the left hand axis. The relationship between qualities and functions is designated with a symbol such as ++ if they are highly correlated, a + if slightly so, a minus if negatively so, etc. (Having children might decrease companionship, for example). The ranking of suitors A, B, and C for example would be plotted on the right hand side, and as before with evaluation charts, a current "winner" (B) might be declared. Alternatively, a goal may be set for each quality and plotted on the same section of the graph and the process continued. This continuation (not done) would involve listing values for the current product(s) or competitors in terms of their numerical values for the

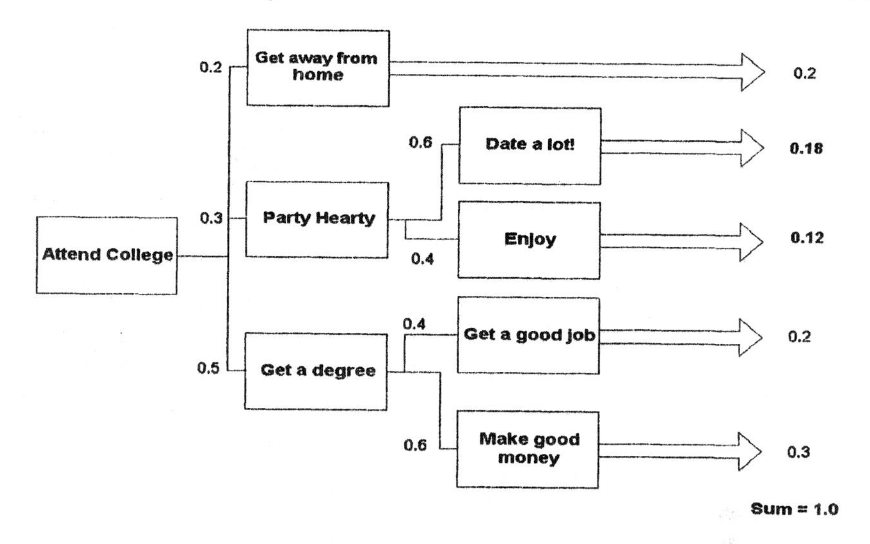

Figure 2.8 Objectives tree for the process of attending college.

functions listed. A listing of technical difficulty, relative costs, and target goals would complete the rows in this section.

Interactions between functions, both positive and negative are also noted on this diagram. For this example, there is a positive correlation between column one and three on the functions. This interaction between functions often lends a "house-like" shape to the diagram, thus this figure if often called the "House of Quality". Interactions between qualities may be plotted in a similar fashion, but without a special label being attached to the shape (lean-to might work).

Negative correlations between functions (aka contradictions) give rise to design considerations in the overall process and indicate that there may be a problem to be solved. This approach will be covered in the next section.

2.7 Introduction to TRIZ

It was mentioned earlier that the patent database is a site for initial idea solution searches using keyword searches. An alternate method would be to look

QFD Example – Marriage Partner Selection

Quality	Legal Sex	Companionship	Reproduction	*Weight*	1 2 3 4 5
	Function				
Likes to eat out		++		5	B A C
Likes travel		+	+	2	C AB
Wants kids	+	–	+	5	A B C
Same religion		++		3	AB C
Intelligent		+	+	3	C AB
Good looking		+		2	BCA
Good job	-	+		3	C AB
...					B=61, A=60, C=54
Stated values A					
B					
C					

Figure 2.9 QFD diagram for the process of marriage partner selection.

for distillations of patent materials in terms of methods for solving design problems. Such a method was developed initially in the late 1940s by Genrich Altshuller in the USSR, this method has been continually upgraded and added to in the intervening years. Altshuller held the position of patent clerk in the Russian Navy patent office, his work allowed him to study and distil design solution methodologies from inspection of thousands of patents. His work formed the basis for a series of papers on the theory of inventive problem solving; the Russian acronym for this is TRIZ[6].

Alshuller's goals were to codify what knowledge he could from the patent database and reduce the design process as much as possible to a step-by-step procedure. Some of his accomplishments are briefly listed below:

1. Altshuller recognized that problem solving ranged from the application of methodology that is commonly used in whatever specialty one is

working in to true discovery entailing the development of new science or discovery of new principals. As the level of difficult increased, the number of solutions to be examined increased. Highly difficult problems generally involved the use of material outside of one's own specialty.

2. He recognized that most inventions went through different stages of development with a finite number of variations on different themes of transition. One such theme is that systems tend toward increasing ideality, another that systems tend toward Microsystems, another is that systems tend to less need human involvement.
3. Altshuller's first major observation was that most inventive problems involved solution of technical contradictions (negative interaction between desired functions or between desired qualities). This work gave rise to two useful devices, an inventive principles listing (aka engineering parameters) and a technical contradiction matrix. The principles list (Appendix 3) listed 40 different parameters that can be applied in the design of a system. This initial listing includes such terms as segmentation, asymmetry, extraction, nesting, and so forth. The technical contradiction matrix is a 39 by 39 matrix of contradictions (Appendix 3), one axis lists all features that conceivably could be changed in a system (such as the weight of a moving object), the other axis repeats this list but is now labeled undesired result. The intersection of two features lists suggested solutions from the principles list. An example intersection point is weight of moving object (say an airplane wing, row 1) where increasing weight compromises strength (column 14) one solution technique is to use composites (solution 40), which is in fact in practice.
4. Altshuller went well beyond this level of work, studying and developing advanced inventive problem solving techniques that are more algorithmic in nature. Object-action diagramming techniques and directed product evolution arose from this work. These subjects will be included later as specific topics in Chapter 6.

2.8 Summary

This chapter was aimed at the introduction of several simple design tools prior to an in-depth study of the overall process of design as applied to medical devices and processes. As such, it is generic in nature and may be applied to many design processes both in a engineering design environment and in personal decision making.

Homework Exercises

1. Do a web search with the search term "Brainstorming". Evaluate several of the sites, try some of the software available and report on the usefulness of the program.
2. Do a web search with the term concept map. Find and explore one or more example concept maps.
3. Draw a process diagram for the process of taking hamburger meat, grinding it, then flattening it and cutting out presized hamburger patties. The meat that is in between the patties is reinserted into the process just after the incoming meat is ground. What is wrong with this process? If necessary do a web search to answer this question.
4. Visit the web site www.jellybelly.com and find their process listing. Do a flowchart of this process, specifically identifying delays. Discuss means to speed up this process. Extra credit, request that samples be sent to your instructor.
5. Visit any web site that has an example concept map that is of interest to you, print out the map, and comment on the value of it.
6. Pick two design terms or terms relating to a project you have worked on. Pick two different search engines and search on these two terms. What are the differences in yield? Would you recommend one search engine over the other? Why?
7. Do a web search on the term Biomimetics, find a good example of this as applied to a design problem, print it out and discuss it.
8. Generate a simple process chart for the process of brushing teeth.
9. Generate a flow chart for the process of obtaining breakfast. Be sure to indicate delays and make suggestions to decrease same.
10. Generate a simple selection diagram to determine whom you will date for a formal dance.
11. Generate an evaluation chart to assist you in the determination between camping in the mountains or going to the beach for your vacation this year.
12. Generate a simple QFD chart for the selection of an automobile.
13. Generate a QFD diagram to help design a better device for closure of an atrial septal defect.

14. A problem that arose in the early use of long-barreled cannons was that they "wilted" during repeated use due to heating and uneven cooling, especially during rainstorms. Use brainstorming with one or two friends to help solve this problem. Reference the TRIZ contradiction matrix and attempt to find a solution. Document your choices.

References

MindManager business edition, Mindjet LLC, Sausalito, CA.

Pahl, G., Beitz, W., Engineering Design, A Systematic Approach, Springer-Verlag, London, 1988.

de Bono, E., Six Thinking Hats, Little Brown and Company, New York, 1985.

Ball, P., "Life's lessons in design," Nature 409, 413-416 (2001).

John Terninko, Step-by-Step QFD, Customer-Driven Product Design, 2nd Edition, St Lucie Press, Boca Raton, FL, 1997.

Clarke, D. TRIZ: Through the Eyes of an American TRIZ Specialist, Ideation International (www.ideationtriz.com), 1997.

Chapter 3

Design Management, Documentation, and Reporting

"Never tell people how to do things. Tell them what to do and they will surprise you with their ingenuity."
George S. Patton, Jr.

Design management is a multi-step process that is a necessary part of every product development process. Design management consists of:

- design team construction and management
- documentation techniques and requirements
- reporting techniques.

All form an integral part of success in developing a product. All are interrelated and interdependent. All will be audited by the FDA and Quality System auditors.

3.1 Design Team Construction and Management

The team is a basic unit of performance for most organizations. A team melds together the skills, experiences, and insights of several people. It is the natural complement to individual initiative and achievement because it engenders higher levels of commitment to common ends. Increasingly, management looks to teams throughout the organization to strengthen performance capabilities.

In any situation requiring the real-time combination of multiple skills, experiences, and judgments, a team inevitably gets better results than a collection of individuals operating within confined job roles and responsibilities. Teams are more flexible than larger organizational groupings because they can be more quickly assembled, deployed, refocused, and disbanded, usually in ways that enhance rather than disrupt more permanent structures and processes. Teams are more productive than groups that have no clear performance objective because their members are committed to deliver tangible performance results. Teams invariably contribute significant achievements in all areas of a business.

3.1.1 Definition of a team

At the heart of a definition of *team* is the fundamental premise that teams and performance are inextricably connected. The truly committed team is the most productive performance unit management has at its disposal, provided there are specific results for which the team is collectively responsible, and provided the performance ethic of the company demands those results.

Within an organization, no single factor is more critical to the generation of effective teams than the clarity and consistency of the company's overall performance standards – or performance ethic. Companies with meaningful, strong performance standards encourage and support effective teams by helping them both tailor their own goals and understand how the achievement of those goals will contribute to the company's overall aspirations. A company's performance ethic provides essential direction and meaning to the team's efforts.

This crucial link between performance and teams is the most significant piece of wisdom learned from teams. It leads directly to the definition:

A team is a small number of people with complementary skills that are committed to a common purpose, performance goals, and approach for which they hold themselves mutually accountable.

3.1.2 Characteristics of teams

There are six basic characteristics of successful teams, including:

- small number
- complementary skills
- common purpose
- common set of specific performance goals
- commonly agreed-upon working approach
- mutual accountability.

The majority of teams who are successful have their membership range from two to twenty-five people. The most successful have numbered approximately twelve. A larger number of people can theoretically become a team, but they usually break into subteams, rather than function as a single team. The main reason for this is that large numbers of people, by virtue of their size, have trouble interacting constructively as a group, much less agreeing on actionable specifics. Large groups also face logistical issues like finding enough physical space and time to meet together. They also confront more complex constraints like crowd or herd behaviors that prevent the intense sharing of viewpoints needed to build a team.

Teams must develop the right skills, that is, each of the complementary skills necessary to do the team's job. These team skill requirements fall into three categories:

- technical or functional expertise
- problem-solving and decision-making skills
- interpersonal skills.

A team cannot get started without some minimum complement of skills, especially technical and functional ones. No team can achieve its purpose without developing all the skill levels required. The challenge for any team is in striking the right balance of the full set of complementary skills needed to fulfill the team's purpose over time.

A team's purpose and performance goals go together. The team's near-term performance goals must always relate directly to its overall purpose. Otherwise, team members become confused, pull apart, and revert to mediocre performance behaviors. Successful teams have followed the following premises:

- a common, meaningful purpose sets the tone and aspiration
- specific performance goals are an integral part of the purpose
- the combination of purpose and specific goals is essential to performance.

Teams also need to develop a common approach – that is, how they will work together to accomplish their purpose. Teams should invest just as much time and effort crafting their working approach as shaping their purpose. A team's approach must include both an economic and administrative aspect as well as a social aspect. To meet the economic and administrative challenge, every member of the team must do equivalent amounts of real work that goes beyond commenting, reviewing, and deciding.

Team members must agree on who will do particular jobs, how schedules will be set and adhered to, what skills need to be developed, how continuing membership is earned, and how the group will make and modify decisions, including when and how to modify its approach to getting the job done. Agreeing on the specifics of work and how it fits together to integrate individual skills and advance team performance lies at the heart of shaping a common approach. Effective teams always have team members who, over time, assume important social as well as leadership roles such as challenging, interpreting, supporting, integrating, remembering, and summarizing. These roles help promote the mutual trust and constructive conflict necessary to the team's success.

No group ever becomes a team until it can hold itself accountable as a team. Like common purpose and approach, this is a stiff test. Team accountability is about the sincere promises team members make to themselves and others, promises that underpin two critical aspects of teams:

- commitment
- trust.

By promising to hold themselves accountable to the team's goals, each member earns the right to express their own views about all aspects of the team's effort and to have their views receive a fair and constructive hearing. By following through on such a promise, the trust upon which any team must be built is preserved and extended.

3.1.3 Team success factors

There are six team success factors inherent to any effective team:

1. multifunctional involvement
2. simultaneous full-time involvement
3. co-location
4. communication
5. shared resources
6. outside involvement.

Multifunctional involvement means representation at least of the following stakeholders:

- customers
- dealers
- suppliers
- marketers
- lawyers
- manufacturing personnel
- engineers
- designers
- managers
- nonmanagers.

All personnel should be involved with the team from its inception.

Key team members – design, manufacturing, and marketing – must be represented full time from the start. The involvement of others should be full time for the duration of the most intense activity. Rewards should go to teams as a whole. Evaluation, even for members who are only full time for a short time, should be based principally on team performance.

Numerous studies indicate the astonishing exponential decrease in communication that ensues when thin walls or some distance exists between team members. For the most effective environment, team members must be in close proximity.

Communication is everyone's panacea for everything – but nowhere more than in teams. Examination of successful teams has shown that the most important element in ensuring a team's effectiveness and success is the constant communication across functional boundaries. Regular meetings with all functional areas represented and written status reports circulated to everyone are the norm for effective teams.

Duplication of every resource for every development project is not always a true possibility. However, team research has reported that the sharing of resources between new product/service teams and main-line activities, including manufacturing, marketing, and sales, is a leading cause of delayed product development and introduction efforts. One option is to devote areas of laboratories or manufacturing areas for the new product development efforts.

Suppliers, distributors, and ultimate customers must become partners in the development process from the start. Much, if not most, innovation will come from these constituents, if the team trusts them and they trust the team

3.1.4 The team leader

Successful team leaders instinctively know that their primary goal is team performance results instead of individual achievement, including their own. Unlike working groups, whose performance depends solely on optimizing individual contributions, real team performance requires impact beyond the sum of the individual parts. Hence, it requires a complementary mix of skills, a purpose that goes beyond individual tasks, goals that define joint work products, and an approach that blends individual skills into a unique collective skill, all of which produces strong mutual accountability.

Team leaders act to clarify purpose and goals, build commitment and self-confidence, strengthen the teams collective skills and approach, remove externally imposed obstacles, and create opportunities for others. Most important, like all members of the team, team leaders do real work themselves. They also believe that they do not have all the answers – so they do not insist on providing them. They believe they do not need to make all key decisions – so they do not do so. They believe they cannot succeed without the combined contributions of all the other members of the team to a common end – so they avoid any action that might constrain inputs or intimidate anyone on the team.

Team leaders must work hard to do the seven things necessary to good team leadership:

1. keep the purpose, goals, and approach relevant and meaningful
2. build commitment and confidence
3. strengthen the mix and level of skills
4. monitor timing and schedules for planned activities
5. manage relationships with outsiders, including removing obstacles
6. create opportunities for others
7. do real work.

A team leader critically influences whether a potential team will mature into a real team or even a high-performance team. Unless a leader believes in a team's purpose and the people on the team, they cannot be effective.

3.1.5 The design team

The typical product design team is a collection of individuals from various departments within a company who come together for the specific purpose of designing and developing a new medical device. The design team is composed of two subteams:

- the core team
- the working team.

3.1.5.1 The core product team

The core product teams are responsible for performing the research required to reduce risks and unknowns to a manageable level, to develop the Product Specification, and to prepare the Project Plan. They are responsible for all administrative decisions for the project, regulatory and standards activity, as well as planning for manufacturing and marketing the device.

The core product team is composed of individuals representing the following functions:

- Marketing
- Engineering
- Electrical
- Mechanical
- Biomedical
- Chemical
- Software
- Reliability Engineering
- Safety Engineering
- Manufacturing
- Service
- Regulatory
- Quality Assurance
- Finance.

The leader of the core team is usually from Engineering or Marketing. The leader is responsible for conducting periodic team meetings, ensuring minutes of such meetings are recorded and filed, establishing and tracking time schedules, tracking expenses and comparing then to budgeted amounts, presenting status reports to the senior staff, and ensuring sufficient resources in all areas are supplied. The leader will also provide performance evaluation of each member of the team to line managers.

The approximate amount of time required of each participant as well as incremental expenses, such as: model development, simulation software, travel for customer verification activities, laboratory supplies, market research, and project status reviews, should also be estimated.

3.1.5.2 The working design team

The members of the working team, primarily engineers, take the Product Specification and develop the more detailed Design Specification. Working teams exist in all areas of engineering, including electrical, mechanical, and software. Working team member are responsible for developing designs from the Design Specification, ensuring all requirements are verified through testing, providing test reports. Certain members may also be responsible for validating the system as a whole. Individual working teams may be divided into subteams to address individual design assignments.

3.2 Documentation Techniques and Requirements

As medical products encompass more features and technology, they will grow in complexity and sophistication. The hardware and software for these products will be driven by necessity to become highly synergistic and intricate which will in turn dictate tightly coupled designs. The dilemma is whether to tolerate longer development schedules in order to achieve the features and technology, or to pursue shorter development schedules. There really is no choice given the competitive situation of the marketplace. Fortunately, there are several possible solutions to this difficulty. One solution that viably achieves shorter development schedules is a reduction of the quantity of requirements that represent the desired feature set to be implemented. By documenting requirements in a simpler way, the development effort can be reduced by lowering the overall product development complexity. This would reduce the overall hardware and software requirements which in turn reduces the overall verification and validation time.

The issue is how to reduce the number of documented requirements without sacrificing feature descriptions. This can be achieved by limiting the number of product requirements, being more judicious about how the specified requirements are defined, or by recognizing that some requirements are really design specifications. A large part of requirements definition should be geared toward providing a means to delay making decisions about product feature requirements that are not understood until further investigation is carried out.

As stated above, verification and validation must test the product to assure that the requirements have been met and that the specified design has been implemented. At worst, every requirement will necessitate at least one test to demonstrate that it has been satisfied. At best, several requirements might be grouped such that at least one test will be required to demonstrate that they all have been satisfied. The goal for the design engineer is to specify the requirements in such a manner as to achieve as few requirements as are absolutely necessary and still allow the desired feature set to be implemented. Several methods for achieving this goal are refinement of requirements, assimilation of requirements and requirements versus design.

3.2.1 Refinement of requirements

As an example, suppose a mythical device has the requirement "the output of the analog to digital converter (ADC) must be accurate to within plus or minus 5%." Although conceptually this appears to be a straightforward requirement, to the software engineer performing the testing to demonstrate satisfaction of this requirement, it is not as simple as it looks. As stated, this requirement will necessitate at least three independent tests and most likely five tests. One test must establish that the ADC is outputting the specified nominal value. The second and third tests will be needed to confirm that the output is within the plus or minus 5% range. Being a good software engineer, the 5% limit is not as arbitrary as it may seem due to the round off error of the percent calculation with the ADC output units. Consequently, the fourth and fifth test will be made to ascertain the sensitivity of the round off calculation.

A better way to specify this requirement is to state "the output of the analog to digital converter (ADC) must be between X and Y," where X and Y values correspond to the original requirement of "plus or minus 5%." This is a better requirement statement because it simplifies the testing that occurs. In this case, only two tests are required to demonstrate satisfaction of this requirement. Test one is for the X value and test two is for the Y value. The requirement statements are equivalent but the latter is more effective because it has reduced the test set size, resulting in less testing time and consequently a potential for the product to reach the market earlier.

3.2.2 Assimilation of requirements

Consider the situation where several requirements can be condensed into a single equivalent requirement. In this instance, the total test set can be reduced through careful analysis and an insightful design. Suppose that the user interface of a product is required to display several fields of information that indicate various parameters, states and values. It is also required that the user be able to interactively edit the fields, and that key system critical fields must flash or blink so that the user knows that a system critical field is being edited. Further assume that the software requirements document specifies that "all displayed fields can be edited. The rate field shall flash while being edited. The exposure time shall flash while being edited. The volume delivered field shall flash while being edited."

These statements are viable and suitable for the requirements specification but they may not be optimum from an implementation and test point of view. There are three possible implementation strategies for these requirements. First, a "monolithic" editor routine can be designed and implemented that handles all aspects of the field editing, including the flash function. Second, a generic field editor can be designed which is passed a parameter that indicates whether or not the field should flash during field editing. Third, an editor executive could be designed such that it selects either a non-flashing or flashing field editor routine depending on whether the field was critical or not. Conceptually, based on these requirements statements, the validation team would ensure that 1) only the correct fields can be displayed, 2) the displayed fields can be edited, 3) critical fields blink when edited, and 4) each explicitly named field blinks.

The first "monolithic" design option potentially presents the severest test case load and should be avoided. Since it is monolithic in structure and performs all editing functions, all validation tests must be performed within a single routine in order to determine whether the requirements are met. The validation testing would consist of the four test scenarios presented above.

The second design option represents an improvement over the first design. Because the flash/no flash flag is passed as a parameter into the routine, the testing internally to the routine is reduced because part of the testing burden has been shifted to the interface between the calling and called routines. This is easier to test because the flash/no flash discrimination is made at a higher level. It is an inherent part of the calling sequence of the routine and therefore can be visually verified without formal tests. The validation testing would consist of test situations 1, 2, and 4 as presented above.

The third design option represents the optimum from a test stand point because the majority of the validation testing can be accomplished with visual inspections. This is possible because the flash/no flash discrimination is also implemented at a higher level and the result of the differentiation is a flashing field or a non-flashing field. The validation testing would consist of test situations 2 and 4 as presented above.

Based on the design options, the requirements could be rewritten in order to simplify testing even further. Assume that the third design option in fact requires less testing time and is easier to test. The requirement statements can then be written in order to facilitate this situation even more. The following requirements statements are equivalent to those above and in fact tends to drive the design in the direction of the third design option. "All displayed fields can be edited. All critical items being edited shall flash to inform the user that editing is in progress." In this instance, the third design can be augmented by creating a list or look-up table of the fields required to be edited and a flag can be associated with each that indicates whether the field should flash or not. this approach allows a completely visual inspection to replace the testing because the field is either in the edit list or it is not, and if it is, then it either flashes or it does not. testing within the routine is still required, but it now is associated with debug testing during development and not with formal validation testing after implementation.

3.2.3 Requirements versus design

There is agreement that there is a lot of overlap between requirements and design, yet the division between these two is not a hard line. Design can itself be considered a requirement. Many individuals, however, do not appreciate that the distinction between them can be used to simplify testing and consequently shorten overall software development times. Requirements and their specification concentrate on the functions that are needed by the system or product and the users. Requirements need to be discussed in terms of what has to be done, and not how it is to be done.

The requirement "hardcopy strip chart analysis shall be available" is a functional requirement. The requirement "hardcopy strip chart analysis shall be from a pull down menu" has design requirements mixed with the functional requirements. Consequently, there may be times when requirements specifications will contain information that can be construed as design. When developing a requirements specification, resist placing the "how to" design requirements in the system requirements specification and concentrate on the underlying "what" requirements.

As more "how" requirements creep into the requirements specification, more testing must occur on principally two levels. First, there is more detail to test for and second, but strategically more important, there is more validation than verification that needs to be done. Since verification is qualitative in nature and ascertains that the process and design were met, low-key activities have been transferred from the visual and inspection methods into validation testing which is more rigorous and requires formal proof of requirements fulfillment. The distinction of design versus requirements is difficult, but a careful discrimination of what goes where is of profound benefit. As a rule of thumb, if it looks like a description of "what" needs to be implemented, then it belongs in the requirements specification. If it looks like a "how to" description, if a feature can be implemented in two or more ways and one way is preferred over another, or if it is indeterminate as to whether it is a requirements or design, then it belongs in the design specification.

There is another distinct advantage to moving as many "how" requirements to design as possible. The use of computer aided software engineering (CASE) tools has greatly automated the generation of code from design. If a feature or function can be delayed until the design phase, it can then be implemented in an automated fashion. This simplifies the verification of the design because the automation tool has been previously verified and validated so that the demonstration that the design was implemented is simple.

3.3 Introduction to Databases

Throughout the design process data will be generated that may need to be managed in one of two ways – storage in an Excel spreadsheet for later documentation or analysis purposes or storage in a Database for similar purposes. Design projects may indeed involve the design of such a spreadsheet and an overlay of software for data analysis, or design of a database for data storage and subsequent data querying and reporting. At the graduate level, this analysis may include such techniques as Knowledge Discovery, an assembly of techniques used to derive rules from data collected in an environment.

3.3.1 Excel spreadsheets

Excel spreadsheets are useful in situations where data fields are essentially "flat", data can be managed adequately in a simple two dimensional array or arrays (aka multiple worksheets). Data that is non-repetitive can be easily managed using a spreadsheet; data that is repetitive, such as an individual patients demographics for each clinic visit is better handled with a database. Excel spreadsheets are useful for data sets that do not exceed 32,000 data points in length, after this typically data must be chunked in multiple spreadsheets or put into databases. Excel spreadsheets are optimized for simple statistical and other analysis of data and for easily generated plots of data sets. With the use of the Visual Basic editor, some very useful data entry/calculation programs may be generated.

Such programs may include: Elementary electrocardiogram analyses, simple lab test statistics and documentation, real-time display of data, clinic utilization statistics, what-if analyses, etc. More mundane applications include the storage of design specifications and change orders, verification and validation documentation, and straightforward safety process documentation.

3.3.2 Databases

Databases are very much in use in the field of design; modern society probably could not junction without this invention. Databases are simply a convenient and (should be an) efficient method of storing data, with a high level language that allows convenient manipulation of the data. Properly designed databases are efficient in storage of data and in fact can reduce costs due to rapid retrieval of data. Redundant entry of information, such as the address of a supplier, is entered only once in a table, rather than in multiple occurrences when the supplier is referenced. Commercial databases include DB2, SQL (Structured Query Language) server, FoxPro, Access, Oracle, Sybase, Informix, and Paradox. With competition, this field will likely narrow in the near future. Each has advantages, dependent on your background and the size of the problem you are trying to solve. Access, for example, might work well in an initial design for a small clinic database, but growth to a larger clinic or the use of multiple simultaneous data entry points would push a designer to SQL server systems.

Most databases have the following in common. Data that would otherwise be repeated is keyed in once into a structure termed a table. Data that is entered in a table column (field) generally has a given structure (date, alphanumeric, number, etc.), this can be checked for integrity as well as check for reality during entry. The structure of the database allows for relationships between tables, for example one table may link to several others (one patient links to multiple cases) or may link to only one other table (one patient, one home address). Tables link through "keys", such a key might be a patient's social security number, or a patient encounter number generated by a clinic. Data entry techniques can involve the generation and utilization of forms. Data extraction techniques involve the use of a query and the reporting using another form generated for this use.

Data from databases may be exported for use in spreadsheets, and vice versa, thus mastery of databases is not necessary for some work in data analysis.

3.3.3 Example: database development

In the early 1990s the Pain clinic in a major hospital was simply using paper forms for capture of all information. The forms were used for an initial patient interaction/interview/evaluation (5 pages), subsequent psychological patient evaluations if needed (1 page each), and subsequent physical/medical evaluations as needed (multiple pages). The initial interaction form held the expected patient demographics information, hospital identification number, referring physician information, pain history, and medical examination information, assessment, diagnosis, and plan of treatment. The psychological assessment plan included a current psychological evaluation, testing results, treatment plan, and other activities. The medical follow-up paperwork included an evaluation of the pain history since the initial visit, treatment for the pain (such as injections, medications, counseling, physical or occupational therapy, biofeedback, relaxation technique training, biofeedback, or transcutaneous electrical nerve stimulation), effects of the treatment, drugs prescribed, pain evaluation, diagnosis, and follow-up plans.

As is common in a circumstance such as this, three main influences pushed this clinic toward the use of a database. The first driving force was that their record-keeping system was entirely dependent on preserving and accessing the paper records that they were generating, lost or incomplete paperwork meant lost revenue. Secondly, the patient population in the clinic was gradually increasing, putting more of a demand on the one secretary/filing clerk available. Third, and most important, was the pressure from insurers to adequately document and report consistently all interventions performed and the reasons for the interventions, at the risk of non-payment of billed services.

The above scenario led to the initial development of an Access database. Three tables were created, one for the initial visit record system, one for all psychological evaluation/treatment interventions, and one for all medical treatment interventions. The link between all three tables (key) was set to be the patient identifier, the second identifier to keep visits unique was set to be the date of service. An initial system was developed with a paper form tool for data entry (Teleforms) such that information was entered using block letters and numbers, fill in the blank, etc. A later version was based upon the same information layout, but using a direct computer entry method. The disadvantage of the paper based forms were the need for a paper intermediate step to data entry, and the resultant errors due to lack of data entry and misread data forms due to sloppy form copying techniques. The direct terminal entry of data allows the programmer to validate each data entry field as entered and to warn of incomplete data entry on a given patient.

Two main advantages can be gained by development of this database. All insurance information can be adequately entered, documented, and billed for using the report functions in Access. Patient summary letters can be generated for the referring physician also using the report writing functions of Access.

3.4 Reporting Techniques: Presentations, Posters, and Reports

Reporting methods vary considerably dependent on the nature of the project (industrial versus academic), the size of the team and of the project, and the expectations of the person(s) to whom the report is being made. Typical reporting techniques involve oral presentations using transparencies or PowerPoint Slides, Poster presentations (especially in academic settings), and formal reports of progress or results (web or hard copy).

3.4.1 Progress reports: written

Progress reports, at the lowest level, are fairly simple documentation, generally on paper or in a web section, listing the following items: current status, work completed, current work, and future work. An example progress report might read like the following:

Progress Report: EKG Transmitter Project - Week 7 of 11
Current Status: We recently completed our library and web search for applicable EKG transmitter designs. It appears that the transmitter system designed by Goldman et al (see references) is both out of patent and a prime candidate for reverse engineering.
Work Completed: We were able to x-ray the transmitter we borrowed from Dr. Sachs, we were able to do a component count and figure out what brand of battery system they used.
Current Work: B. will meet with EE Prof. Heller this week and go over a chip level redesign of the amplifier system. C. will review chip level transmitter systems, and encapsulation materials.
Future Work: We appear to be on schedule for the planned end date of next month. Our earlier request for funding has been adequate to obtain the necessary supplies and equipment.

An example progress report (NOT!) follows as an antithesis:

Progress Report: Transmitter Project, Week 12 of 11 (sorry this is late!)
Current Status: We have been unable to meet with Dr. Wilson as he is out of town. We came by your office but did not find you in to explain our problem. It

will not be our fault if we do not complete this project!
Work Completed: We had exams last week and next week we have spring break so we have not had time to do anything on this project. It can wait.
Current Work: Packing my bags for spring break.
Future Work: We will place our order for parts when we get back. We are sure X University will quickly get the purchase order in the mail and that the advertised 6-week delivery time is a gimmick. Got to go catch some rays!

Obviously, this is fairly low level reporting, and should serve as a minimum reference. More elaborate reporting schemes would involve additional line items from the original listing of the problem specification (the who, what, where, why ... list) and elaborations on the details of current budget levels, current interactions with all interested parties (design, manufacturing, sales, etc.) and a good discussion of status with respect to the original detailed timelines and specifications.

3.4.2 Oral reporting

Oral reporting of progress will include the above terms at whatever level of complexity is required to convey the information to the audience. PowerPoint presentations will generally convey information better than those using transparencies if and only if they are properly done. Some general rules to follow are:

- Use your slide area well, but place no more than 6-8 lines of information on a page. Text needs to be used sparingly; your job is to fill in the blanks, not read material to your audience.
- Use color and specific colors judiciously. If possible, use color to make a point.
- Use motion (PowerPoint) sparingly. Overuse of materials "flying in" from different areas will quickly lose an audience.
- Learn your style of lecturing; determine if you are a one slide per minute or a one slide per three-minute speaker. Any faster than two to three slides a minute tends to be

irritating, and likely will lose the audience.

- Use graphics if they assist in understanding the talk.
- If your talk is more than 15 minutes long, consider some way to interest (awaken) the group, via a personal account or a clean joke.
- Be sure you tell the group what you are going to tell them, then tell them, then summarize what you said. (Someone may have slept through two of the three)!
- Be sure that you cover your bases, double check that you have done the who/what/why... material.
- Practice your talk. Do not over-practice your talk. Give a dry run if possible in front of a co-worker or fellow student that you can trust to give you valid feedback.
- Consider whether or not to give your audience handouts of your slides in order to retain your message(s).
- If necessary, to avoid nervousness, visualize your audience in their underwear. They are now the ones to be embarrassed!

3.4.3 Poster presentations

In academic circles, if you really want to meet people that are interested in your work, and want a one-to-one discussion with them, poster presentations are a good method. For reporting of student work in an academic environment, there seems to be about an even split in the reporting schemes used in courses. Some general rules for poster presentations follow:

- Know the size of the poster you are going to place your work on. Typically, a board will be provided which measures 6 or 8 feet wide by 4 feet tall, elevated so that the bottom of the board is approximately 2 feet off the ground. However, if you are reporting in a foreign country, sizes may be 1 meter wide by 2 meters high. Plan ahead and lay out your poster presentation on a marked off floor area before packing it!
- Check to see what method of attachment is allowed. Some situations call for pushpins, others for double sided tape, etc. Bring your own if unsure.
- The title of your poster should appear at the top in large

letters, at least 4 to 6 inches in height, readable at a distance of 6 feet. Use upper and lower case, block lettering using all caps is not good form. If you can do so, put the title on a continuous sheet of paper, rather than on pasted together single sheets. Author names and affiliations are best placed below this banner, using a slightly smaller font, and perhaps italics.

- Subsections should also be legible at a distance and should be abstractions of the primary points of the poster, rather than a text or textbook presentation. Be sure all key points are covered (abstract, introduction, ... conclusion, references) as necessary.
- Bolded text is generally easier to read, but check this, as not all fonts are easy to read bolded.
- Use color in your text to make a point, if appropriate.
- Your poster should "read" from the top left, in vertical columns, to the bottom right. If you need to change this, be sure to use arrows to interconnect your panels.
- Color highlighting of your text blocks, which may also be on colored paper, will make your poster more attractive, if the colors are complementary.
- Use pictures, diagrams, cartoons, figures, etc., rather than text wherever possible. If you are allowed to do so, prepare handout material to supplement your poster. Be sure to include contact information.
- Your poster should be self-explanatory. You may be talking with one person, another can be reading and deciding if they wish to wait to get additional information.
- If appropriate and allowed, bring in additional materials, such as a computer to give a visual demonstration of your work. Use sound appropriately, if at all. Do not induce headaches in yourself and the adjacent poster presenters with inappropriately loud or obnoxious sounds.
- Prepare brief comments for questioners.
- Retrieve your materials at the time stated; otherwise you may lose the effort put into their development.
- As appropriate, carry and hand out your business card. Your next job may come of your interactions here.

Homework Exercises

1. Take the material written just above on the rules for a poster session; generate a PowerPoint presentation that conveys the same thoughts in a more vital fashion.

2. For the material on PowerPoint presentations, demonstrate several of the points made using a PowerPoint presentation.

3. Perform a web search for optical character recognition (OCR). Comment on the range of uses for this method of data entry. Comment on some of the disadvantages of this method.

4. Draft a design for a computer method that would contain the relevant information needed to catalog equipment used in a medium sized biomedical engineering department. At what point would you consider the use of Access over Excel?

5. You are in charge of developing a database for a drop-in clinic for a medium sized city. What would be some of the key parameters you would need to enter on every patient? Discuss this briefly.

6. Construct a "design team" exercise during or after class to tackle a design exercise. Reporting will be done orally by one of the team members. Members must take one of the following roles: Marketing. Manufacturing/distribution, Legal/Safety, Engineering, or team leader, members are responsible for assuming their "roles" on the design team. Design topics could include any one of the following:

   - Design a device to detect SIDS in an infant.
   - Design an automated EEG electrode placement system.
   - Design a device to track Alzheimer's patients locations.
   - Design a system to track asthmatics location and sample the environment for noxious stimuli.
   - Design a head restraint system for race car drivers
   - Design a pain clinic database.
   - Design a system to quantify male or female arousal in an MRI machine.
   - ...any other design suggested by your instructor.

References

Chevlin, David H. and Joseph Jorgens III, "Medical Device Software Requirements: Definition and Specification," *Medical Instrumentation* Volume 30, Number 2, March/April, 1996.

Davis, Alan M. and Pei Hsia, "Giving Voice to Requirements Engineering," in *IEEE Software.* Volume 11, Number 2, March, 1994.

Dubnicki, Carol, "Building High-Performance Management Teams," *Healthcare Forum Journal.* May-June, 1991.

Fairly, Richard E., *Software Engineering Concepts.* New York: McGraw-Hill Book Company, 1985.

Fries, Richard C., *Reliable Design of Medical Devices.* New York: Marcel Dekker, Inc., 1997.

Gause, Donald C. and Gerald M. Weinberg, *Exploring Requirements: Quality Before Design.* New York: Dorset House Publishing, 1989.

Goodman, Paul A. and Associates, *Designing Effective Work Groups.* San Francisco: Jossey-Bass. 1986.

Hackman, J. Richard, ed., *Groups That Work (And Those That Don't).* San Francisco: Jossey-Bass. 1990.

Hirschhorn, Larry, *Managing in the New Team Environment.* Reading, MA.: Addison-Wesley, 1991.

Hoerr, John, "The Payoff from Teamwork," *Business Week.* July 10, 1989.

House, Charles H., "The Return Map: Tracking Product Teams," *Harvard Business Review.* January-February, 1991.

Katz, Ralph, "High Performing Research Teams," *Wharton Magazine.* Spring, 1982.

Katzenbach, Jon R. and Douglas K. Smith, *The Wisdom of Teams.* New York: Harper Collins Publishers, Inc., 1999.

Kidder, Tracy, *The Soul of a New Machine.* Boston: Atlantic-Little, Brown, 1981.

Kotkin, Joel, "The Smart Team at Compaq Computer," *Inc.* magazine, February, 1986.

Larson, Carl E. and Frank M. LaFasto, *Teamwork: What Must Go Right/What Can Go Wrong.* Newbury Park, CA: Sage Publications, 1989.

Pantages, Angeline, "The New Order at Johnson Wax," *Datamation.* March 15, 1990.

Peters, Tom, *Thriving on Chaos.* New York: Alfred A. Knopf, 1988.

Potts, Colin, Kenji Takahashi, and Annie I. Anton, "Inquiry-Based Requirements Analysis," in *IEEE Software.* Volume 11, Number 2, March, 1994.

Smith, Preston G. and Donald G. Reinert, *Developing Products in Half the Time.* New York: Van Nostrand Reinhold, 1991.

Weisbord, Marvin R., *Productive Workplaces.* San Francisco: Jossey-Bass. 1989.

Chapter 4

Product Definition

"Abstract art: a product of the untalented,
sold by the unprincipled, to the utterly bewildered."
Al Capp

New product ideas are not simply born. New product ideas come from examining the needs of hospitals, nurses, respiratory therapists, physicians and other medical professionals, as well as from sales and marketing personnel. It is also important to talk with physicians and nurses and determine what their problems are and how they can be addressed. Often needs are based upon personal experiences and dislike of the performance of a current product. Some product development is the direct result of legal cases wherein a defect is identified in a product. These problems generally represent product opportunities. A successful new product demands that it meet the end user's needs. It must have the features and provide the benefits the customer expects.

The multiphased process of defining a product involves the customer, the company, potential vendors, and current technologies. The result is a clear definition of what the product is, and is expected to do, included in a Business Proposal. The first inputs to the process are the needs of the customer and the needs of the company.

The customer's needs and expectations are the primary source of information when defining a device. If the new product does not meet the customer's needs or expectations, there is no market for the device. In addition, the needs of the company are important in defining the device. Issues such as market need, product niche, etc., must be considered in the definition process.

The company's competencies must also be taken into consideration. What are they, how do they match the customer's and company's needs, what is required outside of the company's competencies, and is it easily available? In addition, the competencies of potential vendors or other companies in alliance or partnership with the original company must be considered.

Once a rough idea of the potential device is taking shape, the next consideration is technology. What technologies are appropriate for the proposed device, how available are they, are they within the company's competency, are resources readily available?

Finally, the type of proposed device or process must be decided. Is it a new application for older devices, is it a new platform, or is it an enhancement to an older device or process? Establishing answers in these areas leads to the definition of a device that leads to the development of a product specification. Let's look at each area in more detail.

4.1 The Product Definition Process

Numerous methods of obtaining new product information exist. They include various ways of collecting data, such as internal sources, industry analysis, and technology analysis. Then the information is screened and a business analysis is conducted. Regardless of the method of obtaining the information, there are certain key questions:

- Where are we in the market now?
- Where do we want to go?
- How big is the potential market?
- What does the customer really want (demands vs. wishes)?
- How feasible is technical development?

- How do we get where we want to go?
- What are the chances of success?

4.1.1 Surveying the customer

The customer survey is an important tool in changing an idea into a product. The criticality of the survey is exhibited by an estimate that, on the average, it takes 58 initial ideas to get one commercially successful new product to market. It is therefore necessary to talk with various leaders in potential markets to build a credible database of product ideas.

The goal of the customer survey is to match the needs of the customer with the product concept. Quality has been defined as meeting the customer needs. So a quality product is one that does what the customer wants it to do. The objective of consumer analysis is to identify segments or groups within a population with similar needs so that marketing efforts can be directly targeted to them. Several important questions must be asked to find that market which will unlock untold marketing riches:

- What is the *need* category?
- Who is buying and who is using the product?
- What is the *buying* process?
- Is the device a high- or low-involvement product?
- How can the market be segmented?

4.1.2 Defining the company's needs

While segmentation analysis focuses on consumers as individuals, market analysis takes a broader view of potential consumers to include market sizes and trends. Market analysis also includes a review of the competitive and regulatory environment. Three questions are important in evaluating a market:

- What is the *relevant* market?
- Where is the product in its product life cycle?
- What are the key *competitive* factors in the industry?

4.1.3 What are the company's competencies?

Once a market segment has been chosen, a plan to beat the competition must be chosen. To accomplish this, a company must look at itself with the same level of objectivity it looks at its competitors. Important questions to assist in this analysis include:

- What are our core competencies?
- What are our weaknesses?
- How can we capitalize on our strengths?
- How can we exploit the weaknesses of our competitors?
- Who are we in the marketplace?
- How does my product map against the competition?

4.1.4 What are the outside competencies?

Once a company has objectively looked at itself, it must then look at others in the marketplace:

- What are the strengths of the competition?
- What are their weaknesses?
- What are the resources of the competition?
- What are the market shares of the industry players?

4.1.5 Completing the product definition

There are many other questions that need to be answered in order to complete the product definition. In addition to those mentioned above, an organization needs to determine:

- How does the potential product fit with our other products?
- Do our current technologies match the potential product?
- How will we differentiate the new product?
- How does the product life cycle affect our plans?

It is also important to consider the marketing mix of products, distribution networks, pricing structure, and the overall economics of the product plan. These are all important pieces of the overall product plan as developed in a Business Proposal. However, the needs and wants of the customer remain the most important information to be collected. One method of obtaining the required customer requirements is Quality Function Deployment.

4.2 Overview of Quality Function Deployment

Quality Function Deployment (QFD) is a process in which the "voice of the customer" is first heard and then deployed through an orderly, four-phase process in which a product is planned, designed, made and then made consistently. It is a well-defined process which begins with customer requirements and keeps them evident throughout the four phases. The process is analytical enough to provide a means of prioritizing design trade-offs, to track product features against competitive products, and to select the best anufacturing process to optimize product features. Moreover, once in production, the process affords a means of working backwards to determine what a prospective change in the manufacturing process or in the product's components may do to the overall product attributes.

The fundamental insight of QFD from an engineering perspective is that customer wants and technical solutions do not exist in a one-to-one correspondence. Though this sounds simplistic, the implications are profound. It means that product "features" are not what customers want; instead, they want the "benefits" provided by those features. To make this distinction clear, QFD explicitly distinguishes between customer attributes that the product may have and technical characteristics which may provide some of the attributes the customer is looking for. Taking a pacemaker as an example, the customer attribute might be that the patient wants to extend their life, while the technical characteristic is that the pacemaker reduces arrhythmias.

4.3 The QFD Process

The QFD process begins with the wants of the customer, since meeting these is essential to the success of the product. Product features should not be defined by what the developers think their customers want. For clear product definition that will lead to market acceptance, manufacturers must spend both time and money learning about their customer's environments, their constraints, and the obstacles they face in using the product. By fully understanding these influences, a manufacturer can develop products that are not obvious to its customers or competitors at the outset, but will have high customer appeal.

Quality Function Deployment should be viewed from a very global perspective as a methodology that will link a company with its customers and assist the organization in its planning processes. Often, an organization's introduction to QFD takes the form of building matrices. A common result is that building the matrix becomes the main objective of the process. The purpose of QFD is to get in touch with the customer and use this knowledge to develop products which satisfy the customer, not to build matrices.

QFD uses a matrix format to capture a number of issues pertinent and vital to the planning process. The matrix represents these issues in an outline form which permits the organization to examine the information in a multidimensional manner. This encourages effective decisions based on a team's examination and integration of the pertinent data.

The QFD matrix has two principal parts:

- the voice of the customer
- technical information.

4.3.1 The voice of the customer

The voice of the customer is the basic input required to begin a QFD project. The customer's importance rating is a measure of the relative importance that customers assign to each of the voices. The customer's competitive evaluation of the company's products or services permits a company to observe how its customers rate its products or services on a numerical scale. Any complaints that customers have personally registered with the company serve as an indication of dissatisfaction.

4.3.2 Technical information

The first step in developing the technical portion of the matrix is to determine how the company will respond to each voice. The technical or design requirements that the company will use to describe and measure each customer's voice are placed across the top of the matrix. For example, if the voice of the customer stated "want the control to be easy to operate," the technical requirement might be "operating effort." The technical requirements represent how the company will respond to its customers' wants and needs.

The center of the matrix, where the customer and technical portion intersect, provides an opportunity to record the presence and strength of relationships between these inputs and action items. Symbols may be used to indicate the strength of these relationships. The information in the matrix can be examined and weighed by the appropriate team. Goals or targets can be established for each technical requirement.

Tradeoffs can be examined and by comparing each technical requirement against the other technical requirements. Each relationship is examined to determine the net result that changing one requirement has on the others.

4.3.3 Overview of the QFD process

The Quality Function Deployment process consists of 9 steps:

1. determining the voice of the customer
2. customer surveys for importance ratings and competitive evaluation
3. developing the customer portion of the matrix
4. developing the technical portion of the matrix
5. analyzing the matrix and choosing priority items
6. comparing proposed design concepts and synthesizing the best
7. developing a part planning matrix for priority design requirements
8. developing a process planning matrix for priority process requirements
9. developing a manufacturing planning chart.

In planning a new project or revisions to an old one, organizations need to be in touch with the people who buy and use their products and services. This is vital for hard issues, such as a product whose sales are dependent on the customers' evaluation of how well their needs and wants are satisfied. It is equally crucial for softer issues, such as site selection and business planning.

Once the customers' wants and needs are known, the organization can obtain other pertinent customer information. Through surveys, it can establish how its customers feel about the relative importance of the various wants and needs. It can also sample a number of customers who use its products and competitors' products. This provides the customers evaluation of both the organization's performance and that of its chief competitors.

Records can be examined to determine the presence of any customer complaint issues. This can be the result of letters of complaint, phone complaints, reports to the FDA, or other inquiries and comments.

Once this information is available, it can be organized and placed in the horizontal customer information portion of the QFD matrix. The voices of the customers represent their wants and needs: their requirements or qualities demanded. These are the inputs to the matrix, along with importance ratings, competitive evaluations, and complaints.

The appropriate team can then begin developing the technical information portion of the matrix. The customers' voices must be translated into items that are measurable and actionable within the organization. Companies use a variety of names to describe these measurable items, such as design requirements, technical requirements, product characteristics, and product criteria or functions.

The relationship between the inputs and the actionable items can then be examined. Each technical requirement is analyzed to determine if action on the item will affect the customer's requirements. A typical question may be: "Would the organization work on this technical requirement to respond favorably to the customers' requirements?"

For those items in which a relationship is determined to exist, the team then must decide on the strength of the relationship. Symbols are normally used to denote a strong, moderate, or weak relationship. Some of the symbols commonly used are a double circle, single circle, and a triangle, respectively. The symbols provide a quick visual impression of the overall relationship strengths of the technical requirements and the customers' wants and needs.

The team must instigate testing to develop technical data showing the performance of the parent company and its competitors for each of the technical requirements. Once this information is available, the team can begin a study to determine the target value that should be established for each technical requirement. The objective is to ensure that the next-generation product will be truly competitive and satisfy its customers' wants and needs. A comparison of the customers' competitive ranges and the competitive technical assessments helps the organization determine these targets.

Additional information can be added to the matrix depending on the team's judgment of value. Significant internal and regulatory requirements may be added. Measure of organizational difficulty can be added. Column weights can be calculated. These can serve as an index for highlighting those technical requirements that have the largest relative effect on the product.

Once this matrix is complete, the analysis stage begins. The chief focus should be on the customer portion of the matrix. It should be examined to determine which customer requirements need the most attention. This is an integrated decision involving the customers' competitive evaluation, their importance ratings, and their complaint histories. The number of priority items selected will be a balance between their importance and the resources available within the company.

Items selected for action can be treated as a special project or can be handled by use of the QFD matrix at the next level of detail. Any items so selected can become the input to the new matrix. Whereas the first matrix was a planning matrix for the complete product, this new matrix is at a lower level. It concerns the subsystem or assembly that affects the requirement.

The challenge in the second-level matrix is to determine the concept that best satisfies the deployed requirement. This requires evaluation of some design concept alternatives. Several techniques are available for this type of comparative review. The criteria or requirements for the product or service are listed at the left of the matrix. Concept alternatives are listed across the top.

The results of the evaluation of each concept versus the criteria can be entered in the center portion.

Once the best concept alternative is selected, a QFD part planning matrix can be generated for the component level. The development of this matrix follows the same sequence as that of the prior matrix. Generally, less competitive information is available at this level and the matrix is simpler. The technical requirements from the prior matrix are the inputs. Each component in the selected design concept is examined to determine its critical part requirements. These are listed in the upper portion. Relationships are examined and symbols are entered in the center portion. The specifications are then entered for these selected critical part requirements in the lower portion of the matrix.

The part planning matrix should then be examined. Experience with similar parts and assemblies should be a major factor in this review. The analysis should involve the issue of which of the critical part requirements listed are the most difficult to control or ensure continually. This review will likely lead to the selection of certain critical part requirements that the team believes deserve specific follow-up attention.

If a team believes the selected critical part characteristics are best handled through the QFD process, a matrix should be developed for process planning. The critical part concerns from the Part Planning matrix should be used as inputs in the left area of the matrix. The critical process requirements are listed across the top. Relationships are developed and examined in the central area. The specification for operating levels for each process requirement are recorded in the lower area of the matrix. For example, if a critical part requirement was spot-weld strength, one critical process parameter would be weld current. The amount of current would be a critical process parameter to ensure proper spot weld strength. The specification for this critical process requirement would be the amperes of current required to ensure the weld strength.

Upon completion of the planning at the part and process levels, the key concerns should be deployed to the manufacturing level. Most organizations have detailed planning at this level and have developed spreadsheets and forms for recording their planning decisions. The determinations from the prior matrices should become inputs to these documents. Often, the primary document at this level is a basic planning chart. Items of concern are entered in the area farthest left. The risk associated with these items is assessed and recorded in the next column. In typical risk assessments, the level of the concern and the probability of its occurrence are listed, as are the severity of any developing problems and the probability of detection. These items, along with other concerns, can be used to develop an index to highlight items of significant concern. Other areas in the chart can be use to indicate issues such as the general types of controls, frequency of checking, measuring devices, responsibility, and timing.

4.4 Summary of QFD

The input to the QFD Planning Matrix is the voice of the customer. The matrix cannot be started until the customers' requirements are known This applies to internal planning projects as well as products and services that will be sold to marketplace customers. Use of the QFD process leads an organization to develop a vital customer focus.

The initial matrix is usually the planning matrix. The customers' requirements are inputs. Subsequent matrices may be used to deploy or flow down selected requirements from the product planning matrix for part planning and process planning. Some forms of a manufacturing chart or matrix can be used to enter critical product and process requirements from prior matrices.

The principal objective of the QFD process is to help a company organize and analyze all the pertinent information associated with a project and to use the process to help it select the items demanding priority attention. All companies do many things right. The QFD process will help them focus on the areas that need special attention.

Homework Exercises

1. Do a web search on QFD, report the number and geographical distribution of the information found, comment on these results.
2. QFD can be used for technical as well as social system development. Find and report on an example of an improved clinic or other system based on QFD principles.

3. A related technique is called six-sigma. Do a web search to define this term, then comment on its relationship with QFD.
4. Find and report on any QFD application to a technical problem.
5. Develop the first level QFD diagram for your next car purchase.
6. You are an employee of Datex-Ohmeda, you are charged with the development of an inexpensive anesthesia machine for use in third world countries. Develop a QFD matrix for this task.
7. Do a QFD matrix for your current design project.
8. Find and report on the use of QFD for purchase decisions (web or textbook search).
9. Find and report on the use of QFD applied to customer satisfaction (web or textbook search).

References

Brodie, Christina Hepner and Gary Burchill, *Voices Into Choices – Acting on the Voice of the Customer.* Madison: Joiner Associates, Inc., 1997.

Cohen, L. "*Quality Function Deployment: How to Make QFD Work for You*" Addison Wesley, 1995.

Day, Ronald G., *Quality Function Deployment - Linking a Company with Its Customers.* Milwaukee, WI: ASQC Quality Press, 1993.

Eureka, William, Ryan, Nancy, *The Customer-Driven Company: Managerial Perspectives on Quality Function Deployment*, ASI Press, Dearborn MI 1994

Fries, Richard C., *Reliable Design of Medical Devices.* New York: Marcel Dekker, Inc., 1997.

Gause, Donald C. and Gerald M. Weinberg, *Exploring Requirements: Quality Before Design.* New York: Dorset House Publishing, 1989.

Guinta, Lawrence R. and Nancy C. Praizler, *The QFD Bool: The Team Approach to Solving Problems and Satisfying Customers Through Quality Function Deployment.* New York: AMACOM Books, 1993.

Kriewall, Timothy J. and Gregory P. Widin, "An Application of Quality Function Deployment to Medical Device Development," in *Case Studies in Medical Instrument Design*. New York: The Institute of Electrical and Electronics Engineers, Inc., 1991.

Potts, Colin, Kenji Takahashi, and Annie I. Anton, "Inquiry-Based Requirements Analysis," in *IEEE Software*, Volume 11, Number 2, March, 1994.

Silbiger, Steven, *The Ten Day MBA*. New York: William Morrow and Company, Inc., 1993.

Taylor, J. W. *Planning Profitable New Product Strategies*. Radnor, PA: Chilton Book Company, 1984.

Terninko, John, *Step-by-Step QFD, Customer-Driven Product Design, 2nd Edition*, St. Lucie Press, Boca Raton, FL, 1997.

Chapter 5

Product Documentation

"I love being a writer, what I can't stand is the paperwork."
Peter de Vries

All documents and records required by the Quality System Regulation and the Medical Device Directives must be maintained at the manufacturing establishment or other location that is reasonably accessible to responsible officials of the manufacturer and to auditors. They must be legible and stored so as to minimize deterioration and to prevent loss. Those stored in computer systems must be backed up.

Documents and records deemed confidential by the manufacturer may be marked in order to aid the auditor in determining whether information may be disclosed. All records must be retained for a period of time equivalent to the design and expected life of the device, but not less than two years from the date of release of the product by the manufacturer.

There are several types of documents which must be kept by every medical device manufacture. These types include:

- Business Proposal
- Product Specification
- Design Specification
- Software Quality Assurance Plan (where applicable)
- Software Requirements Specification (where applicable)
- Software Design Description (where applicable).

There are four primary types of records which must be kept by every medical device manufacturer. These types are:

- Design History File (DHF)
- Device Master Record (DMR)
- Device History Record (DHR)
- Technical Documentation File (TDF).

Each type of record is discussed in the following sections.

5.1 Documents

5.1.1 The business proposal

The purpose of the Business Proposal is to identify and document market needs, market potential, the proposed product and product alternatives, risks and unknowns, and potential financial benefits. The Business Proposal also contains a proposal for further research into risks and unknowns, estimated project costs, schedule, and a request to form a core team to carry out needed research, to define the product and to prepare the project plan.

The Business Proposal usually contains:

- Project Overview, Objectives, Major Milestones, Schedule
- Market Need and Market Potential
- Product Proposal
- Strategic Fit

- Risk Analysis and Research Plan
- Economic Analysis
- Recommendation to Form a Core Project Team
- Supporting Documentation.

5.1.1.1 Project overview, objectives, major milestones, and schedule

This portion of the Business Proposal contains a statement of overall project objectives and major milestones to be achieved. The objectives clearly define the project scope and provide specific direction to the project team.

The Major Milestones and Schedule follow the statement of objectives. The Schedule anticipates key decision points and completion of the primary deliverables throughout all phases of development and implementation. The Schedule contains target completion dates, however, it must be stressed that these dates are tentative and carry an element of risk. Events contingent upon achievement of the estimated dates should be clearly stated. Examples of milestones include:

- design feasibility
- patent search completed
- product specification verified by customers
- design concept verified through completion of sub-system functional model completed
- process validation completed
- regulatory approval obtained
- successful launch into Territory A
- project assessment complete, project transferred to manufacturing and sustaining engineering.

5.1.1.2 Market need and market potential

This section of the Business Proposal defines the customer and clinical need for the product or service and, identifies the potential territories to be served. Specific issues which are to be addressed include, but should not be limited, to the following:

- What is the market need for this product, i.e., what is the problem to be solved?
- What clinical value will be delivered?
- What incremental clinical value will be added over existing company or competitive offerings?
- What trends are occurring that predict this need?
- In which markets are these trends occurring?
- What markets are being considered, what is the size of the market and what are the competitive shares?
- What is the market size and the estimated growth rate for each territory to be served?
- What are the typical selling prices and margins for similar products?
- When must the product be launched to capture the market opportunity?
- If competitors plan to launch similar products, what is our assessment of their launch date?
- Have competitors announced a launch date?
- What other similar products compose the market?
- Will the same product fit in all markets served? If not, what are the anticipated gross differences and why? What modifications will be required?
- Is the target market broad-based and multifaceted or a focused niche?
- What are the regulatory requirements, standards and local practices which may impact the product design for every market to be served?

5.1.1.3 Product proposal

The Product Proposal section proposes the product idea that fulfills the market need sufficiently well to differentiate its features and explain how user and/or clinical value will be derived. The product specification is not written nor does design commence during this phase. It may be necessary to perform some initial feasibility studies, construct non-working models, perform simulations and conduct research in order to have a reasonable assurance that the product can be designed, manufactured, and serviced. Additionally, models, simulations, and product descriptions will be useful to verify the idea with customers. It is also recommended that several alternative product ideas be evaluated against the "base case" idea. Such evaluation will compare risks, development timelines, costs and success probabilities.

5.1.1.4 Strategic fit

This section discusses how the proposed product conforms with (or departs from) stated strategy with respect to product, market, clinical setting, technology, design, manufacturing and service.

5.1.1.5 Risk analysis and research plan

This section contains an assessment of risks and unknowns, an estimate of the resources needed to reduce the risks to a level whereby the product can be designed, manufactured, and serviced with a reasonable high level of confidence. The personnel resource requirement should be accompanied by the plan and timetable for addressing, researching and reducing the risks.

The following categories of risks and unknowns should be addressed. Not all of these categories apply for every project. Select those which could have a significant impact on achieving project objectives.

- Technical
    - Feasibility (proven, unknown, or unfamiliar?)
    - New technology
    - Design
    - Manufacturing process
    - Accessibility to technologies
    - Congruence with core competencies
    - Manufacturing process capability
    - Cost constraints
    - Component and system reliability
    - Interface compatibility
- Market
    - Perception of need in market place
    - Window of opportunity; competitive race
    - Pricing

  - Competitive positioning and reaction
  - Cannibalization of existing products
  - Customer acceptance
- Financial
  - Margins
  - Cost to develop
  - Investment required
- Regulatory
  - Filings and approvals (IDE, PMA, 510k, CE, TUV, etc.)
  - Compliance with international standards
  - Clinical studies; clinical trials
  - Clinical utility and factors, unknowns
- Intellectual property
  - Patents
  - Licensing agreements
  - Software copyrights
- Requisite skill sets available to design and develop
  - Electrical
  - Mechanical
  - Software
  - Industrial Design
  - Reliability
- Manpower availability
- Vendor selection
  - Quality system
  - Documentation controls
  - Process capability
  - Component reliability
  - Business stability
- Schedule
  - Critical path
  - Early or fixed completion date
  - Resource availability
- Budget.

5.1.1.6 Economic analysis

This section includes a rough estimate of the costs and personnel required to specify, design, develop, and launch each product variant into the market place.

5.1.1.7 Core project team

This section discusses the formation of a core project team to perform the research required to reduce risks and unknowns to a manageable level, to develop and verify the User Specification. and to prepare the project plan

The requisite skills of the proposed team members should also be outlined. To the extent possible, the following functions should be involved in research, preparation of the User Specification, and the preparation of the project plan.

- Marketing
- Engineering
- Manufacturing
- Service
- Regulatory
- Quality Assurance
- Finance.

The approximate amount of time required of each participant as well as incremental expenses should also be estimated. Some examples of incremental expenses include: model development, simulation software, travel for customer verification activities, laboratory supplies, market research, and project status reviews.

5.1.2 Product specification

The Product Specification is the first step in the process of transforming product ideas into approved product development efforts. It details the results of the customer survey and subsequent interface between the Marketing, Design Engineering, Reliability Assurance and Regulatory Affairs personnel. It specifies what the product will do, how it will do it and how reliable it will be. To be effective, it must be as precise as possible.

The product specification should be a controlled document, that is, subject to revision level control, so that any changes that arise are subjected to review and approval prior to implementation. It prevents the all too typical habit of making verbal changes to the specification, without all concerned personnel informed. This often leads to total confusion in later stages of development, as the current specification is only a figment of someone's imagination or a pile of handwritten papers in someone's desk.

The specification should also have joint ownership. It should only be written after all concerned departments have discussed the concept and its alternatives and have agreed on the feasibility of the design. Agreement should come from Marketing, Design Engineering, Manufacturing, Customer Service, Reliability Assurance and Regulatory Affairs.

The specification is a detailed review of the proposed product and includes:

- the type of product
- the market it addresses
- the function of the product
- the product parameters necessary to function effectively
- accuracy requirements
- tolerances necessary for function
- the anticipated environment for the device
- cautions for anticipated misuse
- safety issues
- human factors issues
- the anticipated life of the product
- the reliability goal
- requirements from applicable domestic or international standards.

Each requirement should be identified with some form of notation, such as brackets and a number. For traceability purposes, each numbered subsection of the specification should start numbering its requirements with the number 1. For example:

5.3.1 Analog to Digital Converter

The output of the analog to digital converter must be between X and Y [1].

In parsing the requirements, this particular one would be referred to as 5.3.1-1. Subsequent requirements in this paragraph would be numbered in consecutive order. Requirements in the next paragraph would restart the numbering with #1.

Software programs are available to assist in the parsing process. The software establishes a database of requirements for which a set of attributes are developed that help trace each requirement. Some attributes which might be established include:

- Paragraph number
- Requirement number
- Author of the requirement
- System or subsystem responsible for the requirement
- Type of verification or validation test.

5.1.3 Design specification

The Design Specification is a document that is derived from the Product Specification. Specifically, the requirements found in the Product Specification are partitioned and distilled down into specific design requirements for each subassembly. The Design Specification should address the following areas for each subsystem:

- the reliability budget
- service strategy
- manufacturing strategy
- hazard consideration
- environmental constraints
- safety
- cost budgets
- standards requirements
- size and packaging
- the power budget

- the heat generation budget
- industrial design/human factors
- controls/adjustments
- material compatibility.

In addition, all electrical and mechanical inputs and outputs and their corresponding limits under all operating modes must be defined.

Each performance specification should be listed with nominal and worst case requirements under all environmental conditions. Typical performance parameters to be considered include:

- gain
- span
- linearity
- drift
- offset
- noise
- power dissipation
- frequency response
- leakage
- burst pressure
- vibration
- long term stability
- operation forces/torques.

As in the Product Specification, the requirements in the Design Specification should be identified by a notation such as a bracket and numbers. The parsing tool works well for focusing on these requirements.

5.1.4 Software quality assurance plan (SQAP)

The term *Software Quality Assurance* is defined as a planned and systematic pattern of activities performed to assure the procedures, tools and techniques used during software development and modification are adequate to provide the desired level of confidence in the final product. The purpose of a

Software Quality Assurance program is to assure the software is of such quality that it does not reduce the reliability of the device. Assurance that a product works reliably has been classically provided by a test of the product at the end of its development period. However, because of the nature of software, no test appears sufficiently comprehensive to adequately test all aspects of the program. Software Quality Assurance has thus taken the form of directing and documenting the development process itself, including checks and balances.

Specifying the software is the first step in the development process. It is a detailed summary of what the software is to do and how it will do it. The specification may consist of several documents, including the Software Quality Assurance Plan, the Software Requirements Specification and the Software Design Specification. These documents serve not only to define the software package, but are the main source for requirements to be used for software verification and validation.

A typical Software Quality Assurance Plan includes the following sections.

5.1.4.1 Purpose

This section delineates the specific purpose and scope of the particular SQAP. It lists the names of the software items covered by the SQAP and the intended use of the software. It states the portion of the software life cycle covered by the SQAP for each software item specified.

5.1.4.2 Reference documents

This section provides a complete list of documents referenced elsewhere in the text of the SQAP.

5.1.4.3 Management

This section describes the organizational structure that influences and controls the quality of the software. It also describes that portion of the software life cycle covered by the SQAP, the tasks to be performed with special emphasis on software quality assurance activities, and the relationships between these tasks and the planned major checkpoints. The sequence of the tasks shall be indicated as well as the specific organizational elements responsible for each task.

5.1.4.4 Documentation

This section identifies the documentation governing the development, verification and validation, use, and maintenance of the software. It also states how the documents are to be checked for adequacy.

5.1.4.5 Standards, practices, conventions, and metrics

This section identifies the standards, practices, conventions and metrics to be applied as well as how compliance with these items is to be monitored and assured.

5.1.4.6 Review and audits

This section defines the technical and managerial reviews and audits to be conducted, states how the reviews and audits are to be accomplished, and states what further actions are required and how they are to be implemented and verified.

5.1.4.7 Test

This section identifies all the tests not included in the Software Verification and Validation Plan and states how the tests are to be implemented.

5.1.4.8 Problem reporting and corrective action

This section describes the practices and procedures to be followed for reporting, tracking, and resolving problems identified in software items and the software development and maintenance processes. It also states the specific organizational responsibilities.

5.1.4.9 Tools, techniques, and methodologies

This section identifies the special software tools, techniques, and methodologies that support SQA, states their purpose, and describes their use.

5.1.4.10 Code control

This section defines the methods and facilities used to maintain, store, secure and document controlled versions of the identified software during all phases of the software life cycle.

5.1.4.11 Media control

This section states the methods and facilities used to identify the media for each computer product and the documentation required to store the media and protect computer program physical media from unauthorized access or inadvertent damage or degradation during all phases of the software life cycle.

5.1.4.12 Supplier control

This section states the provisions for assuring that software provided by suppliers meets established requirements. It also states the methods that will be used to assure that the software supplier receives adequate and complete requirements.

5.1.4.13 Records collection, maintenance, and retention

This section identifies the SQA documentation to be retained, states the methods and facilities to be used to assemble, safeguard, and maintain this documentation, and designates the retention period.

5.1.4.14 Training

This section identifies the training activities necessary to meet the needs of the SQAP.

5.1.4.15 Risk management

This section specifies the methods and procedures employed to identify, assess, monitor, and control areas of risk arising during the portion of the software life cycle covered by the SQAP.

5.1.4.16 Additional sections as required

Some material may appear in other documents. Reference to these documents should be made in the body of the SQAP. The contents of each section of the plan shall be specified either directly or by reference to another document.

5.1.5 Software requirements specification (SRS)

The SRS is a specification for a particular software product, program, or set of programs that perform certain functions. The SRS must correctly define all of the software requirements, but no more. It should not describe any design, verification, or project management details, except for required design constraints. A good SRS is unambiguous, complete, verifiable, consistent, modifiable, traceable, and usable during the Operation and Maintenance phase.

Each software requirement in an SRS is a statement of some essential capability of the software to be developed. Requirements can be expressed in a number of ways:

- through input/output specifications
- by use of a set of representative examples
- by the specification of models.

A typical Software Requirements Specification includes the following sections.

5.1.5.1 Purpose

This section should delineate the purpose of the particular SRS and specify the intended audience.

5.1.5.2 Scope

This section should identify the software product to be produced by name, explain what the software product will, and if necessary, will not do, and describe the application of the software being specified.

5.1.5.3 Definitions, acronyms, and abbreviations

This section provides the definitions of all terms, acronyms, and abbreviations required to properly interpret the SRS.

5.1.5.4 References

This section should provide a complete list of all documents referenced elsewhere in the SRS or in a separate specified document. Each document should be identified by title, report number if applicable, date, and publishing organization. It is also helpful to specify the sources from which the references can be obtained.

5.1.5.5 Overview

This section should describe what the rest of the SRS contains and explain how the SRS is organized.

5.1.5.6 Product perspective

This section puts the product into perspective with other related products. If the product is independent and totally self-contained, it should be stated here. If the SRS defines a product that is a component of a larger system, then this section should describe the functions of each subcomponent of the system, identify internal interfaces, and identify the principal external interfaces of the software product.

5.1.5.7 Product functions

This section provides a summary of the functions that the software will perform. The functions should be organized in a way that makes the list of functions understandable to the customer or to anyone else reading the document for the first time. Block diagrams showing the different functions and their relationships can be helpful. This section should not be used to state specific requirements.

5.1.5.8 User characteristics

This section describes those general characteristics of the eventual users of the product that will affect the specific requirements. Certain characteristics of these people, such as educational level, experience, and technical expertise impose important constraints on the system's operating environment. This section should not be used to state specific requirements or to impose specific design constraints on the solution.

5.1.5.9 General constraints

This section provides a general description of any other items that will limit the developer's options for designing the system. These can include regulatory policies, hardware limitations, interfaces to other applications, parallel operation, control functions, higher-order language requirements, criticality of the application, or safety and security considerations.

5.1.5.10 Assumptions and dependencies

This section lists each of the factors that affect the requirements stated in the SRS. These factors are not design constraints on the software, but include any changes to them that can affect the requirements.

5.1.5.11 Specific requirements

This section contains all the details the software developer needs to create a design. The details should be defined as individual specific requirements. Background should be provided by cross referencing each specific requirement to any related discussion in other sections. Each requirement should be organized in a logical and readable fashion. Each requirement should be stated such that its achievement can be objectively verified by a prescribed method.

The specific requirements may be classified to aid in their logical organization. One method of classification would include:

- functional requirements
- performance requirements
- design constraints
- attributes
- external interface requirements.

This section is typically the largest section within the SRS.

5.1.6 Software design description (SDS)

A software design description is a representation of a software system that is used as a medium for communicating software design information. The Software Design Description is a document that specifies the necessary information content and recommended organization for a software design description. The SDD shows how the software system will be structured to satisfy the requirements identified in the software requirements specification. It is a translation of requirements into a description of the software structure, software components, interfaces, and data necessary for the implementation phase. In essence, the SDD becomes a detailed blueprint for the implementation activity. In a complete SDD, each requirement must be traceable to one or more design entities.

The SDD should contain the following information:

- Introduction
- References

- Decomposition description
- Dependency description
- Interface description
- Detailed design.

5.1.6.1 Decomposition description

The decomposition description records the division of the software system into design entities. It describes the way the system has been structured and the purpose and function of each entity. For each entity, it provides a reference to the detailed description via the identification attribute.

The decomposition description can be used by designers and maintainers to identify the major design entities of the system for purposes such as determining which entity is responsible for performing specific functions and tracing requirements to design entities. Design entities can be grouped into major classes to assist in locating a particular type of information and to assist in reviewing the decomposition for completeness. In addition, the information in the decomposition description can be used for planning, monitoring and control of a software project.

5.1.6.2 Dependency description

The dependency description specifies the relationships among entities. It identifies the dependent entities, describes their coupling, and identifies the required resources. This design view defines the strategies for interactions among design entities and provides the information needed to easily perceive how, why, where, and at what level system actions occur. It specifies the type of relationships that exist among the entities.

The dependency description provides an overall picture of how the system works in order to assess the impact of requirements and design changes. It can help maintenance personnel to isolate entities causing system failures or resource bottlenecks. It can aid in producing the system integration plan by identifying the entities that are needed by other entities and that must be developed first. This description can also be used by integration testing to aid in the production of integration test cases.

5.1.6.3 Interface description

The entity interface description provides everything designers, programmers, and testers need to know to correctly use the functions provided by an entity. This description includes the details of external and internal interfaces not provided in the Software Requirements Specification.

The interface description serves as a binding contract among designers, programmers, customers, and testers. It provides them with an agreement needed before proceeding with the detailed design of entities. In addition, the interface description may be used by technical writers to produce customer documentation or may be used directly by customers.

5.1.6.4 Detailed design description

The detailed design description contains the internal details of each design entity. These details include the attribute descriptions for identification, processing, and data.

The description contains the details needed by programmers prior to implementation. The detailed design description can also be used to aid in producing unit test plans.

5.2 Records

5.2.1 The design history file

The Design History File (DHF) is a compilation of records which describes the design history of a finished device. It covers the design activities used to develop the device, accessories, major components, labeling, packaging and production processes.

The Design History File contains or references the records necessary to demonstrate that the design was developed in accordance with the approved design plans and the requirements of the Quality System Regulation.

The design controls in CFR 21 820.30(j) require that each manufacturer establish and maintain a DHF for each type of device. Each type of device means a device or family of devices that are manufactured according to one DMR. That is, if the variations in the family of devices are simple enough that they can be handled by minor variations on the drawings, then only one DMR exists. It is common practice to identify device variations on drawings by dash numbers. For this case, only one DHF could exist because only one set of related design documentation exists. Documents are never created just to go into the DHF.

The QS regulation also requires that the DHF shall contain or reference the records necessary to demonstrate that the design was developed in accordance with the approved design plan and the requirements of this part. As noted, this requirement cannot be met unless the manufacturer develops and maintains plans that meet the design control requirements. The plans and subsequent updates should be part of the DHF. In addition, the QS regulation specifically requires that:

- the results of a design review, including identification of the design, the date, and the individual(s) performing the review, shall be documented in the DHF
- design verification shall confirm that the design output meets the design input requirements. The results of the design verification, including identification of the design, method(s), the date, and the individual(s) performing the verification, shall be documented in the DHF.

Typical documents that may be in, or referenced in, a DHF include:

- design plans;
- design review meeting information;
- sketches;
- drawings;
- procedures;

- photos;
- engineering notebooks;
- component qualification information;
- biocompatibility (verification) protocols and data;
- design review notes;
- verification protocols and data for evaluating prototypes;
- validation protocols and data for initial finished devices;
- contractor / consultants information;
- parts of design output/DMR documents that show plans were followed; and
- parts of design output/DMR documents that show specifications were met.

The DHF contains documents such as the design plans and input requirements, preliminary input specs, validation data and preliminary versions of key DMR documents. These are needed to show that plans were created, followed and specifications were met. The DHF is not required to contain all design documents or to contain the DMR, however, it will contain historical versions of key DMR documents that show how the design evolved.

The DHF also has value for the manufacturer. When problems occur during re-design and for new designs, the DHF has the "institutional" memory of previous design activities. The DHF also contains valuable verification and validation protocols that are not in DMR. This information may be very valuable in helping to solve a problem; pointing to the correct direction to solve a problem; or, most important, preventing the manufacturer from repeating an already tried and found-to-be-useless design.

5.2.1 The device master record

The Device Master Record (DMR) is a compilation of those records containing the specifications and procedures for a finished device. It is set up to contain or reference the procedures and specifications that are current on the manufacturing floor. The Device Master Record for each type of device should include or refer to the location of the following information:

- device specifications including appropriate drawings, composition, formulation, component specifications, and software specifications

- production process specifications including the appropriate equipment specifications, production methods, production procedures, and production environment specifications
- quality assurance procedures and specifications including acceptance criteria and the quality assurance equipment used
- packaging and labeling specifications, including methods and processed used
- installation, maintenance, and servicing procedures and methods.

It is more important to construct a document structure that is workable and traceable than to worry about whether something is contained in one file or another.

5.2.2 The device history record

The Device History Record (DHR) is the actual production records for a particular device. It should be able to show the processes, tests, rework, etc. that the device went through from the beginning of its manufacture through distribution. The Device History Record should include or refer to the location of the following information:

- the dates of manufacture
- the quantity manufactured
- the quantity released for distribution
- the acceptance records which demonstrate the device is manufactured in accordance with the Device Master Record
- the primary identification label and labeling used for each production unit
- any device identification and control numbers used.

5.2.3 The technical documentation file

The Technical Documentation File (TDF) contains all the relevant design data by means of which the product can be demonstrated to satisfy the essential safety requirements which are formulated in the Medical Device Directives. In the case of liability proceedings or a control procedure, it must be possible to turn over the relevant portion of this file. For this reason, the file must be compiled in a proper manner and must be kept for a period of 10 years after the production of the last product.

The Technical Documentation File must allow assessment of the conformity of the product with the requirements of the Medical Device Directives. It must include:

- a general description of the product, including any planned variants
- design drawings, methods of manufacture envisaged and diagrams of components, sub-assemblies, circuits, etc.
- the descriptions and explanations necessary to understand the above mentioned drawings and diagrams and the operations of the product
- the results of the risk analysis and a list of applicable standards applied in full or in part, and descriptions of the solutions adopted to meet the Essential Requirements of the Directives if the standards have not been applied in full
- in the case of products placed on the market in a sterile condition, a description of the methods used
- the results of the design calculations and of the inspections carried out. If the device is to be connected to other device(s) in order to operate as intended, proof must be provided that it conforms to the Essential Requirements when connected to any such device(s) having the characteristics specified by the manufacturer
- the test reports and, where appropriate, clinical data
- labels and instructions for use.

The manufacturer must keep copies of EC type-examination certificates and/or the supplements thereto in the Technical Documentation File. These copies must be kept for a period ending at least five years after the last device has been manufactured.

5.3 A Comparison of the Medical Device Records

A manufacturer will accumulate a large amount of documentation during the typical product development process. The primary question then becomes which documentation is kept and where is it kept? Table 5-1 is an attempt to summarize the typical types of documentation and where they are kept. This is not an exclusive list, but serves only as guidance.

Table 5-1 Comparison of Record Storage

Record	Inclusion			
	Design History File	Device Master Record	Device History Record	Technical File
Agency submittals		X		X
Assembly inspection records		X	X	
Bills of material		X		
Calibration instructions/records		X		
Certificate of Vendor Compliance			X	
Certificates of compliance	X			X
Check sheets			X	
Clinical trial information	X			X
Combined product analysis				X
Component specifications		X		
Declarations of Conformity				X
Design Review records	X			
Design specification	X	X		
Design test protocols	X			
Design test results	X			X
Design validation plans	X			
Design validation protocols	X			
Design validation results	X	X		
Design verification plans	X			
Design verification protocols	X			

Record	Inclusion			
	Design History File	Device Master Record	Device History Record	Technical File
Design verification results	X			X
Engineering drawings	X	X		
Essential Requirements checklists				X
Evaluations of potential vendors	X			
Evaluations of contractors	X			
Evaluations of consultants	X			
Field action reports			X	
Field service reports			X	
Final inspection instructions		X		
Incoming material Quality Records		X		
Inspection instructions		X		
Inspection plans		X		
Installation instructions		X		
Labeling requirements	X	X		X
Lab notebooks	X	X		
Letters of transmittal		X		
Listings of applicable standards				X
Machining inspection records			X	
Maintenance procedures		X		
Maintenance service reports			X	
MDD design specifications				X
Medical Device Reports (MDRs)			X	
Medical Device Vigilance Reports			X	
Nonconforming material reports			X	
Packaging instructions		X		
Packaging specifications		X		
Post-release design control change records		X		
Pre-release design control change records	X			
Primary inspection records		X		
Process change control records		X		
Process validation records		X		
Product complaints			X	

Record	Inclusion			
	Design History File	Device Master Record	Device History Record	Technical File
Product descriptions		X		X
Product environmental specs		X		
Product manuals		X		
Product routings		X		
Product specifications	X	X		
Product test specifications	X	X		
Production release documentation		X		
Project plans	X			
Project team minutes	X			
Promotional materials		X		
Purchase orders			X	
Quality inspection audit reports		X		
Quality problem reporting sheets			X	
Quality memorandums		X		
Rationale for deviation from standards/regulations				X
Receipt vouchers			X	
Regulatory submittals		X		
Rework plans	X			
Risk analysis	X			X
Sales order reports			X	
Service specifications		X		
Shipping orders			X	
Software source code	X	X		
Tooling specs/revision log		X		
Work orders			X	

Table 5-1 Comparison of Record Storage (Continued)

Homework Exercises

1. Write a one page business proposal for your design project. Rough out a product specification page and design specification page if applicable.

2. You are going into competition with Johnson and Johnson; you plan to capture 30% of the market for band-aids. Do the needed web search to determine your market potential in terms of the US market.

3. The web sites medicaldata.com and medicaldesignonline.com both have daily columns discussing new medical developments. Go to one of the web sites (or a related one) and peruse the industry news section. For one of the recent developments listed, discuss and document the market need. Identify what was obtained from this site versus what you obtain from other site searches.

4. Improper record keeping and other poor practices have bankrupted several medically related firms. Do a web or library search to find such a case. Briefly discuss the case.

5. You are assigned to investigate the consequences of prostectomy. Identify the current market for this operation and the consequences of the operation. Identify a need for improvement relating to your observations.

6. Do a web search using the term "medical device ". Detail how many hits are really consulting firms that assist in the structuring of a business proposal or product specification. Print out documentation on two or three of these companies and discuss what the product really is in terms of this chapter. The use of a good search engine (such as Go Network) is recommended, most of the single search engines are not powerful enough.

7. There are a few web sites that specialize in determining the market for devices or treatments that target a complex of consequences of lung disease or the like. Most charge a high fee for identifying opportunities for entrepreneurship in the field. Find such a site, document it, and discuss the perceived value of the information.

References

ANSI/IEEE Standard 730, *IEEE Standard for Software Quality Assurance Plans*. New York: The Institute of Electrical and Electronics Engineers, Inc., 1989.

ANSI/IEEE Standard 830, *IEEE Guide to Software Requirements Specifications*. New York: The Institute of Electrical and Electronics Engineers, Inc., 1984

ANSI IEEE Standard 1016, *IEEE Recommended Practice for Software Design Descriptions*. New York: The Institute of Electrical and Electronics Engineers, Inc., 1987.

Brodie, Christina Hepner and Gary Burchill, *Voices Into Choices – Acting on the Voice of the Customer*. Madison: Joiner Associates, Inc., 1997.

Chevlin, David H. and Joseph Jorgens III, "Medical Device Software Requirements: Definition and Specification," *Medical Instrumentation* Volume 30, Number 2, March/April, 1996.

Davis, Alan M. and Pei Hsia, "Giving Voice to Requirements Engineering," in *IEEE Software*. Volume 11, Number 2, March, 1994.

Day, Ronald G., *Quality Function Deployment - Linking a Company with Its Customers*. Milwaukee, WI: ASQC Quality Press, 1993.

Fairly, Richard E., *Software Engineering Concepts*. New York: McGraw-Hill Book Company, 1985.

Fries, Richard C., *Reliable Design of Medical Devices*. New York: Marcel Dekker, Inc., 1997.

Gause, Donald C. and Gerald M. Weinberg, *Exploring Requirements: Quality Before Design*. New York: Dorset House Publishing, 1989.

Guinta, Lawrence R. and Nancy C. Praizler, *The QFD Bool: The Team Approach to Solving Problems and Satisfying Customers Through Quality Function Deployment*. New York: AMACOM Books, 1993.

Higson, Gordon R., *The Medical Devices Directives – A Manufacturer's Handbook.* Brussles: Medical Technology Consultants Europe Ltd., 1993.

Keller, Marilyn and Ken Shumate, *Software Specification and Design: A Disciplined Approach for Real-Time Systems.* New York: John Wiley & Sons, Inc., 1992.

Kriewall, Timothy J. and Gregory P. Widin, "An Application of Quality Function Deployment to Medical Device Development," in *Case Studies in Medical Instrument Design.* New York: The Institute of Electrical and Electronics Engineers, Inc., 1991.

Potts, Colin, Kenji Takahashi, and Annie I. Anton, "Inquiry-Based Requirements Analysis," in *IEEE Software*, Volume 11, Number 2, March, 1994.

Pressman, Roger S., *Software Engineering: A Practitioner's Approach.* New York: McGraw-Hill Book Company, 1987.

Schoenmakers, C.C.W., *CE Marking for Medical Devices.* New York: The Institute of Electrical and Electronic Engineers, 1997.

Siddiqi, Jawed and M. Chandra Shekaran, "Requirements Engineering: The Emerging Wisdom," in *Software.* Volume 13, Number 2, March, 1996.

Silbiger, Steven, *The Ten Day MBA.* New York: William Morrow and Company, Inc., 1993.

Taylor, J. W. *Planning Profitable New Product Strategies.* Radnor, PA: Chilton Book Company, 1984.

Trautman, Kimberly A., *The FDA and Worldwide Quality System Requirements Guidebook for Medical Devices.* Milwaukee: American Society for Quality Press, 1997.

21 CFR §820. Washington DC: Food and Drug Administration, 1996.

Chapter 6

Product Development

"America's abundance was not created by public sacrifices to the common good, but by the productive genius of free men who pursued their own personal interests and the making of their own private fortunes."
Ayn Rand

Design input provides the foundation for product development. The objective of the design input process is to establish and document the design input requirements for the device. The design input document is as comprehensive and precise as possible. It contains the information necessary to direct the remainder of the design process. It includes design constraints, but does not impose design solutions.

Once the documentation describing the design and the organized approach to the design is complete, the actual design work begins. As the design activity proceeds, there are several failure-free or failure-tolerant principles that must be considered to make the design more reliable. Each is important and has its own place in the design process.

6.1 Hardware and Software Techniques

6.1.1 Block diagram

The first step in an organized design is the development of a block diagram of the device (see Figure 6-1). The block diagram is basically a flow chart of the signal movement within the device and is an aid to organizing the design. Individual blocks within the block diagram can be approached for component design, making the task more organized and less tedious. Once all blocks have been designed, their connections are all that remain.

6.1.2 Redundancy

One method of addressing the high failure rate of certain components is the use of redundancy, that is, the use of more than one component for the same purpose in the circuit. The philosophy behind redundancy is if one component fails, another will take its place and the operation will continue. An example would be the inclusion of two reed switches in parallel where if one fails because the reeds have stuck together, the other is available to continue the operation.

Redundancy may be of two types:

- Active
- Standby.

6.1.2.1 Active redundancy

Active redundancy occurs when two or more components are placed in parallel, with all components being operational. Satisfactory operation occurs if at least one of the components functions. If one component fails, the remaining parts will function to sustain the operation. Active redundancy is important in improving the reliability of a device. Placing components redundantly increases the MTBF of the circuit, thus improving reliability. Consider the following example.

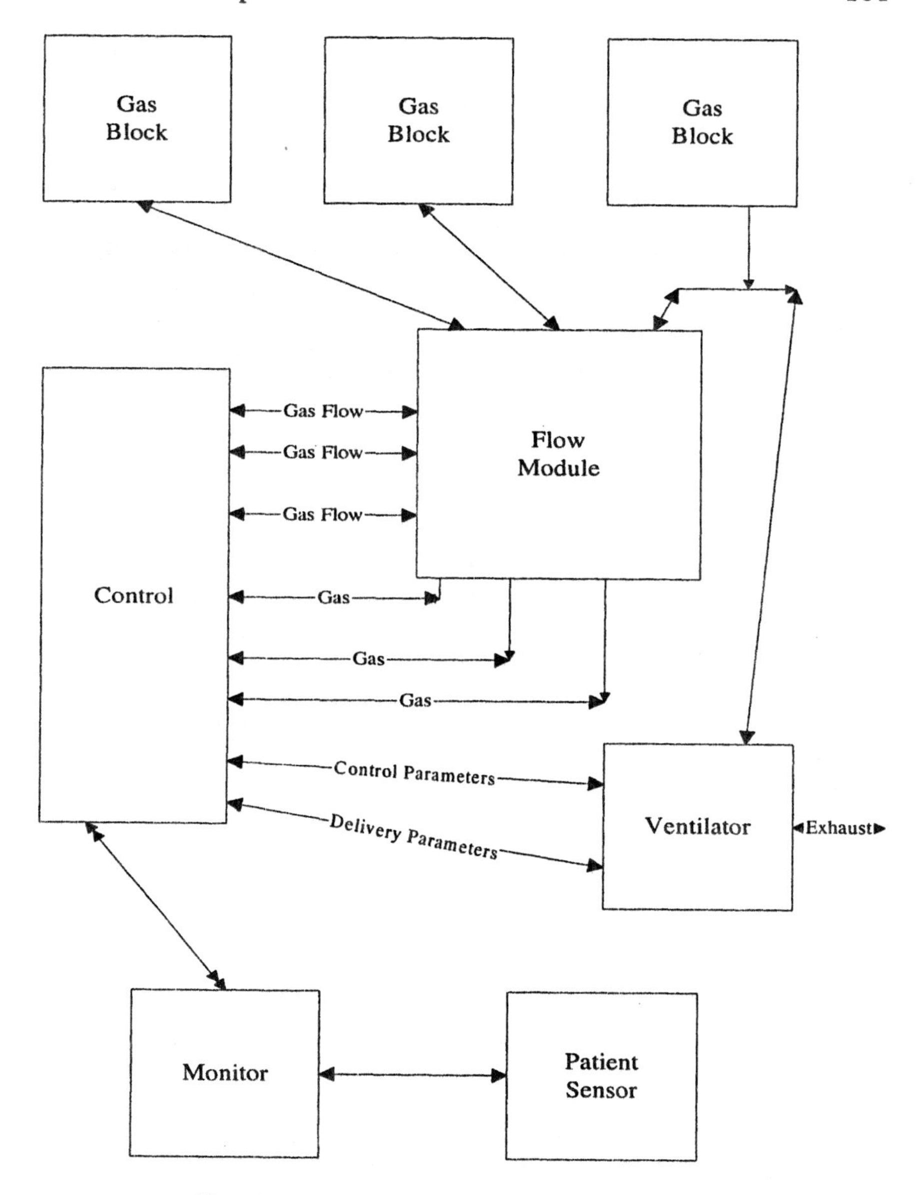

Figure 6-1 Block diagram. (From Fries, 1997.)

Figure 6-2 shows a circuit for an amplifier. Let's use the component U1 as our candidate for redundancy. The failure rate for the component in MIL-HDBK-217 gives a value for our intended use of 0.320 failures/million hours. The failure rate assumption is that the component was in its useful life period. Therefore, the reciprocal of the failure rate is the Mean Time Between Failure (MTBF). When calculating the MTBF, the failure rate must be specified in failures per hour. Therefore, the failure rate, as listed in the handbook or in vendor literature must be divided by one million.

$$
\begin{aligned}
\text{MTBF} &= 1/\lambda \\
&= 1/0.00000032 \\
&= 3{,}125{,}000 \text{ hours}
\end{aligned}
$$

Let's assume for our particular application, this MTBF value is not acceptable. Therefore, we decide to put two components in parallel (Figure 6-3). Again, we assume the useful life period of the component. For this case:

$$
\begin{aligned}
\text{MTBF} &= 3/2\lambda \\
&= 3/2(0.00000032) \\
&= 3/0.00000064 \\
&= 4{,}687{,}500 \text{ hours}
\end{aligned}
$$

By putting two components in active redundancy, the MTBF of the circuit has increased by 50%.

6.1.2.2 Standby redundancy

Standby redundancy occurs when two or more components are placed in parallel, but only one component is active. The remaining components are in standby mode.

Returning to our previous example, we have decided to use standby redundancy to increase our reliability (Figure 6-4). Again assuming the useful life period and ignoring the failure rate of the switch,

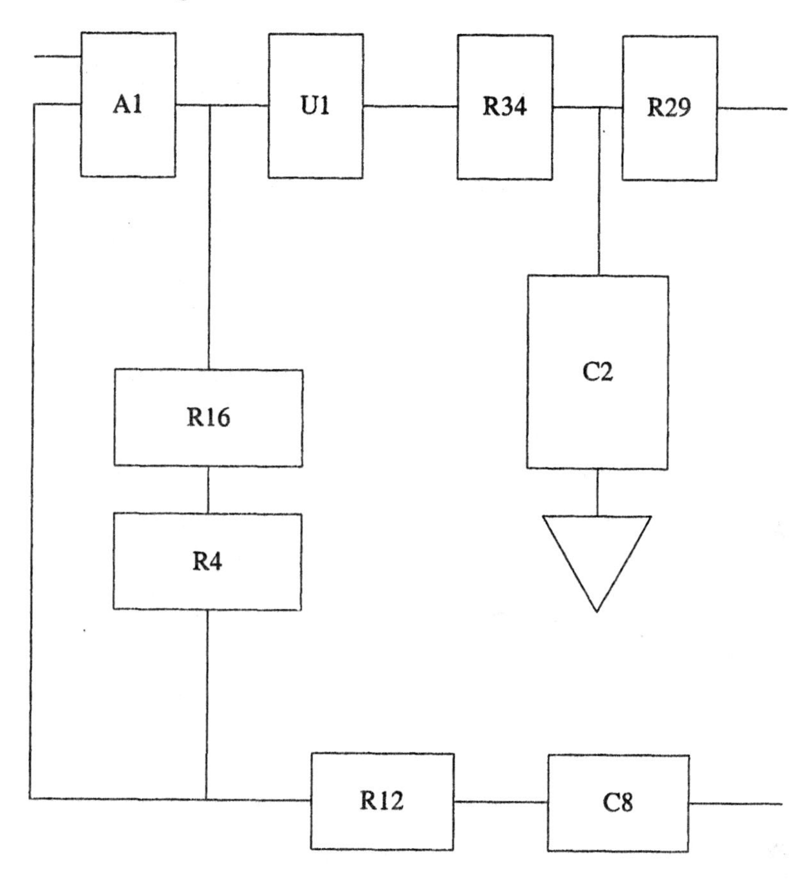

Figure 6-2 Circuit example. (From Fries, 1997.)

$$\begin{aligned} \text{MTBF} &= 2/\lambda \\ &= 2/0.00000032 \\ &= 6{,}250{,}000 \text{ hours} \end{aligned}$$

By using standby redundancy, the MTBF has increased by 100% over the use of the single component and by 33% over active redundancy.

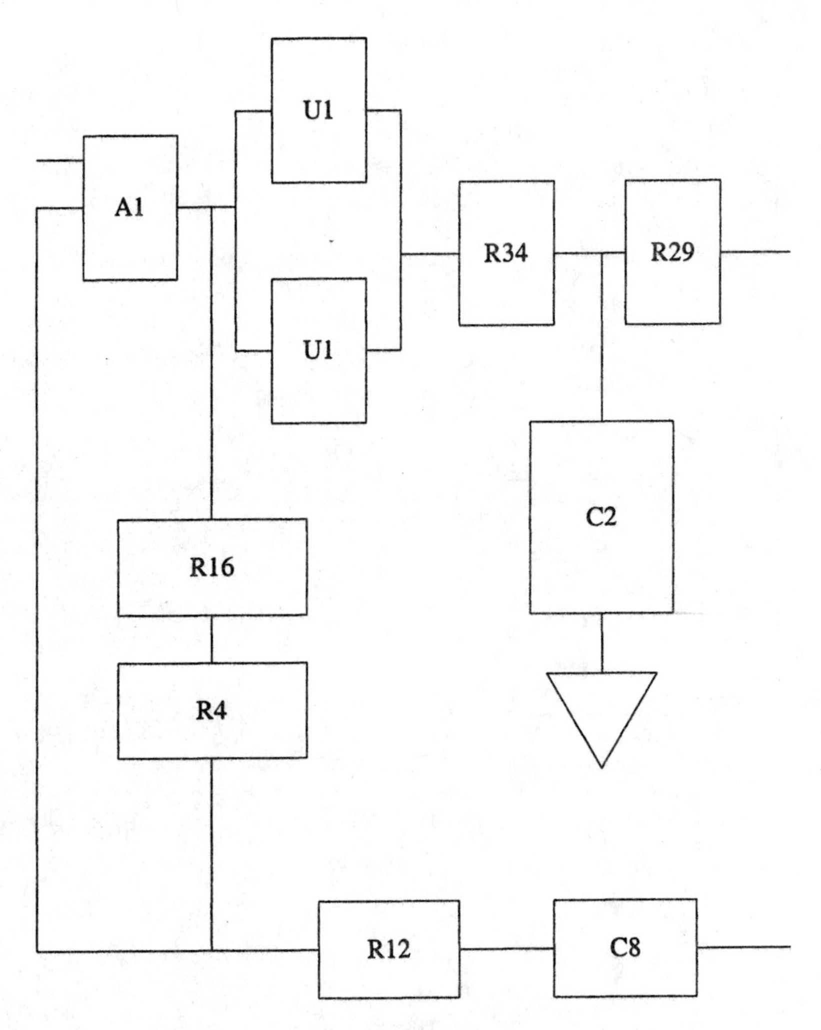

Figure 6-3 Active redundancy. (From Fries, 1997.)

Obviously, the use of redundancy is dependent upon the circuit and the failure rates of the individual components in the circuit. However, the use of redundancy definitely increases the reliability of the circuit. What type of redundancy is used again depends on the individual circuit and its intended application.

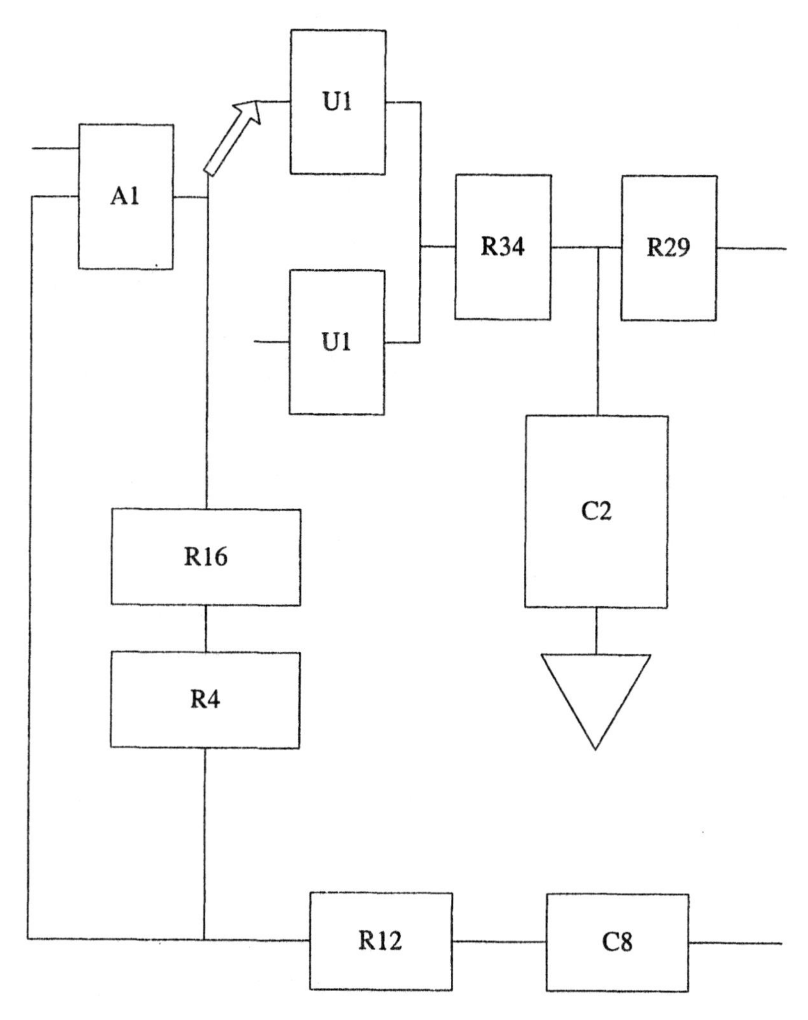

Figure 6-4 Standby redundancy. (From Fries, 1997.)

6.1.3 Component selection

As certain portions of the design become firm, the job of selecting the proper components becomes a primary concern, especially where there are long lead times for orders. How are the vendors for these components chosen? If one is honest in looking back at previous design developments and honest in listing the three main criteria for choosing a component vendor, they would be:

Lowest cost
Lowest cost
Lowest cost.

The only other parameter which may play a part in choosing a vendor is loyalty to a particular vendor, no matter what his incoming quality may be. Obviously, these are not the most desirable parameters to consider if the design is to be reliable. The parameters of choice include:

- Fitness for use
- Criticality versus non-criticality
- Reliability
- History
- Safety.

6.1.3.1 Component fitness for use

Fitness for use includes analyzing a component for the purpose to which it was designed. Many vendors list common applications for their components and tolerances for those applications. Where the desired application is different than that listed, the component must be analyzed and verified in that application. This includes specifying parameters particular to its intended use, specifying tolerances, inclusion of a safety margin and a review of the history of that part in other applications.

For components being used for the first time in a particular application and for which no history or vendor data is available, testing in the desired application should be conducted. There is more about this in the chapter on validation (Chapter 16).

6.1.3.2 Component reliability

The process of ensuring the reliability of a component is a multi-step procedure, including:

- Initial vendor assessment
- Vendor audit
- Vendor evaluation
- Vendor qualification.

The initial vendor assessment should be a review of any past history of parts delivery, including on time deliveries, incoming rejection rate, willingness of the vendor to work with the company and handling of rejected components. The vendor should also be questioned as to the nature of his acceptance criteria, what type of reliability tests were performed and what the results of the tests were. It is also important to determine whether the nature of the test performed was similar to the environment the component will experience in your device.

Once the initial vendor assessment is satisfactorily completed, an audit of the vendor's facility is in order. The vendor's processes should be reviewed, the production capabilities assessed, rejection rates and failure analysis discussed. Sometimes the appearance of the facility provides a clue as to what type of vendor you are dealing with. A facility that is unorganized or dirty may tell you about the quality of the work performed.

Once components are shipped, you need to ensure that the quality of the incoming product is what you expect. A typical approach to the evaluation would be to do 100% inspection on the first several lots to check for consistent quality. Once you have an idea of the incoming quality and you are satisfied with it, components can be randomly inspected or inspected on a skip-lot basis.

Many companies have established a system of qualified vendors to determine what components will be used and the extent of incoming inspection. Some vendors qualify through a rigorous testing scheme that determines the incoming components meet the specification. Other companies have based qualification on a certain number of deliveries with no failures at incoming. Only components from qualified vendors should be used in any medical device. This is especially important when dealing with critical components.

6.1.3.3 Component history

Component history is an important tool in deciding what components to use in a design. It is important to review the use of the component in previous products, whether similar or not. When looking at previous products, the incoming rejection history, performance of the component in field use and failure rate history need to be analyzed.

A helpful tool in looking at component history is the use of available data banks of component information. One such data bank is MIL-HDBK-217. This military standard lists component failure rates based upon the environment in which they are used. The information has been accumulated from the use of military hardware. Some environments are similar to that seen by medical devices and the data is applicable. MIL-HDBK-217 is discussed in greater detail later in this chapter.

Another component data bank is a government program named GIDEP. The only cost for joining this group is a report listing failure rates of components in your applications. You receive reports listing summaries of other reports the group has received. It is a good way to get a history on components you intend to use. More information may be obtained by writing to:

GIDEP Operations Center
Department of the Navy
Naval Weapons Station
Seal Beach, Corona Annex
Corona, CA 91720

A good source for both mechanical and electrical component failure rates is the books produced by the Reliability Analysis Center. They may be contacted at:

Reliability Analysis Center
P. O. Box 4700
Rome, NY 13442-4700
Telephone: +1+800+526-4802

6.1.3.4 Component safety

The safety of each component in your application must be analyzed. Do this by performing a fault tree analysis, where possible failures are traced back to the components causing them.

A failure mode analysis can be performed that looks at the results of single point failures of components. Unlike the fault tree, which works from the failure back to the component, failure mode analysis works from the component to the resultant failure. This is also discussed in more detail later in the chapter.

6.1.4 Component derating

Component failure in a given application is determined by the interaction between the strength and the stress level. When the operational stress levels of a component exceed the rated strength of the component, the failure rate increases. When the operational stress level falls below the rated strength, the failure rate decreases.

With the various ways for improving the reliability of products, derating of components is an often-used method to guarantee the good performance as well as the extended life of a product. Derating is the practice of limiting the stresses, which may be applied to a component, to levels below the specified maximum.

Derating enhances reliability by:

- reducing the likelihood that marginal components will fail during the life of the system
- reducing the effects of parameter variations
- reducing the long-term drift in parameter values
- providing allowance for uncertainty in stress calculations
- providing some protection against transient stresses, such as voltage spikes.

An example of component derating is the use of a 2 watt resistor in a 1 watt application. It has been shown that derating a component to 50% of its operating value generally decreases its failure rate by a factor greater than 30%. As the failure rate is decreased, the reliability is increased.

Components are derated with respect to those stresses to which the component is most sensitive. These stresses fall into two categories, operational stresses and application stresses. Operational stresses include:

- temperature
- humidity
- atmospheric pressure.

Application stresses include:

- voltage
- current
- friction
- vibration.

These latter stresses are particularly applicable to mechanical components.

Electrical stress usage rating values are expressed as ratios of Maximum Applied Stress to the Component's Stress Rating. The equation for table guidelines is:

Usage Ratio = Maximum Applied Stress/Component Stress Rating

For most electronic components, the usage ratio varies between 0.5 and 0.9.

Thermal derating is expressed as a maximum temperature value allowed or as a ratio of "actual junction temperature" to "maximum allowed junction temperature" of the device. The standard expression for temperature measurement is the Celsius scale.

Derating guidelines should be considered to minimize the degradation effect on reliability. In examining the results from a derating analysis, one often finds that a design needs less than 25 components aggressively derated to greatly improve its reliability. And, depending on the design of the product, these components often relate to an increase in capacitance voltage rating, a change of propagation speed, an increase in the wattage capacity of a selected few power resistors, etc.

6.1.5 Safety margin

Components or assemblies will fail when the applied load exceeds the strength at the time of application. The consideration of the load should take into account combined loads, such as voltage and temperature or humidity and friction. Combined loads can have effects that are out of proportion to their separate contributions, both in terms of instantaneous effects and strength degradation effects.

Establishing tolerances is an essential element of assuring adequate safety margins. Establishing tolerances, with appropriate controls on manufacturing provides control over the resulting strength distributions. Analysis should be based on worst case strength or distributional analysis, rather than on an anticipated strength distribution.

Safety margin is calculated as follows:

$$\begin{aligned}\text{Safety Margin} &= (\text{Mean safety factor}) - 1 \\ &= (\text{Mean strength/mean stress}) - 1\end{aligned}$$

An example illustrates the concept:

> A structure is required to withstand a pressure of 20,000 psi. A safety margin of 0.5 is to be designed into the device. What is the strength that must be designed in?

$$\begin{aligned}\text{Safety Margin} &= (\text{strength/stress}) - 1 \\ 0.5 &= (\text{strength}/20{,}000) - 1 \\ 1.5 &= \text{strength}/20{,}000 \\ (20{,}000 \times 1.5) &= \text{strength} \\ 30{,}000 \text{ psi} &= \text{strength}\end{aligned}$$

Most handbooks list a safety margin of 2.0 as the minimum required for high reliability devices. In some cases, this may result in an over-design. The safety margin must be evaluated according to device function, the importance of its application and the safety requirements. For most medical applications, a minimum safety margin of 0.5 is adequate.

6.1.6 Load protection

Protection against extreme loads should be considered whenever practicable. In many cases, extreme loading situations can occur and must be protected against. When overload protection is provided, the reliability analysis should be performed on the basis of the maximum load which can be anticipated, bearing in mind the tolerances of the protection system.

6.1.7 Environmental protection

Medical devices should be designed to withstand the worst case environmental conditions in the product specification, with a safety margin included. Some typical environmental ranges that the device may experience include:

operating temperature	0 to +55 degrees centigrade
storage temperature	-40 to +65 degrees centigrade
humidity	95% RH at 40 degrees centigrade
mechanical vibration	5 to 300 Hz at 2 Gs
mechanical shock	24" to 48" drop
mechanical impact	10 Gs at a 50 msec pulse width
electrostatic discharge	up to 50,000 volts

Electromagnetic compatibility becomes an issue in an environment, like an operating room. Each medical device should be protected from interference from other equipment, such as electrocautery and should be designed to eliminate radiation to other equipment.

6.1.8 Product misuse

An area of design concern that was briefly addressed earlier in this chapter is the subject of product misuse. Whether through failure to properly read the operation manual or through improper training, medical devices are going to be misused and even abused. There are many stories of product misuse, such as the hand held monitor that was dropped into the toilet bowl, the physician who used a hammer to pound a 9-volt battery into a monitor backwards or the user who spilled a can of soda on and into a device.

Practically, it is impossible to make a device completely misuse-proof. But it is highly desirable to design around the ones that can be anticipated.

Some common examples of product misuse include:

- excess application of cleaning solutions
- physical abuse
- spills
- excess weight applied to certain parts
- excess torque applied to controls or screws
- improper voltages, frequencies or pressures
- improper or interchangeable electrical or pneumatic connections.

Product misuse should be discussed with Marketing to define as many possible misuse situations as can be anticipated. The designer must then design around these situations, including a safety margin, which will serve to increase the reliability of the device. Where design restrictions limit the degree of protection against misuse and abuse, the device should alarm or should malfunction in a manner that is obvious to the user.

6.1.9 Design for variation

During design, one may need to deal with the problem of assessing the combined effects of multiple variables on a measurable output or other characteristic of a product, by means of experiments. This is not a problem that is important in all designs, particularly when there are fairly large margins between capability and required performance, or for design involving negligible risk or uncertainty, or when only one or a few items are to be manufactured. However, when designs have to be optimized in relation to variations in parameter values, processes, and environmental conditions, particularly if these variations can have combined effects, it is necessary to use methods that can evaluate the effects of the simultaneous variations.

Statistical methods of experimentation have been developed which enable the effects of variation to be evaluated in these types of situation. They are applicable whenever the effects cannot be theoretically evaluated, particularly when there is a large component of random variation or interactions between variables. For multivariable problems, the methods are much more economical than traditional experiments, in which the effect of one variable is evaluated at a time. The traditional approach also does not enable interactions to be analyzed, when these are not known empirically.

6.1.10 Design of experiments

The statistical approach to design of experiments is a very elegant, economical, and powerful method for determining the s-significant effects and interactions in multivariable situations.

6.1.10.1 The Taguchi method

Genichi Taguchi developed a framework for statistical design of experiments adapted to the particular requirements of engineering design. Taguchi suggested that the design process consists of three phases: system design, parameter design, and tolerance design. In the system design phase, the basic concept is decided, using theoretical knowledge and experience to calculate the basic parameter values to provide the performance required. Parameter design involves refining the values so that the performance is optimized in relation to factors and variation which are not under the effective control of the designer, so that the design is robust in relation to these. Tolerance design is the final stage, in which the effects of random variation of manufacturing processes and environments are evaluated, to determine whether the design of the product and the production processes can be further optimized, particularly in relation to cost of the product and the production processes.

Taguchi separates variables into two types. Control factors are those variables which can be practically and economically controlled, such as a controllable dimensional or electrical parameter. Noise factors are the variables which are difficult or expensive to control in practice, though they can be controlled in an experiment, e.g., ambient temperature, or parameter variation with a tolerance range. The objective is then to determine the combination of control factor settings (design and process variables) which will make the product have the maximum robustness to the expected variation in the noise factors.

6.1.11 Fundamentals of software engineering management

Good management of software development is critical to delivering a high quality, reliable product. There are many skills necessary to be a good manager. The intent here is not to try to describe what is required to be a good manager, but to identify some fundamental management activities that must be accomplished for software developers to be successful in their tasks. These fundamental management activities are:

- Planning
- Estimating
- Tracking progress.

6.1.11.1 Planning software development

After the Normandy invasion, Dwight Eisenhower reportedly said "Plans are worthless, but planning is everything." As soon as the action starts, a plan must start to change. None of us can ever foresee how all the variables in a project will turn out. Our plans can never be entirely correct. If we are to have any hope of keeping control of a project once it is underway, we must have done good planning. Good planning requires a clear understanding of the problem, a recognition of the assumptions being made, a definition of what success will be and an in-depth knowledge of the resources available and their strengths and weaknesses.

Planning encompasses more than just documenting resources needed for the project and creating a schedule. It includes looking at the project from a management view including schedule and resources, as well as looking at how the work will be done. What development model should be used? What methodology? What programming language and tools? Planning also includes identifying how the software will be controlled, and how it will be tested.

A key input to planning for medical device software is safety risk. The most important factor is the greatest severity of injury that can result from a software failure. The United States Food and Drug Administration calls this the "level of concern" of the software. Since the software can pose no greater risk of injury than the medical device it is a part of, the software level of concern cannot be greater than the risk of the device. It can possibly be lower if the software is not used to control critical device functions and if a software failure could only cause a lesser severity of injury than the device itself could. Understanding the software level of concern is important, because some choices in software methods and process are not appropriate for software with a high level of concern.

Often when a software development project is planned, some of the most important considerations aren't even discussed because everyone believes they are so obvious. These are the objectives for the project and the assumptions that the project team is making. Making these explicit and clear allows the project team to recognize when objectives change or assumptions are not being fulfilled. This allows the team to adjust, rather than continuing down a path that is unlikely to succeed.

Another area that good planning addresses is relationships between groups. A project may depend on the work of others. Without thinking through and getting agreement on how knowledge and information will be shared, or how deliverables are to be made available, much time and effort may be used in managing communication breakdowns that have a high level of emotion. Actions as simple as asking questions may become a problem if the person being asked is on the critical path of another project. Thinking through a process for resolving issues between groups before the project gets underway is a beneficial exercise that is too frequently overlooked or left to be thought about "when it gets to be a problem."

Sub-contractors are often used for developing parts of the software. This can be a very useful approach, reducing development time and adding expertise in an area where the development team may not have much experience. On the other hand, managing the contract may not be simple. The developer of the medical device is responsible for all the components used in it, and must make sure that the software being developed by the contractor is of sufficient quality for its intended purpose. Once again, careful planning before the work begins will allow for adjustments to be made when unexpected situations arise.

Project risks are another topic that planning should address. Establishing the four Cs for all significant foreseeable risks will provide a great deal of help should one or more of them become a problem: chronology (when will the risk be quantified), contingencies (what are the possible courses of action that could be followed), consequences (what are the likely results of each action), and criteria (how will the course of action be chosen). Having gone through the process of analyzing potential project risks during the planning phase of the project will also provide help for dealing with unexpected problems that may come up after the project is underway.

6.1.12 Choosing the software development process model

A software development process model is the portion of a software life cycle model that occurs before the first release of the software. For any software development, there are some fundamental activities that always are performed, and some optional activities that are included to improve the likelihood of meeting specific project objectives such as short development schedule, high reliability, or high conformance with customer desires. The sequence in which these activities are performed, and the formality with which they are performed and documented may vary. A software development process describes the activities to be performed and defines the chronological ordering of these activities. In order to define the development schedule, a software development process model must be selected.

There are a number of basically different software development process models, with many variations. Whether a particular model is appropriate depends on the goals of the project and the level of concern of the software.

6.1.12.1 Development process models for high level of concern

If the requirements of the software are established and reliability is a major objective, such as for software with a higher level of concern, these software development process models should be considered.

16.1.12.1.1 Waterfall model

This was the first documented software life cycle model. It divides the development process into steps, each of which reduces the level of abstraction of the solution. Each step includes a verification task and an exit criteria that must be met before moving on to the next step. As much as possible, iterations of a step are performed during the subsequent step.

The waterfall model's advantages are that it helps find errors early and provides a well understood structure. Its difficulties are that the requirements must be fully specified at the beginning of the project, before any design work has started. Finding out that requirements are wrong or incomplete late in the project can lead to extensive rework.

The waterfall model works best for complex systems where the requirements and technical methodologies are well understood. Many variations have been defined, such as overlapping steps, breaking implementation steps into parallel subprojects, and adding an introductory risk analysis step.

6.1.12.1.2 Incremental delivery model

The incremental delivery model is a modification of the waterfall model. It starts like the waterfall by analyzing requirements and creating an architectural design. Instead of delivering all of the software functionality at the end of the project, the functionality is divided up into increments that are delivered successively through out the project. Each increment refines the requirements and architectural design, then does detailed design, implementation, verification and release of its functionality.

This model works well when there is a need to deliver partial functionality before all of the functionality is needed. For example, a new medical device might need some software functionality for early hardware testing, additional functionality for validating expected clinical results in animals, more functionality when a human clinical study is performed, and the complete functionality for the market release of the device.

6.1.12.1.3 Spiral model

The spiral model was developed by Boehm to address some of the difficulties with the waterfall model. The spiral model iterates a set of steps, creating in effect a series of mini projects. Each of these mini projects completes a loop around the spiral. The first step in each of these mini projects is to determine the objectives, alternatives and constraints for the portion of the product being developed. The next step is to determine risks and resolve them.

Then the alternatives are evaluated, the deliverables for the iteration are developed and verified and a plan for the next iteration is created.

The main advantages of the spiral model are its flexibility and that it is risk driven, and as the project progresses and costs increase, the risks decrease. The disadvantage is that the spiral model requires expertise in risk management.

6.1.12.1.4 Cleanroom model

The cleanroom model was created to develop software that has a predictable reliability. It combines a set of techniques that depend on verifying the correctness of each step in the development process model. This results in more formality in specifying requirements, performing design and implementing the design in code. Since each step is verified as correct, cleanroom eliminates structural testing. It uses a statistical approach to functional testing to demonstrate that the requirements were implemented and to measure the software reliability in terms of mean time to failure.

Since the design is verified against the requirements, the requirements specification must be complete before design can begin. The requirements specification must also be written with sufficient formality that functional correctness verification of the design can be supported. This can best be achieved by using a formal specification language. The design must proceed in small steps, each being verified to be equivalent with its predecessor. Verification based inspections, which inspect for correctness rather than defects, are used to provide independent confirmation of the design's correctness.

Software coding proceeds in a similar manner of stepwise implementation and verification using inspections. Since the code is verified for correctness to the design, no developer debugging or unit testing is needed for demonstrating that the code implements the design. Cleanroom eliminates this activity, and the developers do not execute their code.

Cleanroom relies on independent testing to ensure that the requirements were implemented correctly. It also uses statistical testing techniques, sampling inputs based on probability of usage, to determine the software's reliability. It adds a feedback loop driven by continuously measuring reliability to the incremental delivery development process model in order to improve the reliability of each incremental delivery. The result is a final product with very high quality and a predictable reliability.

6.1.13 Development process models for low level of concern

For low level of concern software, where there is no safety risk, other objectives may lead to different development process models. If the requirements are understood, but the primary objective is time to market, the design to schedule development process model may be appropriate. If the requirements are not well understood and the primary objective is to demonstrate functionality, the evolutionary delivery model may be the best choice. These models are probably not acceptable for higher level of concern software.

6.1.13.1 Design to schedule model

This model prioritizes functionality and then develops it incrementally, with the early increments having the highest priority features. The difference between this model and the incremental delivery model is that with the design to schedule model you quit when the deadline is reached no matter how much has been delivered. At the beginning of the project, it is unclear how many of the planned increments will be completed.

6.1.13.2 Evolutionary delivery model

This model is used when requirements are changing rapidly or are not understood very well at the beginning of the project. The portions of the system that are best understood are developed and delivered. Feedback is gathered from users or potential users and the additional understanding is used to evolve the product to another version, which is developed and delivered. This iterative process is repeated until the users are satisfied that the necessary functionality is present in the software.

6.1.13.3 Code and fix model

If no planning is done, the default that gets used is called the code and fix model. It is not really a software development process model, but more the lack of one. With the code and fix model, you start with an idea of what you want to build, maybe write some specifications, then start coding, debugging and testing. As problems are found, they are fixed and sent back for more testing. When the number of problems being found in test falls to an acceptable level, or you run out of time to do more testing and fixing, you release the product. This model is not recommended for any type of software development, and is clearly not acceptable for any development in which software could result in loss of safety.

6.1.14 Choosing a design method

As with development process models, there are a number of basically different software design methods with many variations. They each provide criteria for expressing and refining the principles of good software design. As with life cycle models, each work best for certain types of problems. Whether a particular method is appropriate depends on the characteristics and level of concern of the software.

Most software design methods take one of three approaches:

- Top-down structured analysis and design
- Data-driven analysis and design
- Object-oriented analysis and design.

All these methods use decomposition to divide a complex problem into parts that are small enough to be understood and implemented correctly. They differ in what is being decomposed. Top-down structured analysis and design uses algorithmic decomposition, data-driven analysis and design uses data structure decomposition and object-oriented analysis and design uses object decomposition.

6.1.14.1 Structured analysis and structured design

Structured analysis and structured design grew from the ideas of structured programming and was popularized in the 1970s. It is a top down refinement approach that presents details in a layered fashion, hiding the detailed information regarding the design until the appropriate level. Structured analysis shows how data logically moves through a system being transformed by processes. Each process is decomposed into another set of processes and data flows providing more detail. The logical building blocks are algorithms, and the system is decomposed until the function of each process is a simple algorithm performing a single function.

Structured design partitions the system physically into modules that are organized into hierarchies with defined interfaces. Each module should solve one piece of the problem. Each module should be easy to understand. Connections between the modules should be as simple as possible. Each module has four attributes: input and output, function, internal logic and internal data.

6.1.14.2 Data-driven analysis and design

Data-driven analysis and design derives the structure of the software from the structure of the data that is input to the software and the structure of the data that is output by the software. These input and output structures are first modeled using a graphical notation. They then are converted into a program structure that maps inputs to outputs. The processing necessary to make the transformation from the input to output can be identified and associated with the program structure. The processing can then be decomposed as necessary. Data-driven design has been applied primarily to systems where input and output structures can be well defined and which have little concern for time-critical events, such as information management systems.

6.1.14.3 Object-oriented analysis and design

Object-oriented analysis and design groups data and the functions performed on that data into a single entity called an object. Rather than identifying data structures and process structures separately and then decomposing each, the object-oriented approach models systems in the real world as collections of objects which collaborate to perform some behavior. Objects can be identified, they can take action, and the current values of their properties can be determined. These characteristics are called identity, behavior and state. Objects communicate by messages which cause the receiving object to take an action.

6.1.15 Choosing a programming language

Programming languages are the tools used to transform the software design into executable instructions for the computer. The manner in which the programming language chooses to implement fundamental design concepts impacts the usability of the language. The trade-offs between programming languages are on characteristics such as ease of use, flexibility, performance, size of code generated, ease of maintenance and availability of development tools. The choice of programming language depends on the type of problem, the availability of tools for the target hardware, the design method chosen and the objectives of the project.

There is no such thing as a "safe" programming language. The responsibility for producing safe software rests with the software engineering team. A major consideration in the selection of a programming language is the availability of programmers with experience using the language. Programmers who are experienced with a language are more likely to know the potential problems and avoid them. There are however, some attributes of programming languages that make it easier for experienced programmers to produce dependable code. These include:

- Strong data typing - Will the data typing prevent misuse of variables?
- Exception handling - Do mechanisms exist to recover from runtime malfunctions?
- Separate compilation - Can modules be compiled separately? Is there type checking across module boundaries?
- Exhaustion of memory - Are there ways to guard against running out of memory at runtime?

When available, programming languages that provide these facilities would be a better choice for software which has safety as a primary objective.

6.1.16 Necessary technical software development activities

Software development is done in the context of systems engineering. What the system is to do must be determined first. These system requirements are then used to develop a system architecture, identifying which functions will be performed by which component of the system. The decisions about how to allocate functions to various components are made based on the objectives for the system, such as performance, cost, reliability, weight, power consumption, etc. The functions that are allocated to the software become the starting point for the software requirements analysis.

Technical software development activities produce work products that must be verified. Static analysis techniques such as reviews, walkthroughs and inspections, and dynamic techniques such as unit testing and system testing are used to verify the work products.

6.1.17 Software requirements analysis

This is the first technical step in the software engineering development process. Software requirements analysis refines the system requirements allocated to software to provide a model of the software behavior. The first task in software requirements analysis is to fully understand the basic elements of the problem that the software must solve. This includes identifying the exact purpose of the system, who will use it, and what the constraints are on the possible solutions. Once the problem is completely recognized, the functionality and data necessary for a solution are identified. Various alternative solutions can be analyzed and evaluated based on the criteria most important for the particular application. The results of this analysis is a set of function, data, performance and external interface requirements that define precisely what to build. These requirements make up the software requirements specification. The SRS plays many roles in a large development project.

1. It is the contract between management and the development team on exactly what is to be built.

2. It records the results of the analysis. It shows where the requirements are complete and where additional work is needed.
3. It defines what properties the software must have, and where there are constraints that limit the design choices.
4. It is used for estimating size and determining cost and schedule.

5. It is used by testers to determine acceptable behavior of the software.
6. It provides the standard definition of the expected behavior of the software for the system's maintainers.

If any commercially available off-the-shelf software is being included in the medical device software, it must be fully identified in the software requirements specification.

6.1.18 Software hazard analysis

For medical device software, software requirements analysis must also specify safety requirements. Identified system hazards that have been traced down to software must be mitigated by requirements or constraints on the software's behavior. These requirements and constraints are also documented in the software requirements specification and must be consistent with the rest of the software requirements.

The most direct way to trace system hazards to software is with a top-down fault tree analysis. How the software can contribute to the hazard condition is determined, and then requirements or constraints are identified that will prevent this software condition from occurring. When the software condition can be prevented by adding functionality, a requirement is written. If the software condition can only be prevented by constraining something from happening, a design constraint is written. Requirements are much easier to implement and verify than constraints and should be used to mitigate the software condition if possible. After these safety requirements and constraints are documented, it must be shown that the software requirements specification satisfies them. To do this, the software requirements specification must completely describe the behavior of the software under all conditions. Checking the software requirements specification for completeness requires analysis of states, transitions between states, inputs and outputs, values and timing. Some examples of criteria for checking specification completeness are:

- Every software state must be reachable from the initial software state
- Every software state must have a behavior specified for every possible input
- All information from sensors should be used somewhere in the specification
- Interlock failures should result in the halting of hazardous functions
- All incoming values should be checked and a response specified in the event of an out-of-range or unexpected value
- The response to excessive inputs must be specified
- Safety-critical outputs should be checked for reasonableness and for hazardous values.

6.1.19 Requirements traceability

To ensure that all requirements are implemented in the product, each requirement should be traced to the component of the design where it is implemented. In order to accomplish this, each requirement and each design component must be uniquely identified.

Traceability information can be maintained in traceability tables or in traceability lists. A traceability table is a matrix with requirements on one axis and design components on the other. The cell that is at the intersection of the requirement and the associated design component contains an entry showing the relationship. In a traceability list, each requirement is identified, along with a list of the design components that implement it.

To assure that all hazard mitigations result in requirements that are included in the software requirements specification, the hazard mitigations should be traced to the software requirements specification in the same manner that the requirements are traced to design components. This level of traceability makes it easy to see that each mitigation in the hazard analysis is identified in the software requirements and included in the software design. By extending this traceability to verification, it can be shown that all hazards mitigated by software have been specified, implemented and verified.

6.1.20 Software architectural design

Software architectural design defines the major structural elements of the software, their externally visible properties and the relationship among them. It partitions the real world problem (the software requirements) into elements of a software solution and organizes the relationships between these elements. The primary objective is to achieve an abstract representation of the structure, both of control and data. If the behavior of an element can impact other elements, that behavior should be described in the architecture. A modular program structure defining the control relationships between components and an organization of the logical relationship among the data elements is the starting point for software design. Some rules of thumb for good architectures:

- Well-defined modules with functionality based on the principles of information hiding and separation of concerns
- Hardware specifics should be encapsulated
- Dependencies on commercial tools or products should be encapsulated
- Separate modules that are producers of data from those that are consumers of data
- Modules should be defined so they can be implemented independently.

Safety must be designed into a system. Trying to add safety on at the end of development can increase risk due to added complexity. Architectural decisions are extremely important for implementing safety requirements. The concept of modularity, allocating design decisions into separate components, is a characteristic of a good design that is almost essential to be able to verify that safe operation has been achieved. Without understanding (and documenting) the behavior of a component that may impact other components, it will be nearly impossible to show that the system is safe.

6.1.21 Detailed design

Detailed design refines the abstract architectural design, filling in the details necessary to construct the final product. Detailed design must specify algorithms, data representations, connections between different processing elements and between processing elements and data structures. Detailed design must also be concerned with the packaging of the software product. Detailed design is performed using the chosen methodology. No matter what design methods and techniques are used, there are a number of fundamental design concepts that are important.

Modularity - The design should identify components or modules, and each module should solve one well-defined piece of the problem. The purpose of each module should be well defined. Each module should include the functional processing, data structures and control mechanisms necessary to achieve its purpose. Modules should communicate with each other using well-defined interfaces.

Information hiding - The internal processing details and data used by a module should not be observable from outside the module. The design decisions and their implementation should be hidden from other modules. This allows the detailed design and implementation decisions to be changed without impacting other modules.

Structure - This determines how the processing in a module is organized and controlled. If the software is thought of as a network, made up of processing nodes connected by control or data links, the logical path through the network is the structure. Examples of structure include hierarchical ordering and concurrent ordering. In hierarchically ordered modules, the processing elements are related by "uses" and "is used by" relationships. In a hierarchy, process nodes execute sequentially , the relationships are directed, and a node is not allowed to use a node that precedes it in the sequence. In a concurrent structure, process nodes execute in parallel and control is maintained by use of shared variables and message passing, using mechanisms such as semaphores and queues.

Encapsulation - If a data structure can only be accessed by routines packaged with it in a single module it is said to be encapsulated. Other routines that use the data structure do so by using the access routines. They do not need to know how the data structure is implemented.

Cohesion - This measures the strength of the relatedness of elements within a module. Maximizing cohesion will reduce the number of interconnections between modules. Cohesion is described as (from weakest or least desirable to strongest or most desirable):

1. Coincidental cohesion - elements within the module have no apparent relationship to one another
2. Logical cohesion - elements within the module perform similar functions
3. Temporal cohesion - all elements are executed at the same time
4. Communication cohesion - all elements refer to the same set of input/output data
5. Sequential cohesion - the output of one element is used as the input for the next element
6. Functional cohesion - all elements are related to the performance of a single function
7. Informational cohesion - each element performs a single function and all elements refer to a single data structure.

Coupling - This is the measure of the strength of connections between modules. It measures how well information hiding has been achieved. The stronger the coupling between two modules, the more likely that a change in one of the modules will require a change in the other. Coupling is ranked from strongest (least desirable) to weakest (most desirable).

1. Content coupling - the module modifies internal data or instructions in the other module
2. Common coupling - all modules share global data items
3. Control coupling - a module passes control flags that determine the sequence of processing in another module
4. Stamp coupling - only modules that require the data share global data
5. Data coupling - data items are passed between modules via parameters.

6.1.22 Implementation (coding)

After a module has been designed, the design must be translated into source code. This is a detailed, labor intensive task. The primary goals are to write the code so that its purpose is clear, so that it correctly implements the design, and so that it will integrate easily into the system. Simplicity and clarity are desirable characteristics, complexity and cleverness are to be avoided. This is especially true in any software that is critical to safety. In this case, standard techniques should be used that are easy to understand and are easily documented.

To consistently achieve the desirable code characteristics, coding standards are used to specify a preferred coding style. Coding standards usually include items such as:

1. Naming conventions for variables and functions
2. Guidelines for scope of data
3. Guidelines for using specific types of data
4. Guidelines for control structures
5. Use of assertions and other error detection practices
6. Specific items to be aware of in the particular programming language
7. Documentation conventions.

Documentation that is included with the source code should provide the information necessary to maintain the module. This documentation should address how the module accomplishes its function and illuminate any portion of the code that may not be sufficiently self-documenting. The documentation generally consists of a prologue or header which has a standard format and comments embedded in the code that explain major data manipulations or end cases and exception handling.

6.1.23 Integration

Integration is the combining of code that has been implemented independently into a single system where it must work together. One approach to integration is to have a specific integration phase in the development process model. The individual software modules are built in the previous phases and then combined into a system in the integration phase. This is often referred to as "big bang" integration. While it is possible to wait until all the code has been developed to put it together as a system, the effort required to get everything working may be very great. In practice it is much more efficient to integrate the code a small piece at a time. This approach is called incremental integration, or sometimes continuous integration. Incremental integration requires establishing an initial system and then adding just a little additional code at a time, while making sure that the system continues to operate. This requires careful planning and tight control over the order in which code is added to the system since modules must be integrated after other modules which they depend upon. The integration control process must include criteria for including new code in each version of the system.

Incremental integration has several additional advantages. Each software element can be tested as part of the system, eliminating the need to develop a special testing bed to test the new software element. Incremental integration also provides a focus on the source of problems. If a problem appears, it is probably related to the new module being added to the system, either in the new module itself or in the interfaces between it and the rest of the system. Incremental integration also provides flexibility, since it is possible to easily revert to the previous system if adding a new module results in a problem.

6.2 Structured and Unstructured Design Techniques

The initial part of the design/specify/build/test procedure is the most demanding, if the initial conception of the problem and the consequent design solution is inadequate, the product or solution may be doomed to failure. Chapter two covered some of the fundamental design tools used in initial attempts at a design solution, this section of this chapter is meant to give an overview of some of the more advanced methods. This section will include an extensive example problem "ideation" using a software package called "Innovation Workbench", a software package that is an outgrowth of the basic TRIZ method discussed in chapter 2. It has some properties in common with another package, TechOptimizer, which also evolved from the same roots. A brief overview then will be given of a structured design technique developed by Nam Suh, as well as an overview of a classical design methodology as documented in the text by Pahl and Beitz (*Engineering Design*).

6.2.1 The use of innovation workbench

Innovation Workbench is a software package that guides a designer through the initial design/solution search process by having the designer fill out material in a questionnaire. The questionnaire consists of four main parts. The first part is termed "Innovation Situation Questionnaire", this section consists of nine main sections that serve to document the current situation and the allowable changes that the designer might be able to make. The second section, "Problem Formulator", requires that the designer build a diagram that interrelates the elements of the process/system under study, with an emphasis on the generation of "good" interactions v "detrimental" interactions (in the chart to follow, arrows v arrows with a hatch mark). The detrimental interactions are analogous to the technical contradictions discussed in the section on TRIZ in chapter 2, these interactions and the diagram are used to generate directions for innovation, some of which are then selected for further study in a section titled "prioritize directions". Finally, two sections are devoted to the "development of concepts" and "evaluation of the results", these sections will receive little development here, as the majority of the useful part of this exercise is developed in the first three sections.

In the section to follow, the problem of looking for a method to more accurately measure the CO2 output of a human is addressed. The need for the measurement is for the development of a method for determination of apnea, the cessation of breathing. The technique that is "current", and therefore is to be improved upon, is the measurement of a CO2 detection system with a sampling port 12" away from the patient's nose area. This constraint leads to a decreased timeliness of the measurement, when combined with airflow in the room (a detrimental item) leads to a deceased sensitivity of the measurement (also detrimental).

In the multiple pages to follow, the program prompts will be denoted by underlining and (generally) numbering. Input from the designer will generally be without demarcation, with the exception of dated and timed "idea" capture sections and the diagram. Explanatory sections by the author will be denoted by italics.

Ideation Process

Innovation Situation Questionnaire

1. Brief description of the problem

Current devices for the measurement of CO_2 expired from patient's airways require contact with the patient's mouth or the use of a nasal/oral cannula (tube) for sampling of the air stream.

2. Information about the system

2.1 System name

CO_2 Monitoring of patients at risk.

2.2 System structure

Current system is comprised of a nasal/oral set of tubes that sample air from the areas near the mouth and nose, plus a pump and optical sensing system to determine the CO_2 in the sampled air.

Component list

- tube with nasal tubes and one mouth tube, these tubes intersect...
- pumping system
- optical bench
- sampled air includes CO_2 & moisture
- ambient air includes ambient CO_2
- power
- mouth
- nose
- patient
- nafion tubing (moisture leaking tube)
- subsystems interconnections...

Patient expires air.
Pump samples air (some fraction of expired air) from the combination of nasal and airway openings, this air varies as a combination of patient expired air and ambient air.
The sampled air passes through the nafion tubing, which assists in lowering the moisture content to approximately that of the environment

5/10/01 11:34:39 AM Idea:
Moisture content could be useful.

The sampled air then goes through the optical bench. The optical properties measured relate to CO_2 concentration, which relates to patient expired air. This measurement is continuous, thus we also have information regarding CO_2 concentration and the timing of this information, meaning respiration rate... The expired and sampled air is dumped into the environment.

2.3 Functioning of the system

tube with nasal tubes and one mouth tube, these tubes intersect...
strap holds the cannula on to the patient
pumping system
optical bench
sampled air includes CO_2 & moisture
ambient air includes ambient CO_2
power
mouth
nose
patient
nafion tubing (moisture leaking tube)

- the nafion tube samples air in the vicinity of the openings
- the tubing allows the moisture in the sampled air to lose moisture to that of the ambient air
- the tubing also allows the sampled air to approximate the temperature of the ambient

subsystems interconnections...

Patient expires air.
Pump samples air (some fraction of expired air) from the combination of nasal and airway openings, this air varies as a combination of patient expired air and ambient air.
The sampled air passes through the nafion tubing which assists in lowering the moisture content to approximately that of the environment

5/10/01 11:34:39 AM Idea:
Moisture content could be useful
SP - may not correlate w CO_2 content *(SP = special problem)*

the sampled air then goes through the optical bench. The optical properties measured relate to CO_2 concentration, which relates to patient expired air. This measurement is continuous, thus we also have information regarding CO_2 concentration and the timing of this information, meaning respiration rate... The expired and sampled air is dumped into the environment.

2.4 System environment

- other systems nearby the system or might often be nearby
  - other humans
  - misc possible other equipment
  - bed & LINENS
  - possible ventilation
  - ? other moisture sources
  - other CO_2 sources
- other systems interacting with the system, especially sources of energy, substances, receivers of waste, etc.
  - other close-by humans
  - ventilation (window, AC, fans,...)
  - trace gasses?
  - electric power
- conditions around the system, both artificial and natural (indoor or outdoor, temperature, humidity, medium, etc.)
  - talking
  - eating
  - snoring
  - mouth breathing
  - laughter
  - major changes in environment
- requirements for the functioning of the system and interactions between the system and environment.
  - proper sampling of some of the expired patient air
  - electrical power
  - non-kinking of the tubing/exhaust system
  - no smoke/other major contaminants
  - FDA approval

3. Information about the problem situation

3.1 Problem that should be resolved

- the need for a direct connection to the patient poses a risk (physical) to the patient
- disconnects may cause false alarms
- the need for the direct connection - at least this formulation of it - leads to crimping of the tubing that connects the patient to the measurement system - when the patient moves to a position that causes the crimping.
- sampling of body fluids may cause blockage of the sample tube

Contradiction: the need to be connected and not connected.

3.2 Mechanism causing the problem

- the need for a direct connection to the patient poses a risk (physical) to the patient
  - direct connect needed to sample expired patient air and environmental air. Closeness here guarantees that we get some expired air to measure with the distant optical bench.
- disconnects may cause false alarms
  - we will alarm if we think the patient is not expiring air containing CO_2.
- the need for the direct connection - at least this formulation of it - leads to crimping of the tubing that connects the patient to the measurement system - when the patient moves to a position that causes the crimping.
- sampling of body fluids may cause blockage of the sample tube
  not known if this is a problem - could be in a long term monitoring situation

3.3 Undesired consequences of unresolved problem

Patients will continue to die.
Alarms will not properly be given.

3.4 History of the problem

There are other methods to determine if a patient is breathing, such as looking at chest expansion (requires a harness), chemical sensors at the mouthpiece (slow, requires transducers), full mouthpiece sampling (inconvenient & more invasive than the tongs, mass spectroscopy, IR sampling (I think), optical sensing using IR sensitive cameras works but is too expensive... These expenses relate to the low temperature needed for high sensitivity... I assume the added costs relate to the complexity of the

IR camera...

3.5 Other systems in which a similar problem exists

Heart monitoring - if we really had to we can implant a transducer (mouse) and monitor transmitted ekg.

Temperature monitoring - IR cameras exist that can monitor temperature gradients on the skin, just not too expensive.
Gas monitoring exists in many monitoring systems, just look at NASA Tech briefs - exhaust plume detection on smokestacks, for example.
Gas monitoring on car exhaust.
The problem with the previous 2 solutions is that the stack & car do not move...
Moisture monitoring (see above) probably has similar drawbacks, need to check on IR or OTHER means of detection.
Slow chemical sensors exist for CO_2. Do they exist for H_2O?

3.6 Other problems to be solved

- Alternate solution - use H_2O sensing
- Alternate solution - go to a neighborhood volume of air to sense the CO_2 emission by putting the patient in a tent or sampling at an air intake and not worrying about being close to real-time on breath detection. 10-20 seconds is OK to wait to detect this second's breath...
- Alt. solution - the above works for moisture detection?
- Improve on the camera solution; build a cheap but sensitive optical system for CO_2 detection.
- Turn the current system inside out, but the current detector system around the patient. Look at a redesign of the current optical bench. Moisture intervening might now actually be valuable.
- Build a cheap system that could measure chest wall expansion & transmit when not activated.
- Improve pulse oximetry to the point that we can look at oscillations that are breath to breath measurements.
- Improve thermal imaging to the point that we can look at the plume of heat that is expired on a breath to breath basis.

4. Ideal vision of solution

A device that samples air near the face is no longer required.
Tubing that potentially harms the patient is no longer required.
The ideal system informs us noninvasively that the patient's metabolism in

terms of measureables such as CO_2 expiration/O_2 intake in the optimal location which probably is between the glottis & the splitting of the airway to R&L lungs.

5. Available resources

CO_2 out, O_2 in, H_2O out, heat out Temp)

5/10/01 2:46:39 PM Idea:

the lost color change CO_2 technology of 10 years ago???
Human metabolic - air transport I/O
Optical dependent on time of day?
Space - can see the patient, area around patient
We have up to 30 sec to detect a problem, we are measuring a process (periodic) which takes ~ 5 sec/breath.
consider parallel measures (pOx)

6. Allowable changes to the system

Small changes are allowed.
No major environmental change for optimal solution. (Cost, practicality)
Nothing major re: invasion of body orifices (legal, health standards, comfort).
"Low Cost" or low rental cost per use.
Almost as accurate as "gold standard" full mask monitoring (Safety for patient).

7. Criteria for selecting solution concepts

Safety, medium cost increase if necessary, long term profit, decrease in deaths....

8. Company business environment

University medical center/Biomedical Engineering operation

9. Project data

This is one of several design projects ongoing...

Problem Formulation

1. Build the Diagram

2. Directions for Innovation

(The following text is generated by the computer program based upon the above system diagram... The sections marked with the double carat (») are those selected by the author for further development).

5/11/01 9:16:03 AM Diagram

1. Find an alternative way to obtain [the] (flow of air in room) that does not influence [the] (sampling at capture site).

2. Try to resolve the following contradiction: The useful factor [the] (flow of air in room) should be in place in order to fulfill useful purpose and should not exist in order to avoid hindering [the] (sampling at capture site).

3. Find an alternative way to obtain [the] (sampling at capture site) that offers the following: provides or enhances [the] (flow of air to measurement device), does not influence [the] (sensitivity of measurement), does not require [the] (flow of air from patient) and (positioning of co2 capture 12" away), is not influenced by [the] (flow of air in room).

4. Try to resolve the following contradiction: The useful factor [the] (sampling at capture site) should be in place in order to provide or enhance [the] (flow of air to measurement device), and should not exist in order to avoid hindering [the] (sensitivity of measurement).

5. Find an alternative way to obtain [the] (flow of air from patient) that provides or enhances [the] (sampling at capture site).

6. Find an alternative way to obtain [the] (flow of air to measurement device) that offers the following: provides or enhances [the] (measurement of CO2), does not require [the] (suction from pump) and (sampling at capture site).

7. Find an alternative way to obtain [the] (suction from pump) that provides or enhances [the] (flow of air to measurement device).

8. Find an alternative way to obtain [the] (positioning of co2 capture 12" away) that offers the following: provides or enhances [the] (sampling at capture site), does not influence [the] (timeliness of measurement).

9. Try to resolve the following contradiction: The useful factor [the] positioning of co2 capture 12" away) should be in place in order to provide or enhance [the] (sampling at capture site), and should not exist in order to avoid

hindering [the] (timeliness of measurement).

10. Find an alternative way to obtain [the] (CO_2 is in the air) that provides or enhances [the] (measurement of CO_2).

11. Find an alternative way to obtain [the] (measurement of CO_2) that offers the following: provides or enhances [the] (evaluation of patient), does not require [the] (flow of air to measurement device), (CO_2 is in the air), (baseline for CO_2/air ratio) and (functioning of optical bench).

12. Find an alternative way to obtain [the] (baseline for CO_2/air ratio) that provides or enhances [the] (measurement of CO_2).

13. Find an alternative way to obtain [the] (functioning of optical bench) that offers the following: provides or enhances [the] (measurement of CO_2), does not require [the] (sensitivity of measurement) and (timeliness of measurement).

14. Find an alternative way to obtain [the] (evaluation of patient) that does not require [the] (measurement of CO_2).

15. Consider transitioning to the next generation of the system that will provide [the] (evaluation of patient) in a more effective way and/or will be free of existing problems.

16. Find an alternative way to obtain [the] (sensitivity of measurement) that offers the following: provides or enhances [the] (functioning of optical bench), is not influenced by [the] (sampling at capture site).

17. Find an alternative way to obtain [the] (timeliness of measurement) that offers the following: provides or enhances [the] (functioning of optical bench), is not influenced by [the] (positioning of co_2 capture 12" away).

Prioritize Directions

1. Directions selected for further consideration

6. Find an alternative way to obtain [the] (flow of air to measurement

device) that offers the following: provides or enhances [the] (measurement of CO_2), does not require [the] (suction from pump) and (sampling at capture site).

5/11/01 2:08:33 PM Idea:
Yes, consider replacement of pump/sampling.

6.1. Improve the useful factor (flow of air to measurement device).

6.2. Obtain the useful result without the use of [the] (flow of air to measurement device).

6.3. Increase effectiveness of the useful action of [the] (flow of air to measurement device).

6.4. Synthesize the new system to provide [the] (flow of air to measurement device).

6.5. Apply universal Operators to provide the useful factor (flow of air to measurement device).

6.6. Consider resources to provide the useful factor (flow of air to measurement device).

8. Find an alternative way to obtain [the] (positioning of co2 capture 12" away) that offers the following: provides or enhances [the] (sampling at capture site), does not influence [the] (timeliness of measurement).

8.1. Improve the useful factor (positioning of co2 capture 12" away).

8.2. Obtain the useful result without the use of [the] (positioning of co2 capture 12" away).

8.3. Increase effectiveness of the useful action of [the] (positioning of co2 capture 12" away).

8.4. Synthesize the new system to provide [the] (positioning of co2 capture 12" away).

8.5. Apply universal Operators to provide the useful factor (positioning of

CO_2 capture 12" away).

8.6. Consider resources to provide the useful factor (positioning of CO_2 capture 12" away).

10. Find an alternative way to obtain [the] (CO_2 is in the air) that provides or enhances [the] (measurement of CO_2).

10.1. Improve the useful factor (CO_2 is in the air).

10.2. Obtain the useful result without the use of [the] (CO_2 is in the air).

10.3. Increase effectiveness of the useful action of [the] (CO_2 is in the air).

10.4. Synthesize the new system to provide [the] (CO_2 is in the air).

10.5. Apply universal Operators to provide the useful factor (CO_2 is in the air).

10.6. Consider resources to provide the useful factor (CO_2 is in the air).

9. Try to resolve the following contradiction: The useful factor [the] (positioning of CO_2 capture 12" away) should be in place in order to provide or enhance [the] (sampling at capture site), and should not exist in order to avoid hindering [the] (timeliness of measurement).

9.1. Apply separation principles to satisfy contradictory requirements related to [the] (positioning of CO_2 capture 12" away).

9.2. Apply 40 Innovation Principles to resolve contradiction between useful purpose of (positioning of CO_2 capture 12" away) and its harmful result.

13. Find an alternative way to obtain [the] (functioning of optical bench) that offers the following: provides or enhances [the] (measurement of CO_2), does not require [the] (sensitivity of measurement) and (timeliness of measurement).

13.1. Improve the useful factor (functioning of optical bench).

5/11/01 11:08:31 AM Idea:
Consider the possibility of introducing adjustable elements or links into the system. Pointable mirror setup?

13.2. Obtain the useful result without the use of [the] (functioning of optical bench).

13.3. Increase effectiveness of the useful action of [the] (functioning of optical bench).

5/11/01 11:08:48 AM Idea:
If an action is insufficiently effective, consider introducing a new field (force, effect, or action) that will intensify the action. Add parabolic mirror or lensing system to setup.

13.4. Synthesize the new system to provide [the] (functioning of optical bench).

5/11/01 11:09:53 AM Idea:
Consider the use of Schlieren photography - is in need of special optics and bench...

13.5. Apply universal Operators to provide the useful factor (functioning of optical bench).

5/11/01 11:29:35 AM Idea:
As above, get rid of tubing, go with an optical setup, take current bench & redo...

13.6. Consider resources to provide the useful factor (functioning of optical bench).

14. Find an alternative way to obtain [the] (evaluation of patient) that does not require [the] (measurement of CO_2).

14.1. Improve the useful factor (evaluation of patient).

14.2. Obtain the useful result without the use of [the] (evaluation of patient).

14.3. Increase effectiveness of the useful action of [the] (evaluation of patient).

14.4. Synthesize the new system to provide [the] (evaluation of patient).

5/11/01 11:36:31 AM Idea:
This is where I am going. Get rid of the tubing and pump, reconfigure the optical bench, amplify the area "seen" by the bench, combine optics to a single system using mirrors & reflected light or use mirror to do absorbance / reflectance.

14.5. Apply universal Operators to provide the useful factor (evaluation of patient).

14.6. Consider resources to provide the useful factor (evaluation of patient).

15. Consider transitioning to the next generation of the system that will provide [the] (evaluation of patient) in a more effective way and/or will be free of existing problems.

15.1. Improve Ideality of your system that provides [the] (evaluation of patient).

15.2. Consider the possibility to transform the existing system that provides [the] (evaluation of patient) into bi- or poly-system.

15.3. Consider segmentation of the existing system that provides [the] (evaluation of patient).

15.4. Consider restructuring the existing system that provides [the] (evaluation of patient).

15.5. Increase dynamism of the existing system that provides [the] (evaluation of patient).

15.6. Increase controllability of the existing system that provides [the] (evaluation of patient).

15.7. Make the existing system that provides [the] (evaluation of patient) and/or its elements more universal.

17. Find an alternative way to obtain [the] (timeliness of measurement) that offers the following: provides or enhances [the] (functioning of optical bench), is not influenced by [the] (positioning of co2 capture 12" away).

17.1. Improve the useful factor (timeliness of measurement).

17.2. Obtain the useful result without the use of [the] (timeliness of measurement).

17.3. Increase effectiveness of the useful action of [the] (timeliness of measurement).

17.4. Synthesize the new system to provide [the] (timeliness of measurement).

17.5. Protect [the] (timeliness of measurement) from the harmful influence of [the] (positioning of co2 capture 12" away).

17.6. Apply universal Operators to provide the useful factor (timeliness of measurement).

17.7. Consider resources to provide the useful factor (timeliness of measurement).

3. Find an alternative way to obtain [the] (sampling at capture site) that offers the following: provides or enhances [the] (flow of air to measurement device), does not influence [the] (sensitivity of measurement), does not require [the] (flow of air from patient) and (positioning of co2 capture 12" away), is not influenced by [the] (flow of air in room).

3.1. Improve the useful factor (sampling at capture site).

3.2. Obtain the useful result without the use of [the] (sampling at capture site).

3.3. Increase effectiveness of the useful action of (sampling at capture site).

3.4. Synthesize the new system to provide [the] (sampling at capture site).

3.5. Protect [the] (sampling at capture site) from the harmful influence of [the] (flow of air in room).

3.6. Apply universal Operators to provide the useful factor (sampling at capture site).

3.7. Consider resources to provide the useful factor (sampling at capture site).

4. Try to resolve the following contradiction: The useful factor [the] (sampling at capture site) should be in place in order to provide or enhance [the] (flow of air to measurement device), and should not exist in order to avoid hindering [the] (sensitivity of measurement).

4.1. Apply separation principles to satisfy contradictory requirements related to [the] (sampling at capture site).

4.2. Apply 40 Innovation Principles to resolve contradiction between useful purpose of (sampling at capture site) and its harmful result.

2. List and categorize all preliminary ideas

CO2

This is where I am going. Get rid of the tubing and pump, reconfigure the optical bench, amplify the area "seen" by the bench, combine optics to a single system using mirrors & reflected light or use mirror to do absorbance / reflectance.

As above, get rid of tubing, go with an optical setup, take current bench & redo...

If an action is insufficiently effective, consider introducing a new field (force, effect, or action) that will intensify the action. Add parabolic mirror or lensing system to setup.

The lost color change CO2 technology of 10 years ago???

The sampled air then goes through the optical bench. The optical properties measured relate to CO_2 concentration, which relates to patient expired air. This measurement is continuous, thus we also have information regarding CO_2 concentration and the timing of this information, meaning respiration rate...

Moisture

Moisture content could be useful, SP - may not correlate w CO_2 content

Thermal

Thermal may be of value...SP - may not correlate w CO_2 content

Turbulence

Consider the use of Schlieren photography - is in need of special optics and bench...

Develop Concepts

1. Combine ideas into concepts

This is the crux of the remaining work to be done on this project…

2. Apply Lines of Evolution to further improve concepts

Give some thought to where this technology will be going in the future. It is highly likely that the above problem will be solved within ten years by the introduction of cheaper infrared camera systems. In the further off time line, overall biosensors will likely be available that are implanted in the subject that will warn of impending problems and call a caregiver if necessary…

Evaluate Results

(This section is intentionally blank, this is an ongoing project…)

1. Meet criteria for evaluating concepts
2. Reveal and prevent potential failures
3. Plan the implementation

Summary: The fairly extensive material in the previous several pages should leave one at least the impression that the overall process is fairly all-encompassing. The crux of a good solution (and solution space) lies in the good development of the system diagram, if the diagram properly captures al the relevant interactions and conflicts in a system design, the patented solution generation algorithm should generate a solution suggestion that will solve the design problem at hand. At the very least, the use of such a program provides a comprehensive structure for consideration of many design problems. Not shown above is the ability to reference patent databases and effects databases, the addition of these data make this a powerful tool.

6.2.2 Axiomatic design

A design approach that is also fairly recent in development is one codified in Axiomatic Design, Advances and Applications (2001), by Nam Suh. This design approach stresses codifying functional requirements (FR), design parameters (DP), process variables (PVs) and customer needs as vectors. In an ideal case, if a diagonal matrix can relate FRs and DPs, a unique solution may be generated that has little, if any, relationship between design parameters (independence). Development of the mathematical relationships based upon such principles as minimizing information content allows the development of several axioms for best designs. This approach has led to the development of a software approach to design that is currently being marketed, similar to the above innovation workbench software. (See Acclaro Software, by Axiomatic Design Software, Inc).

6.2.3 *Engineering Design*, Pahl and Beitz

There exist a number of generic design textbooks for any given field that may be referenced and used as main course textbooks for a design text. The above two approaches carry design to extreme points in the realm of patent and process-assisted design (Innovation Workbench) and mathematically based information extraction design (axiomatic design). For complete coverage, designers should be familiar with the very structured approach by Pahl and Beitz, as translated by Ken Wallace (Springer-Verlag, 1988).

This design approach is extremely structured and systematic in nature, the text builds upon an eight-step method for design: Clarification, Abstraction,

Function Structure Generation, Solution Search, Solution Combination, Combination Selection, Concept Variant Inspection, and End Evaluation. Each of the eight steps are sub detailed and reasonably well illustrated. At several points, the search for sub-solutions becomes one of searching through an extensive listing of solution principles, with the end goal of selection of one of them. At other times, there is a good blending of the need for the use of catalogs and standard part sizes, in order to achieve economy.

No software to automate the design process according to Pahl and Beitz is known to these authors, development of such a tool would be of value, especially in the area of Mechanical Engineering.

6.2.4 Design, redesign, and reverse engineering

With age, the opportunity to gain from reverse engineering of a competitor's product increases. This is because, with time – patents expire, copyrights expire, the competitors company may expire, or the root technology that is imbedded in the competitors' technology has been bettered. Other considerations include cases where the cost to maintain old technology becomes too high for general maintenance or repair when needed. Rarely, a materials embargo due to war or trade restrictions forces a reconsideration of the current technology.

The traditional engineering design process involves a cascade from needs determination to design to prototype/test to product generation (Figure 1-1). Loop backs are done as necessary to improve on design errors as they are caught. Reverse engineering, on the other hand, starts with a product in hand, and an associated list of needs associated with that need. The first step in the reengineering generally involves a disassembly of the product, and generation of a database of parts details. Each of these parts is then measured and tested, and an idea of the original design constraints and goals is generated. With a properly generated parts and assembly listing, a comparison can be quickly generated as to the cost savings that might be made with updated technology. If this initial estimate proves to be beneficial, the entire product can be prototyped with upgraded parts and assembly methods, and tested. If successful, you have generated a reverse engineered product.

For example, several years ago a device that was used in sleep studies was coming out of patent, the manufacturer decided to cease manufacture and maintenance of its devices. The device had a rotary dial to enable data to be transmitted via telephone lines to a central lab for data analysis. The data collected consisted of EEG, EMG, EKG, and respiration waveforms, data was transmitted real time (multiplexed fm converted analog signals) to a central laboratory for transcription to chart recorders to generate a paper record to pass on to physicians for later analysis.

The current device was thoroughly studied, a parts list generated, and an initial listing of relevant new technology generated. A flow chart of the then current study protocol was generated and studied for opportunities for improvement. Current, competing technologies were studied for potential improvements to the reverse engineered system. Other potential improvements were solicited from the owner of the company sponsoring the study. The current patent literature was reviewed to be sure that no infringements were generated.

The final configuration consisted largely of a number of then current off-the shelf technologies, such as utilization of the recently introduced Pentium class computer, use of current technology A/D boards, and direct internet connection to enable high speed digital transmission of data to one of several sites. With a few months of work, the devices were updated by at least a 20-year technology jump. A very good return on investment was also achieved.

Homework Exercises

1. Use the term "reverse engineer" in a web search. Report on the variety of firms offering this service.
2. Use the term "value engineering" in a web search. How does it differ from reverse engineering?
3. Use the term "re-engineering" in a web search. How does this relate to reverse engineering?
4. Perform a web search on the term, *Axiomatic Design*. Print out and summarize an article of interest to you.
5. Pahl and Beitz do discuss idea generation techniques. Find which they stress, and why.

6. Based upon the discussion of this chapter (or via a download) perform an innovation situation questionnaire for your design project.
7. The keeping of a design notebook is considered evidence in patent litigation. How do you prove that your work, done with a computer design tool, actually took place on a given day?

References

Bass, Len, Paul Clements and Rick Kazman, *Software Architecture in Practice.* Reading, Massachusetts: Addison Wesley Longman, Inc., 1998.

Boehm, Barry W., "A Spiral Model of Software Development and Enhancement," *Computer.* May, 1988.

Boehm, Barry W., *Software Engineering Economics.* Englewood Cliffs, New Jersey: Prentice-Hall, Inc. 1981.

Booch, Grady, *Object-Oriented Analysis and Design with Applications - Second Edition.* Redwood City, California: The Benjamin Cummings Publishing Company, Inc. 1994.

Booch, Grady, Ivar Jacobson and James Rumbaugh, *The Unified Modeling Language User Guide.* Reading, Massachusetts: Addison Wesley Longman, Inc., 1998.

Deutsch, Michael S. and Ronald R. Willis, *Software Quality Engineering - A Total Technical and Management Approach.* Englewood Cliffs, New Jersey. Prentice-Hall, 1988.

Dyer, Michael, *The Cleanroom Approach to Quality Software Development.* New York: John Wiley & Sons, Inc., 1992.

Fairley, Richard E., *Software Engineering Concepts.* New York: McGraw-Hill Book Company, 1985.

Fries, Richard C., *Reliable Design of Medical Devices.* New York: Marcel Dekker, Inc., 1997.

Government - Industry Data Exchange Program, *Program Summary*. June, 1979.

Hatley, Derek J. and Imtiaz A. Pirbhai, *Strategies for Real-Time System Specification*. New York: Dorset House Publishing, 1987.

Humphrey, Watts S., *Managing the Software Process*. Reading, Massachusetts: Addison-Wesley Publishing Company, 1989.

Ingle, Kathryn A., *Reverse Engineering*, New York: McGraw-Hill Inc., 1994.

Jensen, F. and N. E. Peterson, *Burn-In*. New York: John Wiley and Sons, 1982.

Kan, Stephen H., *Metrics and Models in Software Quality Engineering*. Reading, Massachusetts: Addison Wesley Longman, Inc., 1995.

Leveson, Nancy G., *Safeware*. Reading, Massachusetts: Addison-Wesley Publishing Company, 1995.

Lloyd, D. K., and M. Lipow, *Reliability Management, Methods and Management*. 2nd Edition. Milwaukee, WI: American Society for Quality Control, 1984.

Logothetis, N. and H. P. Wynn, *Quality Through Design*. London, England: Oxford University Press, 1990.

Mason, R. L., W. G. Hunter, and J. S. Hunter, *Statistical Design and Analysis of Experiments*. New York: John Wiley & Sons, 1989.

McConnell, Steve., *Code Complete*. Redmond, Washington: Microsoft Press, 1993.

McConnell, Steve, *Rapid Development*. Redmond, Washington: Microsoft Press, 1996.

MIL-STD-202, *Test Methods for Electronic and Electrical Component Parts*. Washington, DC: Department of Defense, 1980.

MIL-HDBK-217, *Reliability Prediction of Electronic Equipment.* Washington, DC: Department of Defense, 1986.

MIL-STD-750, *Test Methods for Semiconductor Devices.* Washington, DC: Department of Defense, 1983.

MIL-STD-781, *Reliability Design Qualification and Production Acceptance Tests: Exponential Distribution.* Washington, DC: Department of Defense, 1977.

MIL-STD-883, *Test Methods and Procedures for Microelectronics.* Washington, DC: Department of Defense, 1983.

Montgomery, D. C., *Design and Analysis of Experiments.* 2nd Edition. New York: John Wiley & Sons, 1984.

O'Connor, Patrick D. T., *Practical Reliability Engineering.* 3rd Edition. Chichester, England: John Wiley & Sons, 1991.

Page-Jones, Meilir, *The Practical Guide to Structured Systems Design - Second Edition.* Englewood Cliffs, New Jersey. Prentice-Hall, Inc., 1988.

Pahl, G., Beitz, W. *Engineering Design, A Systematic Approach.* London: Springer-Verlag, 1988.

Pressman, R., *Software Engineering.* New York: McGraw-Hill Book Company, 1987.

Putnam, Lawrence H. and Ware Myers, *Measures for Excellence.* Englewood Cliffs, New Jersey: P T R Prentice-Hall, Inc., 1992.

Rakos, John J., *Software Project Management for Small to Medium Sized Projects.* Englewood Cliffs, New Jersey: Prentice-Hall, 1990.

Reliability Analysis Center, *Nonelectronic Parts Reliability Data: 1995.* Rome, NY: Reliability Analysis Center, 1994.

Ross, P. J., *Taguchi Techniques for Quality Engineering.* New York: McGraw-Hill, 1988.

Rumbaugh, James, et al., *Object-Oriented Modeling and Design.* Englewood Cliffs, New Jersey: Prentice-Hall, 1991.

Rumbaugh, James, Ivar Jacobson and Grady Booch, *The Unified Modeling Language Reference Manual.* Reading, Massachusetts: Addison Wesley Longman, Inc., 1998.

Sommerville, Ian and Pete Sawyer, *Requirements Engineering.* Chichester, England: John Wiley & Sons, Inc., 1997.

Storey, Neil, *Safety-Critical Computer Systems.* Harlow, England: Addison Wesley Longman, 1996.

Taguchi, Genichi, *Introduction to Quality Engineering.* Unipub/Asian Productivity Association, 1986.

Taguchi, Genichi, *Systems of Experimental Design.* Unipub/Asian Productivity Association, 1978.

Thayer, Richard H. and Merlin Dorfman, editors, *Software Requirements Engineering - Second Edition.* Los Alamitos, California: IEEE Computer Society Press, 1997.

Yourdon, Edward, *Modern Structured Analysis.* Englewood Cliffs, New Jersey: Yourdon Press, 1989.

Chapter 7

Computer-Aided Design

"Man is still the most extraordinary computer of all."
John F. Kennedy

Computer-aided design (CAD) or computer-aided design and drafting (CADD), is a form of automation that helps designers prepare drawings, specifications, parts lists, and other design-related elements using special graphics- and calculations-intensive computer programs. The technology is used for a wide variety of products in such fields as architecture, electronics, and aerospace, naval, and biomedical engineering. Although CAD systems originally merely automated drafting, they now usually include three-dimensional modeling and computer-simulated operation of the model.

Rather than having to build prototypes and change components to determine the effects of tolerance ranges, engineers can use computers to simulate operation to determine loads and stresses. For example, an automobile manufacturer might use CAD to calculate the wind drag on several new car-body designs without having to build physical models of each one. In microelectronics, as devices have become smaller and more complex, CAD has become an especially important technology. Among the benefits of such systems are lower product-development costs and a greatly shortened design cycle. While less expensive CAD systems running on personal computers have become available for do-it-yourself home remodeling and simple drafting, state-of-the-art CAD systems running on workstations and mainframe computers are increasingly integrated with computer-aided manufacturing systems.

7.1 Definitions of CAD, CAM, and CAE

Computer-aided design (CAD) is the technology concerned with the use of computer systems to assist in the creation, modification, analysis, and optimization of a design. Thus, any computer program that embodies computer graphics and an application program facilitating engineering functions in the design process is classified as CAD software. In other words, CAD tools can vary from geometric tools for manipulating shapes at one extreme, to customized application programs, such as those for analysis and optimization, at the other extreme. Between these two extremes, typical tools currently available include:

- tolerance analysis
- mass property calculations
- finite-element modeling and visualization.

The most basic role of CAD is to define the geometry of design - a mechanical part, architectural structure, electronic circuit, building layout, and so on - because the geometry of the design is essential to all the subsequent activities in the product cycle. Computer-aided drafting and geometric modeling are typically used for this purpose.

Computer-aided manufacturing (CAM) is the technology concerned with the use of computer systems to plan, manage, and control manufacturing operations through either direct or indirect computer interfaces with the plant's production resources. One of the most mature areas of CAM is numerical control. This is the technique of using programmed instructions to control a machine tool that grinds, cuts, mills, punches, bends, or turns raw stock into a finished part. The computer can generate a considerable amount of numerical control instructions based on geometric data from the CAD database plus additional information supplied by the operator.

Another significant CAM function is the programming of robots, which may operate in a work cell arrangement, selecting and positioning tools and work pieces for numerical control machines. These robots may perform individual tasks such as welding or assembly, or carry equipment or parts around the manufacturing floor.

Computer-aided engineering (CAE) is a technology concerned with the used of computer systems to analyze CAD geometry, allowing the designer to simulate and study how the product with behave so that the design can be refined and optimized. CAE tools are available for a wide range of analyses. Kinematics programs, for example, can be used to determine motion paths and linkage velocities in mechanisms. Large-displacement dynamic analysis programs can be used to determine loads and displacements in complex assemblies. Logic timing and verification software simulates the operation of complex electronic circuits.

Probably the most widely used method of computer analysis in engineering is the finite-element method (FEM). This approach is used to determine stress, deformation, heat transfer, magnetic field distribution, fluid flow, and other continuous field problems that would be impractical to solve with any other approach. In FEM, the structure is represented by an analysis model made up of interconnected elements that divide the problem into manageable parts for the computer.

7.2 The Computer-Aided Design Process

The product development cycle is composed of two main processes: the design process and the manufacturing process. The design process starts from customers' demands that are identified by marketing personnel and ends with a complete description of the product, usually in the form of specifications and drawings. The manufacturing process starts from the design specification and ends with shipping of the actual product.

The activities involved in the design process can be classified largely as two types: synthesis and analysis. The initial design activities, such as identification of the design need, formulation of design specifications, a feasibility study with collecting relevant design information, and design conceptualization, are part of the synthesis subprocess . That is the result of the synthesis subprocess is a conceptual design of the prospective product in the form of a block diagram or a layout drawing that shows the relationships among the various product components. The major financial commitments needed to realize the product idea are made and the functionality of the product is determined during this phase of the cycle. Most of the information generated and handled in the synthesis subprocess is qualitative and consequently is hard to capture in the computer system.

Once the conceptual design has been developed, the analysis subprocess begins with analysis and optimization of the design. An analysis model is derived first because the analysis subprocess is applied to the model rather than to the design itself. Despite the rapid growth in the power and availability of computers in engineering, the abstraction of analysis models will still be with us for the foreseeable future.

The analysis model is obtained by removing from the design unnecessary details, reducing dimensions, and recognizing and employing symmetry. Dimensional reduction, for example, implies that a thin sheet of material is represented by an equivalent surface with a thickness attribute or that a long slender region is represented by a line having cross-sectional properties. Bodies with symmetries in the geometry and loading are usually analyzed by considering a portion of the model.

Once a design has been completed, after optimization or some trade-off decisions, the design evaluation begins. Prototypes may be built for this purpose. The new technology called rapid prototyping is becoming popular for constructing prototypes. This technology enables the construction of a prototype by adding and bonding materials (typically plastics) in layers to form objects. The prototypes are generated from the bottom to the top. Thus it enables the construction of the prototype directly from its design because it requires basically the cross-sectional data of the product. If the design evaluation of the prototype indicates that the design is unsatisfactory, the process is repeated with a new design.

As mentioned above, the computer is not widely used in the synthesis phase of the design process because the computer does not handle qualitative information well. However, in the synthesis subprocess, a designer might well collect the relevant design information for the feasibility study by using a commercial database and collect and catalog information in the same way.

The analysis subprocess is the area where the computer reveals its value. In fact, there are many available software packages for stress analysis, interference checking, and kinematic analysis, to name a few. These software packages are classified as CAE. The analysis subprocess can be imbedded in the optimization iteration to yield the optimal design. Various algorithms for finding the optimal solution have been developed, and many optimization procedures are commercially available. Optimization procedures could be thought of as a component of CAD software.

The design evaluation phase also can be facilitated by used of the computer. If we need a design prototype for the design evaluation, we can construct a prototype of the given design by using software packages that automatically generate the program that drives the rapid prototyping machine. These packages are classified as CAM software.

7.3 Components of CAD/CAM/CAE Systems

Specific types of hardware and software are required for the computer-oriented approach to the design and manufacturing process. Since interactive shape manipulation is key to the CAD/CAM process, the hardware and software enabling interactive shape manipulation would be the major components comprising CAD/CAM/CAE systems. This is shown graphically in Figure 7-1.

Graphic devices and their peripherals for input and output operations, in addition to normal computing machines, comprise the hardware for CAD/CAM/CAE systems. The key software components are packages that manipulate or analyze shapes according to the user's interactions with them, either in two or three dimensions, and update the database.

7.3.1 Hardware components

A graphic device is composed of a display processing unit, a display device (a monitor), and one or more input devices. The display device, or monitor, functions as a screen on which a graphical image appears, but locating a

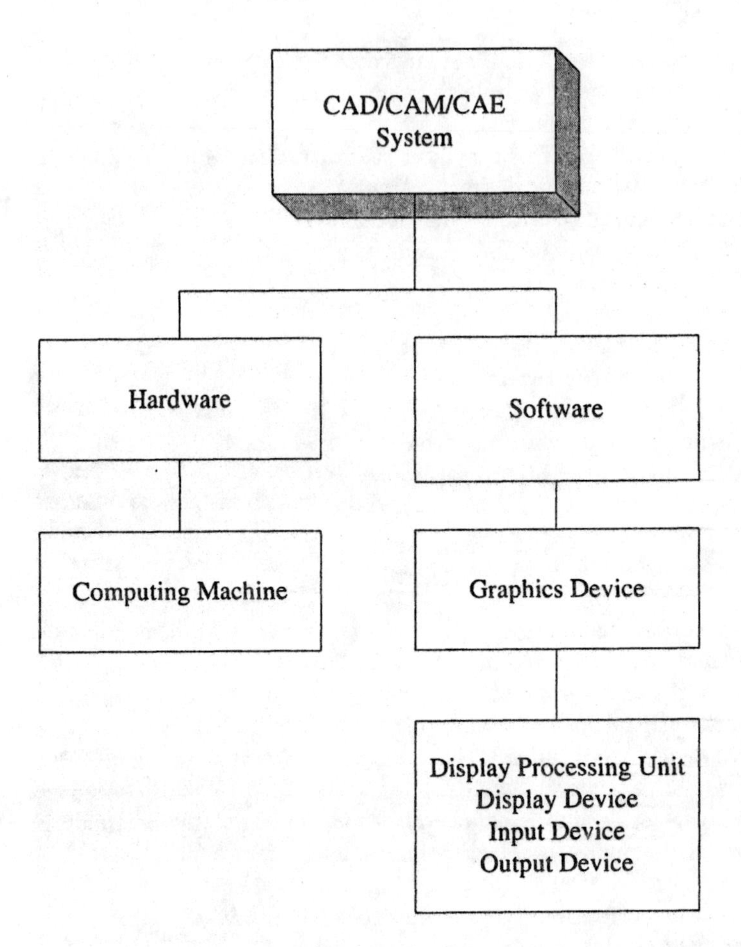

Figure 7-1 Components of a CAD/CAM/CAE system.

specified image on the screen is a function of the display processing unit. In other words, the display processing unit accepts the signals corresponding to the graphics commands, produces electron beams, and transmits them to the proper locations on the monitor to generate the desired image.

A graphics device is usually accompanied by one or a combination of various input devices. These include:

- a mouse
- a space ball
- a data tablet with a puck or stylus
- a keyboard.

These input devices facilitate the interactive shape manipulations by allowing the user to provide graphics inputs directly to the computer. Each graphic device is also usually connected to output devices, such as plotters and a color laser printer. These output devices may be shared with other graphics devices. With these output devices, any image on the display device can be transferred onto paper or other media.

7.3.2 Hardware configuration

The graphics devices described above are not usually used as a single unit, but rather connected to form a cluster to support multiple users. There are three basic configurations.

The first configuration (Figure 7-2) is composed of a mainframe computer and multiple graphics devices. The graphic devices are connected to the mainframe similar to the way alphanumeric terminals are connected to the mainframe in a normal data processing environment. Some output devices, such as plotters, are also connected to the mainframe, as printers are. Because this configuration can be considered as a natural extension of the existing computing environment, it was readily accepted by most of the large companies that already had mainframes. However, there are some disadvantages to this approach. It requires a big initial investment for the hardware and software, and maintenance is expensive. Maintaining a mainframe always involves expansion of the system's memory and hard disk, which is more expensive for a mainframe than for a smaller machine. Furthermore, updating the operating system is not a simple task. Quite often, CAD/CAM/CAE software must be replaced either because much more powerful software has been introduced or because the initial selection of the software was not right. Another serious disadvantage with the mainframe approach is system response time. With a mainframe, all the application programs in each graphics device are competing with each other for the machines computing capability. Thus the system response for any one graphics device varies, depending on the task being ordered by another graphics device.

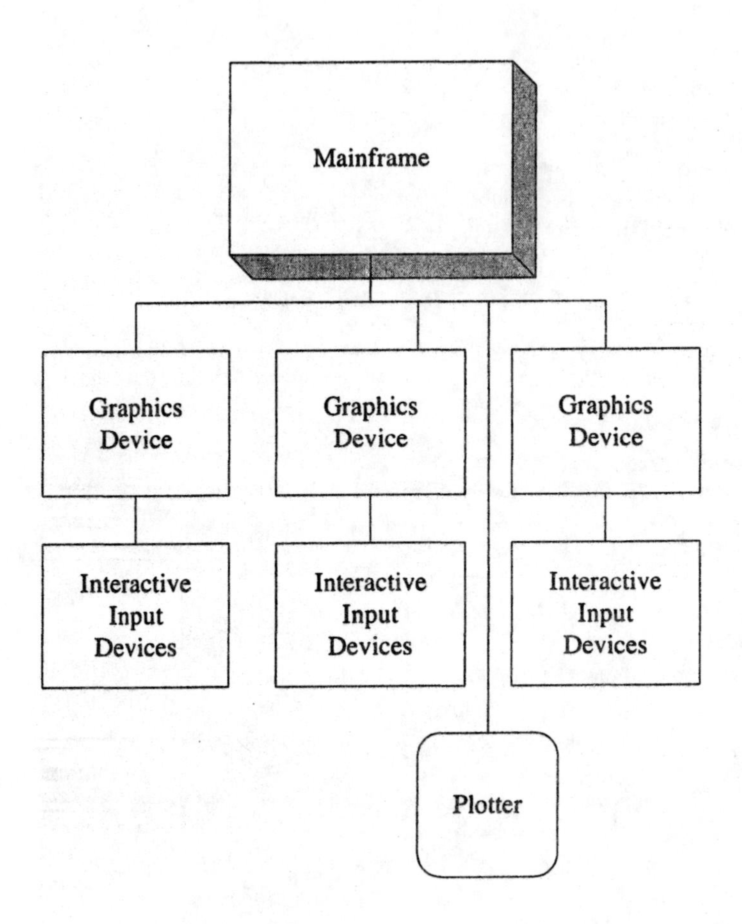

Figure 7-2 Configuration one.

The second configuration (Figure 7-3) is composed of engineering workstations connected in a networked environment. Output devices are also connected to the network. The engineering workstation can be considered a graphics device with its own computing power. This approach is widely used because of rapid progress in workstation technologies and the trend toward distributed computing. In fact, the performance of same-priced engineering workstations has been doubling every year. This approach has several

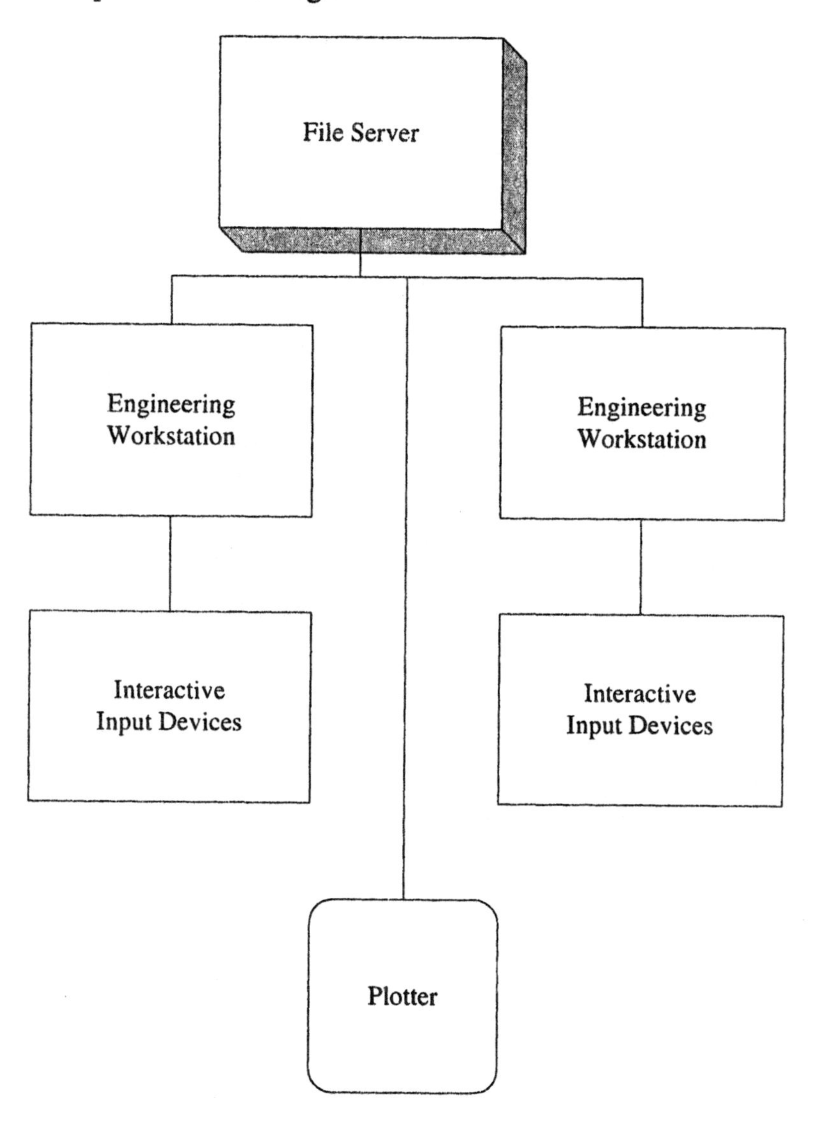

Figure 7-3 Configuration two.

advantages. The user can choose the computing power of any workstation on the network, using the most appropriate workstation for the task, with system response not affected by other people's tasks. Another advantage is the avoidance of a large initial investment. The number of workstations together with the software installation can be increased as the activities related to CAD/CAM/CAE are expanded.

The third configuration is the same as the second, except the engineering workstations are replaced by personal computers that are run by the Microsoft Windows operating systems. A PC-based configuration is popular with small companies, especially where the products being made are composed of small numbers of parts of reasonable complexity. This configuration is also popular with companies whose main purpose is to generate drawings with their CAD/CAM/CAE systems. As the distinction between personal computers and engineering workstations becomes blurred, so does the distinction between the second and third configurations.

7.3.3 Software components

Any software used in the product cycle to reduce the time and cost of product development and to enhance product quality can be classified as CAD/CAM/CAE software. CAD software allows the designer to create and manipulate a shape interactively on the monitor and store it in the database. A typical example of CAD software is a customized application program for automating the design of a specific component or mechanism.

CAM software facilitates the manufacturing process of the product cycle. This software plans, manages, and controls the operations of a manufacturing site through either direct or indirect computer interface with the site's production resources. A typical example of CAM software is the software that generates a part program, simulates the tool motion, and drives a numerical controller machine tool to machine the external surfaces of a component.

CAE software is used to analyze design geometry, allowing the designer to simulate and study how the product will behave. Thus, the design can be refined and optimized. A typical example of CAE software is a finite-element program used to calculate factors such as the stress, deformation, and heat transfer on a component of an assembly.

7.4 Windows-Based CAD Systems

As the CAD/CAM/CAE software market has matured, changes have been radical. First, engineers and manufacturers have become accustomed to the idea that they need more than two-dimensional drafting tools. Fortunately, PC hardware has become incredibly fast and powerful, and many software developers have begun producing good software products that take advantage of the superior graphics environments offered by the Windows operating systems.

These products have the following common features:

- They were developed by exploiting the functions provided by the Windows operating systems to the maximum and thus have user interfaces similar to other Microsoft programs;
- These systems involve the use of the approach called component technology, in which the best key software elements are selected from among available software. Then the system developer can simply assemble proven technologies while focusing on the capabilities that directly facilitate the design process;
- These systems employ object-oriented technology, which means modularizing the program according to its various functions so that each module can be reused later independently;
- The systems provide the capability of either parametric modeling or variational modeling. Both approaches allow the user to define a shape by using constraints instead of manipulating the shapes of elements directly; and
- The systems have Internet support for collaborative engineering. This support allows remotely located users to communicate regarding the same part while making up the part model on the screen. A designer may also check a part by fitting its model to those of other parts designed by other people.

7.5 Rapid Prototyping

Rapid Prototyping refers to the layer-by-layer fabrication of three-dimensional physical models directly from a computer-aided design. This process provides the designers and engineers the capability to literally print out their ideas in three dimensions. The rapid prototyping process provides a fast and inexpensive alternative for producing prototypes and functional models as compared to the conventional methods for part production.

The advantage of building a part in layers is that it allows you to build complex shapes that would be virtually impossible to machine, in addition to the more simple designs. Rapid prototyping can build intricate internal structures, parts inside of parts, and very thin-wall features just as easily as building a simple cube.

All of the rapid prototyping processes construct objects by producing very thin cross sections of the part, one on top of the other, until the solid physical part is completed. This simplifies the intricate three-dimensional construction process in that essentially two-dimensional slices are being created and stacked together.

Rapid prototyping also decreases the amount of operation time required by an engineer to build parts. The rapid prototyping machines, once started, usually run unattended until the part is complete. This comes after the operator spends a small amount of time setting up the control program. Afterwards, some form of clean up operation is usually necessary, generally referred to as post processing.

7.5.1 The rapid prototyping cycle

The rapid prototyping cycle (Figure 7-4) begins with the CAD design and may be repeated inexpensively several times until a model of the desired characteristic is produced.

The first step in the process is the CAD file creation. The final file or files must be in solid model format to allow for a successful prototype build. From the CAD file, an export format called the .STL file must be created. The .STL file, so named by 3D systems for Stereolithography, is currently the

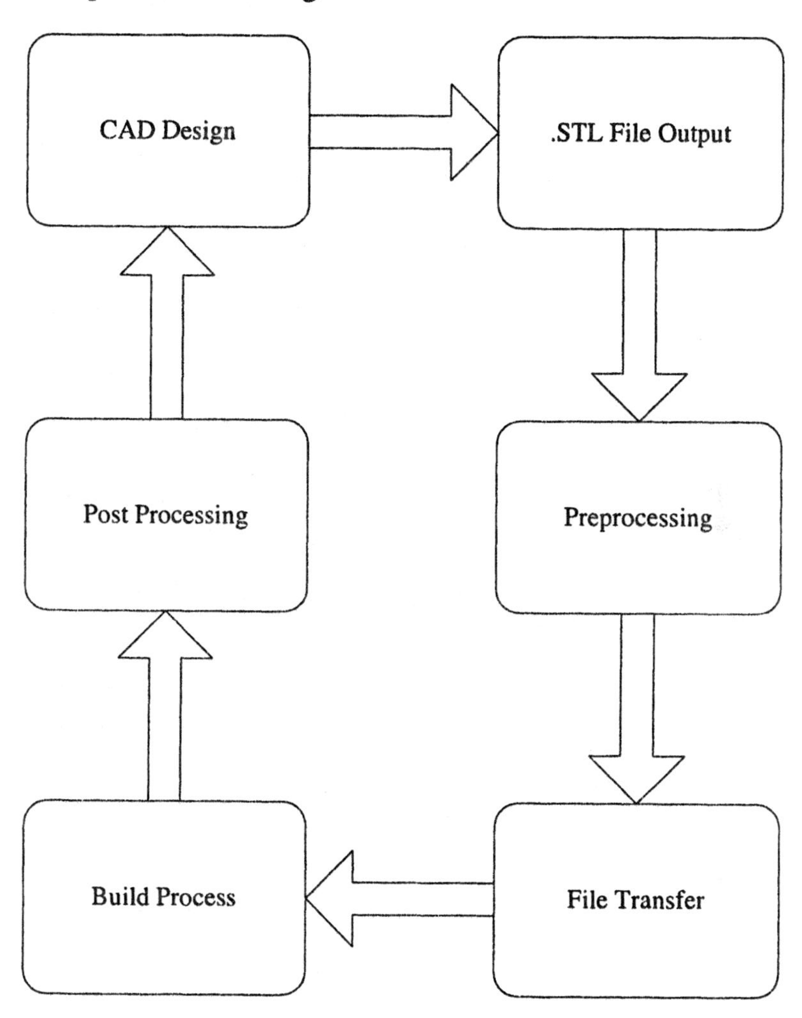

Figure 7-4 The rapid prototyping process.

standard file format for all U.S. rapid prototyping systems. .STL files are triangulated representations of solid models. The individual triangles are represented by simple coordinates in a text file format. .STL files are usually stored in binary format to conserve disk space.

After the .STL file is created, it must be prepared differently for various types of rapid prototyping systems. Some systems can accept the .STL file directly, while others require preprocessing. Preprocesses include verifying the .STL file, slicing, and setting up parameters for machine control. Preprocessing is usually done at a computer separate from the rapid prototyping system to save time and to avoid typing up valuable machine time.

After the .STL file has been preprocessed and saved into a new slice file format, the new file can then be transferred to the rapid prototyping system. File transfer can be done several ways, from manually transferring by disk or tape to a network transfer. Since more complicated files are usually very large, a local area network or Internet connection is now almost essential for easy file transfer.

Once the final file formats are transferred to the rapid prototyping device, the build process occurs. Most rapid prototyping machines build parts within a few hours, but can run unattended for several days for large parts.

Upon completion of the build process, post processing of the part must occur. This includes removal of the part from the machine, as well as any necessary support removal and sanding or finishing. If the finished part meets the necessary requirements, the cycle is complete. Otherwise, iterations can be implemented in the CAD file and the cycle is repeated.

Homework Exercises

1. What are the roles of CAD tools in the design process?
2. What are the roles of CAM tools in the manufacturing process?
3. What is the main advantage of using CAE tools in the design process?
4. List the components if a graphics device and explain the role of each component.
5. List the advantages of a hardware-configuration composed of networked engineering workstations.
6. List the steps in the Rapid Prototyping process.
7. Explain the use of the .STL file.

8. Find information on the following, and list your definitions: Stereolithography, selective laser sintering, fused deposition modeling, and three-dimensional printing.
9. You have been asked to build a model to demonstrate the presence of a brain tumor in a patient. What technologies would you use for this task and why?
10. You are asked to build a model to mimic a hip prosthesis. What technique would you use to do this task?
11. You have designed a small dental prosthesis (under 2" in all dimensions). Find a manufacturer for your device, assuming you would like a prototype as inexpensively as possible.
12. Given the definition of CAD in this chapter, is the Microsoft package "Microsoft Project" a CAD tool? Why or why not?
13. Look up, and discuss, the use of the software package "Working Model 2D" as a design tool.
14. You are concerned with the redesign of an automobile door and the ability of a stocky human being to enter without problem. Find and discuss any software package that might help you simulate this problem.

References

Beaman, J. J., J. W. Barlow, D. L. Bourell, R. H. Crawford, H. L. Marcus, K. P. McAlea, *Solid Freeform Fabrication: A New Direction in Manufacturing.* Boston: Kluwer Academic Press, 1997.

Chen, Li and Simon Li, "A Computerized approach for Concurrent Product and Process Design Optimization," in *Computer-Aided Design*, Volume 34, Number 1, January, 2002.

Cooper, Kenneth G., *Rapid Prototyping Technology: Selection and Application.* New York: Marcel Dekker, Inc., 2001.

Groover, M. P. and E. W. Zimmers, *CAD/CAM: Computer Aided Design and Manufacturing.* Englewood Cliffs, NJ: Prentice-Hall, 1984

Kochan, D., editor, *Solid Freeform M anufacturing: Advanced Rapid Prototyping.* New York: Elsevier Science Publishers, 1993.

Lee, Kunwoo, *Principles of CAD/CAM/CAE Systems.* Reading, MA: Addison Wesley, 1999

McMahon, Chris and Jimmie Browne, *CADCAM: From Principles to Practice.* Wokingham, England: Addison-Wesley Publishing Company, 1993.

Pugh, S. *Total Design.* Wokingham, England: Addison Wesley, 1991.

Salzberg, S. and M. Watkins, "Managing Information for Concurrent Engineering: Challenges and Barriers," in *Research in Engineering Design.* Volume 2, Number 1, 1990.

Wood, Lamont, *Rapid Automated Systems: An Introduction.* New York: Industrial Press, 1993.

Zeid, I., *CAD/CAM Theory and Practice.* New York: McGraw-Hill, 1991.

Chapter 8

Human Factors Issues

"Experience is what causes a person
to make new mistakes instead of old one."
Anonymous

A study conducted at Brigham and Women's Hospital, in Boston, in 1989 attempted to determine the causes of medical device failures within the hospital environment over an eleven month period. The results of the study indicated 41% of device problems or failures were caused by user problems or errors. The use and/or misuse of a medical device is thus seen to have an important impact on the overall reliability of the device. The methodology that addresses such user issues is Ergonomics or Human Factors.

8.1 What Is Human Factors?

Human Factors is defined as the application of the scientific knowledge of human capabilities and limitations to the design of systems and equipment to produce products with the most efficient, safe, effective, and reliable operation. This definition includes several interesting concepts.

Although humans are capable of many highly technical, complex or intricate activities, they also have limitations to these activities. Of particular interest to the medical designer are limitations due to physical size, range of motion, visual perception, auditory perception, and mental capabilities under stress. Although the user may be characterized by these limitations, the designer cannot allow them to adversely affect the safety, effectiveness, or reliability of the device. The designer should therefore identify and address all possible points of interface between the user and the equipment, characterize the operating environment, and analyze the skill level of the intended users.

Interface points are defined as those areas that the user must control or maintain in order to derive the desired output from the system. Interface points include control panels, displays, operating procedures, operating instructions, and user training requirements.

The environment in which the device will be used must be characterized to determine those areas that may cause problems for the user, such as lighting, noise level, temperature, criticality of the operation, and the amount of stress the user is experiencing while operating the system. The design must then be adjusted to eliminate any potential problems.

The skill level of the user is an important parameter to be analyzed during the design process and includes such characteristics as educational background, technical expertise, and computer knowledge. To assure the user's skill levels have been successfully addressed, the product should be designed to meet the capabilities of the least skilled potential user. Designing to meet this worst case situation will assure the needs of the majority of the potential users will be satisfied.

The final and most important activity in Human Factors Engineering is determining how these areas interact within the particular device. The points of interface are designed based on the anticipated operating environment and on the skill level of the user. The skill level may depend not only on the education and experience of the user, but on the operating environment, as well. To design for such interaction, the designer must consider the three elements that comprise human factors: the human element, the hardware element, and the software element.

8.1.1 The human element in human factors engineering

The human element addresses several user characteristics, including memory and knowledge presentation, thinking and reasoning, visual perception, dialogue construction, individual skill level, and individual sophistication. Each is an important factor in the design consideration.

A human being has two types of memory. Short-term memory deals with sensory input, such as visual stimuli, sounds, and sensations of touch. Long term memory is composed of our knowledge database. If the human-machine interface makes undue demands on either short- or long-term memory, the performance of the individual in the system will be degraded. The speed of this degradation depends on the amount of data presented, the rapidity of presentation, the number of commands the user must remember, and/or the stress involved in the activity.

When a human performs a problem-solving activity, they usually apply a set of guidelines or strategies based on their understanding of the situation and their experiences with similar types of problems, rather than applying formal inductive or deductive reasoning techniques. The human-machine interface must be specific in a manner enabling the user to relate to their previous experiences and develop guidelines for a particular situation, i.e. "intuitive".

The physical and cognitive constraints associated with visual perception must be understood when designing the human-machine interface. For example, studies have shown that since the normal line of sight is within 15 degrees of the horizontal line of sight, the optimum position for the instrument face is within a minimum of 45 degrees of the normal line of sight (Figure 8-1). Other physical and cognitive constraints have been categorized and are available in references located at the end of this chapter.

When people communicate with one another, they communicate best when the dialogue is simple, easy to understand, direct, and to the point. The designer must assure device commands are easy to remember, error messages are simple, direct, and not cluttered with computer jargon and help messages are easy to understand and pointed. The design of dialogue should be addressed to the least skilled potential user of the equipment.

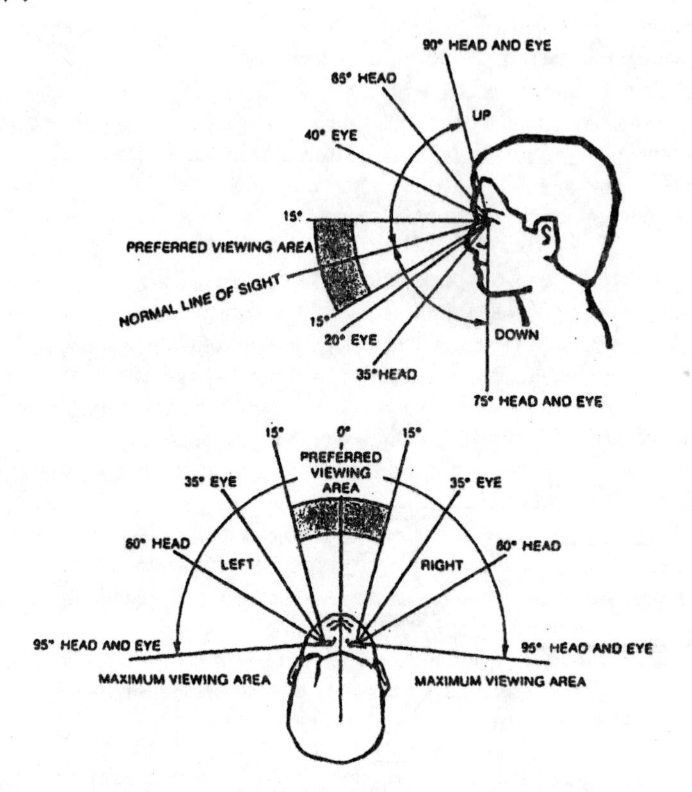

	PREFERRED	MAXIMUM*		
		EYE ROTATION	HEAD ROTATION	HEAD AND EYE ROTATION.
UP	15°	40°	65°	90°
DOWN	15°	20°	35°	75°
RIGHT	15°	35°	60°	95°
LEFT	15°	35°	60°	95°

* Display area on the console defined by the angles measured from the normal line of sight.

Figure 8.1 Normal line of sight. (From Fries, 1997.)

The typical user of a medical device is not familiar with hardware design or computer programming. They are more concerned with the results obtained from using the device, than about how the results were obtained. They want a system that is convenient, natural, flexible and easy to use. They don't want a system that looks imposing, is riddled with computer jargon, requires them to memorize many commands, or has unnecessary information cluttering the display areas.

In summary, the human element requires a device which has inputs, outputs, controls, displays and documentation that reflect an understanding of the user's education, skill, needs, experience, and the stress level when operating the equipment.

8.1.2 The hardware element in human factors

The hardware element considers size limitations, the location of controls, compatibility with other equipment, the potential need for portability, and possible user training. It also addresses the height of the preferred control area and the preferred display area when the operator is standing (Figure 8-2), when the operator is sitting (Figure 8-3) and the size of the human hand in relation to the size of control knobs or switches (Figure 8-4).

Hardware issues are best addressed by first surveying potential customers of the device to help determine the intended use of the device, the environment in which the device will be used, and the optimum location of controls and displays. Once the survey is completed and the results analyzed, a cardboard, foam, or wooden model of the device is built and reviewed with the potential customers. The customer can then get personal, hands-on experience with the controls, displays, the device framework, and offer constructive criticism on the design. Once all changes have been made, the model can be transposed into a prototype, using actual hardware.

8.1.3 Software element in human factors

The software element of the device must be easy to use and understand. It must have simple, reliable data entry, it should be menu driven if there are many commands to be learned, displays must not be over-crowded, and

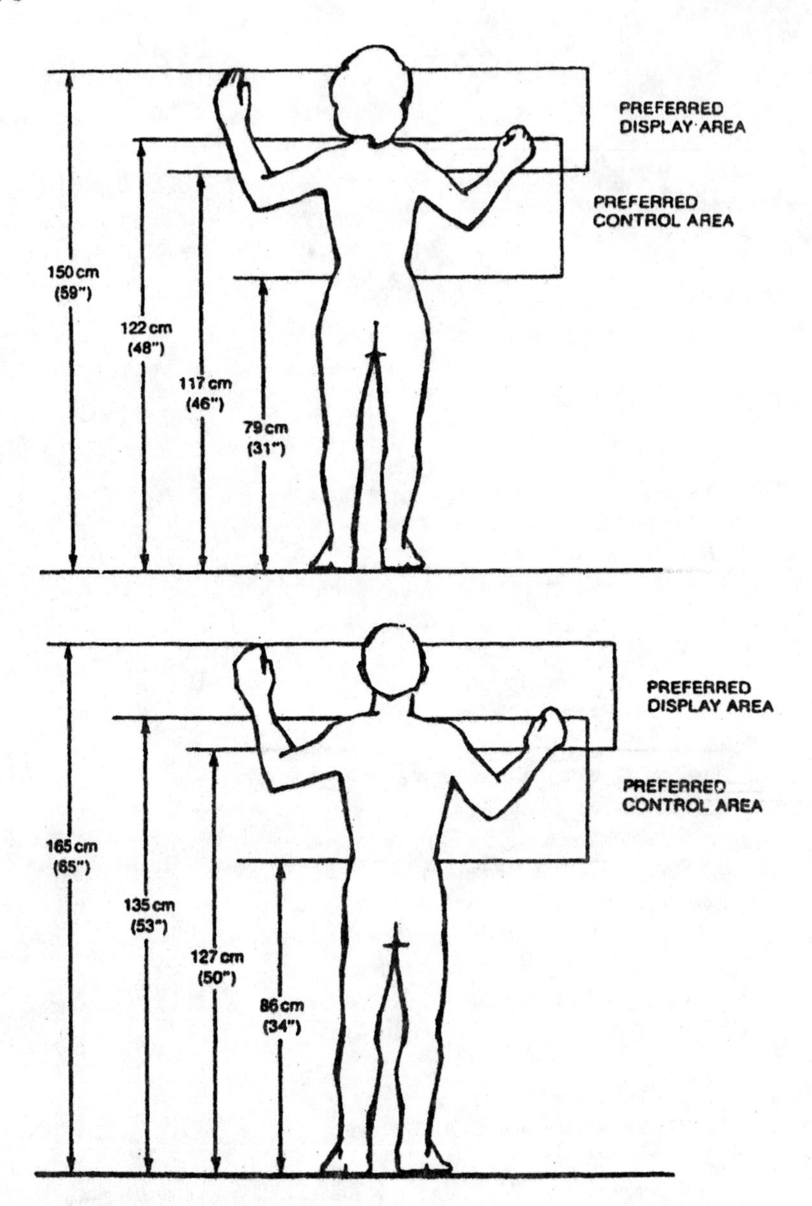

Figure 8-2 Display area when standing. (From Fries, 1997.)

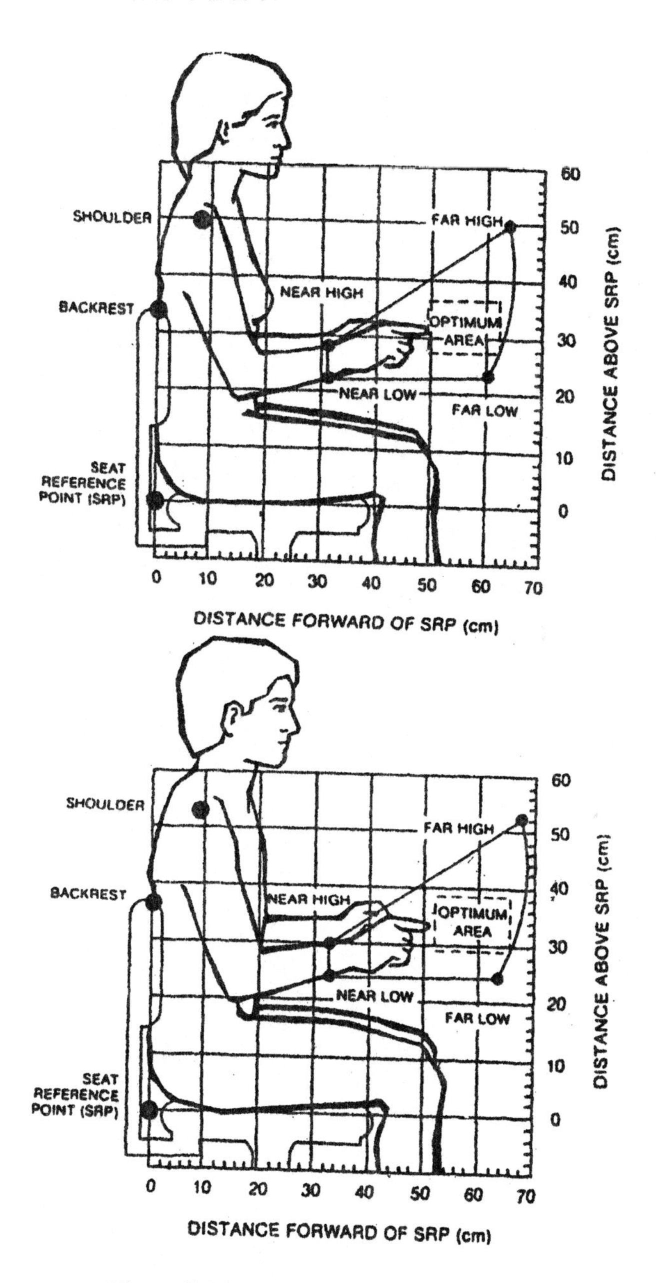

Figure 8-3 Display area when sitting. (From Fries, 1997.)

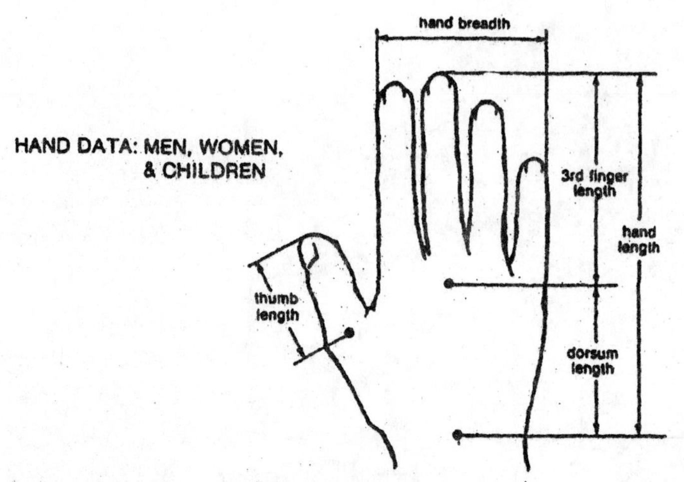

HAND DATA	MEN			WOMEN			CHILDREN			
	2.5% tile	50.% tile	97.5% tile	2.5% tile	50.% tile	97.5% tile	6 yr.	8 yr.	11 yr.	14 yr.
hand length	173mm (6.8")	191mm (7.5")	208mm (8.2")	157mm (6.2")	175mm (6.9")	191mm (7.5")	130mm (5.1")	142mm (5.6")	160mm (6.3")	178mm (7.0")
hand breadth	81mm (3.2")	89mm (3.5")	97mm (3.8")	66mm (2.6")	74mm (2.9")	79mm (3.1")	58mm (2.3")	64mm (2.5")	71mm (2.8")	—
3rd finger lg.	102mm (4.0")	114mm (4.5")	127mm (5.0")	91mm (3.6")	100mm (4.0")	112mm (4.4")	74mm (2.9")	81mm (3.2")	89mm (3.5")	102mm (4.0")
dorsum lg.	71mm (2.8")	75mm (3.0")	81mm (3.2")	66mm (2.6")	74mm (2.9")	79mm (3.1")	56mm (2.2")	61mm (2.4")	71mm (2.8")	75mm (3.0")
thumb length	61mm (2.4")	69mm (2.7")	75mm (3.0")	56mm (2.2")	61mm (2.4")	66mm (2.6")	46mm (1.8")	51mm (2.0")	56mm (2.2")	61mm (2.4")

ADDITIONAL DATA: AVERAGE MAN

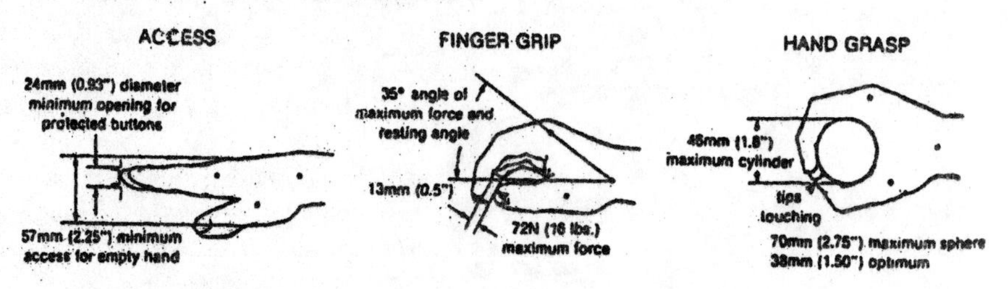

Figure 8.4 Hand sizes. (From Fries, 1997.)

dialogue must not be burdened with computer jargon. The software must provide feedback to the user through error messages and help messages. An indication that the process is involved in some activity is also important, as a blank screen leads to the assumption that nothing is active, and the user starts pushing keys or buttons.

Programmers must consider the environment in which it is to be used, especially with regard to colors of displays, type of data to be displayed, format of the data, alarm levels to be used, etc. Stress and fatigue can be reduced by consideration of color and the intensity of the displayed data. Operator effectiveness can be improved by optimizing the location of function keys, displaying more important data in the primary viewing area, and placing secondary data in the secondary display area. The inclusion of device checkout procedures and menus also improves operator effectiveness and confidence. Application of the KISS principle (Keep It Simple Stupid) is recommended.

8.2 Human Factors Process

Human Factors is the sum of several processes including the analytic process that focuses on the objectives of the proposed device and the functions that should be performed to meet those objectives; the design and development process that converts the results of the analyses into detailed equipment design features; the test and evaluation process which verifies that the design and development process has resolved issues identified in the analytic process.

Human Factors Engineering integrations begins with early device and software planning and may continue throughout the life cycle of the device. As a minimum, Human Factors should continue until the device is introduced commercially. Human Factors efforts following commercial introduction are important to the enhancement of the device and the development of future devices.

8.2.1 Planning

A Human Factors plan should be developed as an integral part of the overall plan for device development. The plan should guide Human Factors efforts in the interrelated processes of analysis, design and development, and test and evaluation. The plan should describe Human Factors tasks necessary to complete each process, the expected results of those tasks, the means of coordinating those tasks with the overall process for device development, and the schedule for that coordination. The plan should address the resources necessary for its accomplishment including levels of effort necessary for its management and coordination as well as for accomplishment of its individual tasks.

The plan should assure that results of Human Factors tasks are available in time to influence the design of the proposed device as well as the conduct of the overall project. Analysis tasks should begin very early. Iterations of analysis tasks that refine earlier products may continue throughout the project. Design and development build on the products of early analysis, and iterations may also continue throughout the project. Test and evaluation should begin with the earliest products of design and development. The results of test and evaluation should influence subsequent iterations of analysis, design and development, and test and evaluation tasks.

8.2.2 Analyses

Successful Human Factors is predicated on careful analyses. Early analyses should focus on the objectives of the proposed device and the functions that should be performed to meet those objectives. Later analysis should focus on the critical human performance required of specific personnel as a means of establishing the Human Factors parameters for design of the device and associated job aids, procedures, and training and for establishing Human Factors test and evaluation criteria for the device. Analyses should be updated as required to remain current with the design effort.

8.2.3 Conduct user studies

The goal of user studies is to learn as much as possible within a reasonable time frame about the customer's needs and preferences as they relate to the product under development. Several methods are available for getting to know the customer.

8.2.3.1 Observations

Observations are a productive first step toward getting to know the user. By observing people at work, a rapid sense for the nature of their jobs is developed, including the pace and nature of their interactions with the environment, co-workers, patients, equipment and documents. Such observations may be conducted in an informal manner, possibly taking notes and photographs. Alternatively, a more formal approach may be taken that includes rigorous data collection. For example, it may be important to document a clinician's physical movements and the time they spend performing certain tasks to determine performance benchmarks. This latter approach is referred to as a time-motion analysis and may be warranted if one of the design goals is to make the customer more productive.

Enough time should be spent observing users to get a complete sense for how they perform tasks related to the product under development. A rule of thumb in usability testing is that 5-8 participants provide 80-90 percent of the information you seek. The same rule of thumb may be applied to observations, presuming that you are addressing a relatively homogenous user population. Significant differences in the user population (i.e., a heterogenous user population) may warrant more extensive observations. For example, it may become necessary to observe people who have different occupational backgrounds and work in different countries, assuming your product will be used internationally.

Designers and engineers should conduct their own observations. For starters, such observations increase empathy for the customer. Also, first-hand experience is always more powerful than reading a marketing report. Place yourself in the position of the customer first, then go to the customer for refinement of the device.

8.2.3.2 Interviews

Similar to observations, interviews provide a wealth of information with a limited investment of time. Structured interviews based on scripted questions are generally better than unstructured interviews (i.e., a free flowing conversation). This is because a structured interview assures that the interviewer will ask everyone the same question, enabling a comparison of answers. Structured interviews may include a few open-ended questions to produce evoke comments and suggestions that could not be anticipated. The interview script should be developed from a list of information needs. Generally, questions should progress from general to more specific design issues. Care should be taken to avoid mixing marketing and engineering related concerns with usability concerns.

Interviews can be conducted just after observations are completed while the experience is "fresh". Conducting the interviews prior to the observations can be problematic, as it tends to alter the way people react.

8.2.3.3 Focus groups

Conducting interviews with people in their working environment (sometimes referred to as contextual interviewing) is generally best. Interviewees are likely to be more relaxed and opinionated. Interviews conducted at trade shows and medical conferences, for example, are more susceptible to bias and may be less reliable. Conference sites are more useful to obtain a "feel for" needs in a market.

Conducting interviews with a group of 5-10 people at a time enables easy determination of a consensus on various design issues. In preparation for such a focus group, a script should be developed from a set of information requirements. Use the script as a guide for the group interview, but feel free to let the discussion take a few tangents if they are productive ones. Also, feel at liberty to include group exercises, such as watching a video or ranking and rating existing products, as appropriate.

Conduct enough focus groups to gain confidence that an accurate consensus has been developed. Two focus groups held locally may be enough if regional differences of opinion are unlikely and the user group is relatively homogenous. Otherwise, it may be appropriate to conduct up to 4 groups each at domestic and international site that provides a reasonable cross section of the marketplace. One result may be, as is the case with anesthesia machine device placement, that European norms are different than U.S. norms, and must be accounted for.

Document the results in a focus groups report. The report can be an expanded version of the script. Begin the report with a summary section to pull together the results. Findings (e.g., answers to questions) may be presented after each question. The findings from various sites may be integrated or presented separately, depending on the design issue and opportunity to tailor the product under development to individual markets. Results of group exercises may be presented as attachments and discussed in the summary.

8.2.3.4 Task analysis

The purpose of task analysis is to develop a detailed view of customer interactions with a product by dividing the interactions into discrete actions and decisions. Typically, a flow chart is drawn that shows the sequence and logic of customer actions and decisions. The task analysis is extended to include tables that define information and control requirements associated with each action and decision. In the course of the task analysis, characterize the frequency, urgency and criticality of integrated tasks, such as "checking the breathing circuit."

8.2.3.5 Benchmark usability test

The start of a new product development effort is a good time to take stock of the company's existing products. An effective way to do this is to conduct a benchmark usability test that yields, in a quantitative fashion, both objective and subjective measures of usability. Such testing will identify the strengths and weaknesses of the existing products, as well as help establish usability goals for the new product.

8.2.3.6 User profile

To culminate the user study effort, write a so-called user profile. A user specification (2-5 pages) summarizes the important things learned about the customers. The profile should define the user population's demographics (age, gender, education level, occupational background, language), product-related experience, work environment and motivation level. The user profile is a major input to the user specification that describes the product under development from the customer's point of view.

8.2.3.7 Setup an advisory panel

To assure early and continued customer involvement, set up an advisory panel that equitably represents the user population. The panel may include 3-5 clinicians for limited product development efforts, or be twice as large for larger efforts. The panel participants are usually compensated for their time. Correspond with members of the panel on an as needed basis and meet with them periodically to review the design in progress. Note that advisory panel reviews are not an effective replacement for usability testing.

8.3 Safety

Medical device design should reflect system and personnel safety factors, including the elimination or minimization of the potential for human error during operation and maintenance under both routine and non-routine or emergency conditions. Machines should be designed to minimize consequence of human error. For example, where appropriate, a design should incorporate redundant, diverse elements arranged in a manner that increases overall reliability when failure can result in the inability to perform a critical function.

Any medical device failure should immediately be indicated to the operator and should not adversely affect safe operation of the device. Where failures can affect safe operation, simple means and procedures for averting adverse effects should be provided. In the vernacular, the device must "fail safe."

When the device failure is life threatening or could mask a life-threatening condition, an audible alarm and a visual display should be provided to indicate the device failure. Wherever possible, explicit notification of the source of failure should be provided to the user. Concise instructions on how to return to operation or how to invoke alternate backup methods should be provided. Where necessary, the appropriate ANSI, AAMI, and/or ISO standards must be met.

8.4 Documentation

Documentation is a general term that includes operator manuals, instruction sheets, online help systems, and maintenance manuals. Many types of users may access these materials. Therefore, the documentation should be written to meet the needs of all target populations.

Preparation of instructional documentation should begin as soon as possible during the specification phase. This assists device designers in identifying critical human factors engineering needs and in producing a consistent human interface. The device and its documentation should be developed together.

During the planning phase, a study should be made of the capabilities and information needs of the documentation users, including:

- the user's mental abilities
- the user's physical abilities
- the user's previous experience with similar devices
- the user's general understanding of the general principles of operation and potential hazards associated with the technology
- the special needs or restrictions of the environment.

As a minimum, the operator's manual should include detailed procedures for setup, normal operation, emergency operation, cleaning and operator troubleshooting.

The operator manual should be tested on models of the device. It is important that these test populations be truly representative of end-users and that they not have advance knowledge of the device.

Maintenance documentation should be tested on devices that resemble production units.

Documentation content should be presented in language free of vague and ambiguous terms. The simplest words and phrases that will convey the intended meaning should be used. Terminology within the publication should be consistent. Use of abbreviations should be kept to a minimum, but defined where they are used. Software exists that can estimate the grade level of the text material you have written, a goal of a 12th grade reader may suffice.

Information included in warnings and cautions should be chosen carefully and with consideration of the skills and training of intended users. It is especially important to inform users about unusual hazards and hazards specific to the device.

8.5 Anthropometry

Anthropometry is the science of measuring the human body and its parts and functional capacities. Generally, design limits are based on a range of values from the 5th percentile female to the 95th percentile male for critical body dimensions. The 5th percentile value indicates that five percent of the population will be equal to or smaller than that value and 95 percent will be larger. The 95th percentile value indicates that 95 percent of the population will be equal to or smaller than that value and five percent will be larger. The use of a design range from the 5th to the 95th percentile values will theoretically accommodate about 90 percent of the user population for that dimension.

8.5.1 Functional dimensions

The reach capabilities of the user population play an important role in the design of the controls and displays of the medical device. The designer should take into consideration both one- and two-handed reaches in the seated and standing positions (Figures 8-5 and 8-6).

Body mobility ranges should be factored into the design process. Limits of body movement should be considered relative to the age diversity and gender of the target user population.

The strength capacities of the device operators may have an impact on the design of the system controls. The lifting and carrying abilities of the personnel responsible for moving and/or adjusting the device need to be considered to assure the device can be transported and adjusted efficiently and safely.

8.5.2 Psychological elements

It is crucial to consider human proficiency in perception, cognition, learning, memory, and judgement when designing medical devices to assure that operation of the system is as intuitive, effective, and safe as possible.

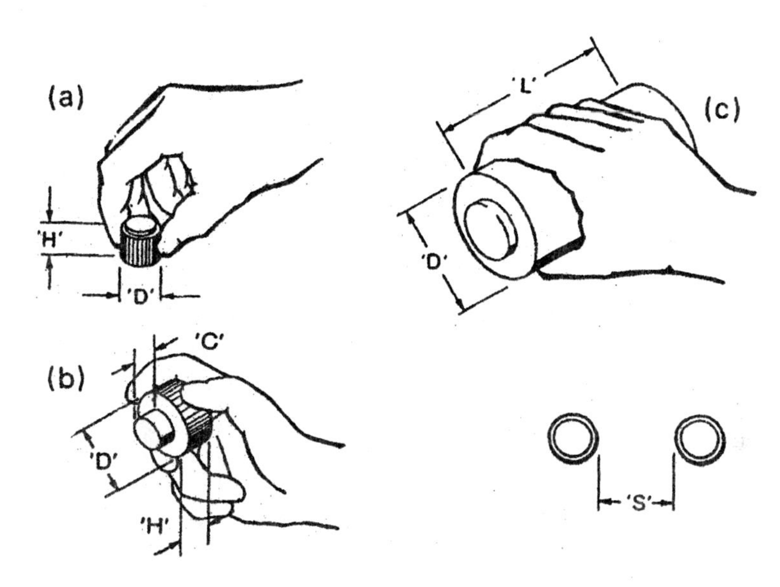

	DIMENSIONS						
	(a) Finger Grasp		(b) Thumb and Fingers Encircled			(c) Palm/Hand Grasp	
	'H' Height	'D' Diameter	'H' Height	'D' Diameter	'C' Clearance	'D' Diameter	'L' Length
Minimum	13 mm (0.5")	10 mm (0.375")	13 mm (0.50")	25 mm (1.0")	16 mm (.625")	38 mm (1.5")	75 mm (3.0")
Maximum	25 mm (1.0")	100 mm (4")	25 mm (1.0")	75 mm (3.0")	—	75 mm (3")	—

	TORQUE		'S' SEPARATION
	*	**	One Hand Individually
Minimum	—	—	25 mm (1.0")
Preferred	—	—	50 mm (2.0")
Maximum	32 mN-m (4.5 in.-oz.)	42 mN-m (6.0 in.-oz.)	—

* To and including 25 mm (1.0") diameter knobs.
** Greater than 25 mm (1.0") diameter knobs.

Figure 8-5 Example of functional dimensions. (From Fries, 1997.)

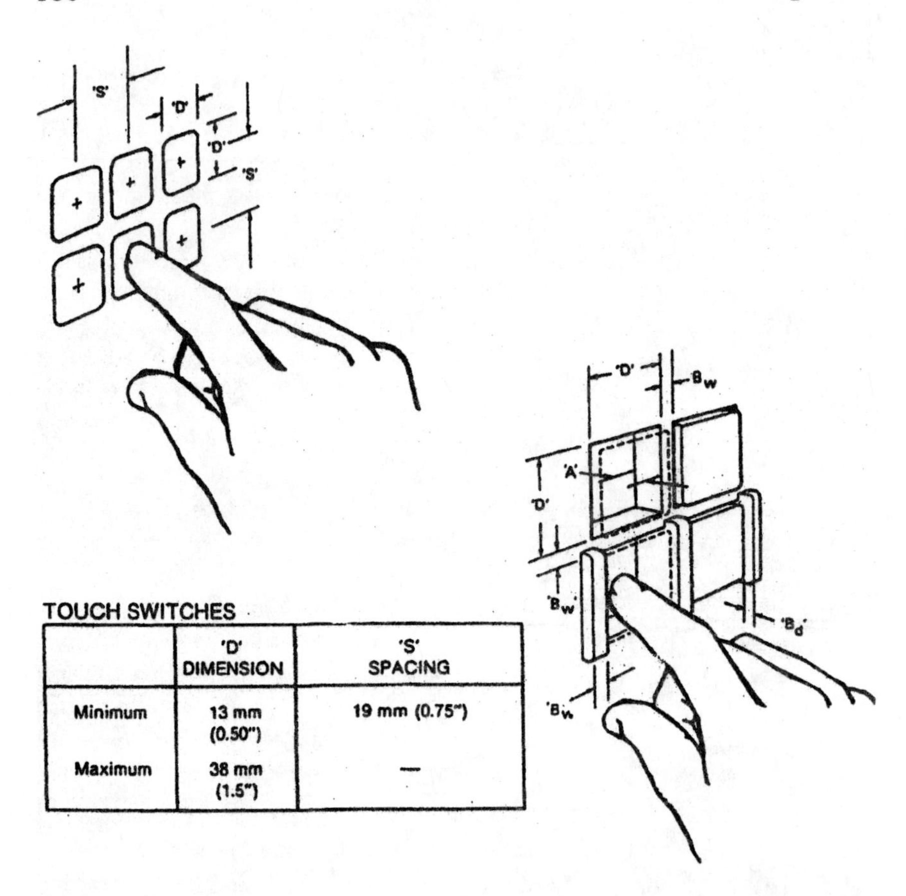

TOUCH SWITCHES

	'D' DIMENSION	'S' SPACING
Minimum	13 mm (0.50")	19 mm (0.75")
Maximum	38 mm (1.5")	—

PUSHBUTTON SWITCHES

	'D' DIMENSION	'A' Displacement	SEPARATION/BARRIERS*		RESISTANCE
			'Bw'	'Bd'	
Minimum	19 mm (0.75")	3 mm** (0.125")	3 mm (0.125")	5 mm (0.187")	280 mN (10 oz.)
Maximum	38 mm (1.5")	6 mm (0.250")	6 mm (0.250")	6 mm (0.250")	16.6 N (60 oz.)

* Barriers shall have rounded edges.
** 5 mm (.188") fof positive position switches.

Figure 8-6 Example of functional dimensions. (From Fries, 1997.)

8.5.3 Workstation design considerations

Successful workstation design is dependent on considering the nature of the tasks to be completed, the preferred posture of the operator, and the dynamics of the surrounding environment. The design of the workstation needs to take into account the adjustability of the furniture, clearances under work surfaces, keyboard and display support surfaces, seating, footrests, and accessories.

The effectiveness with which operators perform their tasks at consoles or instrument panels depends in part on how well the equipment is designed to minimize parallax in viewing displays, allow ready manipulation of controls, and provide adequate space and support for the operator.

A horizontal or nearly horizontal work surface should serve primarily as a work or writing surface or as a support for the operator's convenience items. Certain types of controls, such as joysticks, mousepads, or tracking controls, can also be part of the surface design. Designs must consider the possibility that the user may sit on the surface and/or spill drinks on it.

Controls should have characteristics appropriate for their intended functions, environments, and user orientations, and their movements should be consistent with the movements of any related displays or equipment components. The shape of the control should be dictated by its specific functional requirements. In a bank of controls, those controls affecting critical or life-supporting functions should have a special shape and, if possible, a standard location. ANSI and other standards should be consulted for color requirements.

Controls should be designed and located to avoid accidental activation. Particular attention should be given to critical controls whose accidental activation might injure patients or personnel or might compromise device performance. Feedback on control response adequacy should be provided as rapidly as possible, on anesthesia machines a whistling sound is made immediately to warn the operator that the machine has been switched off. Controls must be properly labeled, if they step through values they must not be able to stop in in-between positions.

8.6 Labeling

Controls, displays, and other equipment items that need to be located, identified, or manipulated should be appropriately and clearly marked to permit rapid and accurate human performance. The characteristics of markings should be determined by such factors as the criticality of the function labeled, the distance from which the labels need to be read, the illumination level, the colors, the time available for reading, the reading accuracy required, and consistency with other markings.

Receptacles and connectors should be marked with their intended function or their intended connection to a particular cable. Convenience receptacles should be labeled with maximum allowable load in amperes or watts. The current rating of fuses should be permanently marked adjacent to the fuse holder. Fuse ratings should be indicated either in whole number, common fractions, or whole number plus common fractions. Labeling of fuses and circuit breakers should be legible in the ambient illumination range anticipated for the maintainer's location.

Operators and maintenance personnel should be warned of possible fire, radiation, explosion, shock, infection or other hazards that may be encountered during the use, handling, storage, or repair of the device. Electromedical instruments should be labeled to show whether they may be used in the presence of flammable gases or oxygen-rich atmospheres. Hazard warnings should be prominent and understandable.

Normally, labels should be placed above panel elements that users grasp, press, or otherwise handle so the label is not obscured by the hand. However, certain panel element positions, user postures, and handling methods may dictate other label placements. Labels should be positioned to ensure visibility and readability from the position in which they should be read.

Labels should be oriented horizontally so that they may be read quickly and easily from left to right. Although not normally recommended, vertical orientation may be used, but only where its use is justified in providing a better understanding of intended function. Vertical labels should be read from top to bottom. Curved labels should be avoided except when they provide setting delimiters for rotary controls.

Labels should not cover any other information source. They should not detract from or obscure figures or scales that should be read by the operator. Labels should not be covered or obscured by other units in the equipment assembly. Labels should be visible to the operator during control activation. All markings should be permanent and should remain legible throughout the life of the equipment under anticipated use and maintenance conditions.

The words employed in the label should express exactly what action is intended. Instructions should be clear and direct. Words that have a commonly accepted meaning for all intended users should be utilized. Unusual technical terms should be avoided. Labels should be consistent within and across pieces of equipment in their use of words, acronyms, abbreviations, and part/system numbers. No mismatch should exist between the nomenclature used in documentation and that printed on the labels.

Symbols should be used only if they have a commonly accepted meaning for all intended users. Symbols should be unique and distinguishable from one another. A commonly accepted standard configuration should be used.

Human Factors Engineering hardware design considerations should include functional dimensions, workstation architecture considerations, alarms and signals, and labeling, and should always take the operator's psychological characteristics into account.

8.7 Software

Computerized systems should provide a functional interface between the system and users of that system. This interface should be optimally compatible with the intended user and should minimize conditions that can degrade human performance or contribute to human error. Thus, procedures for similar or logically related transactions should be consistent. Every input by a user should consistently produce some perceptible response or output from the computer. Sufficient online help should be provided to allow the intended but uninitiated user to operate the device effectively in its basic functional mode without reference to a user's manual or experienced operator. Users should be provided appropriate information at all times on system status either automatically or upon request. Provision of information about system dysfunction is essential.

In applications where users need to log-on to the system, log-on should be a separate procedure that should be completed before a user is required to select among any operational options. Appropriate prompts for log-on should be displayed automatically on the user's terminal with no special action required other than turning on the terminal. Users should be provided feedback relevant to the log-on procedure that indicates the status of the inputs. Log-on processes should require minimum input from the user, consistent with system access security.

In the event of a partial hardware/software failure, the program should allow for orderly shutdown and establishment of a checkpoint so restoration can be accomplished without loss of data and data logging.

Where two or more users need to have simultaneous access to a computer system, under normal circumstances, operation by one person should not interfere with the operations of another person. For circumstances in which certain operators require immediate access to the system, an organized system for insuring or avoiding preemption should be provided. Provisions should be made so that preempted users are notified and can resume operations at the point of interference without data loss.

8.7.1 Data entry

Manual data entry functions should be designed to establish consistency of data entry transactions, minimize user's input actions and memory load, ensure compatibility of data entry with data display, and provide flexibility of user control of data entry. The system should provide feedback to the user about acceptance or rejection of an entry.

When a processing delay occurs, the system should acknowledge the data entry and provide the user with an indication of the delay. If possible, the system should advise the user of the time remaining for process completion.

Data entry should require an explicit completion action, such as the depression of an *ENTER* key to post an entry into memory. Data entries should be checked by the system for correct format, acceptable value, or range of values. Where repetitive entry of data sets is required, data validation for each set should be completed before another transaction can begin.

Data should be entered in units that are familiar to the user. If several different systems of units are commonly used, the user should have the option of selecting the units either before or after data entry. Transposition of data from one system of units to another should be accomplished automatically by the device. When mnemonics or codes are used to shorten data entry, they should be distinctive and have a relationship or association to normal language or specific job-related terminology.

Data deletion or cancellation should require an explicit action, such as the depression of a DELETE key. When a data delete function has been selected by a user, a means of confirming the delete action should be provided, such as a dialogue box with a delete acknowledgement button or a response to a question such as Are you sure? (Y/N). In general, requiring a second press of the DELETE key is not preferred because of the possibility of an accidental double press. Similarly, after data have been entered, if the user fails to enter the data formally, for instance by pressing an ENTER key, the data should not be deleted or discarded without confirmation from the user.

Deleted data should be maintained in a memory buffer from which they can be salvaged, such as the UNDELETE option. The size and accessibility of this buffer should depend on the value of the data that the user can delete from the system.

The user should always be given the opportunity to change a data entry after the data have been posted. When a user requests change or deletion of a data item that is not currently being displayed, the option of displaying the old value before confirming the change should be presented. Where a data archive is being created, the system should record both the original entry and all subsequent amendments. If controlling a device such as a radiation therapy machine, defaults should be programmed into the software so as to not overdose or under dose patients. The device should shut down rather than give potentially fatal doses.

8.8 Feedback

Feedback should be provided that presents status, information, confirmation, and verification throughout the interaction. When system functioning requires the user to standby, WAIT or similar type messages should be displayed until interaction is again possible. When the standby or delay may last a significant period of time, the user should be informed. When a control process or sequence is completed or aborted by the system, a positive indication should be presented to the user about the outcome of the process and the requirements for subsequent user action. If the system rejects a user input, feedback should be provided to indicate why the input was rejected and the required corrective action.

Feedback should be self-explanatory. Users should not be made to translate feedback messages by using a reference system or code sheets. Abbreviations should not be used unless necessary.

8.9 Prompts

Prompts and help instructions should be used to explain commands, error messages, system capabilities, display formats, procedures, and sequences, as well as to provide data. When operating in special modes, the system should display the mode designation and the file(s) being processed. Before processing any user requests that would result in extensive or final changes to existing data, the system should require user confirmation. When missing data are detected, the system should prompt the user. When data entries or changes will be nullified by an abort action, the user should be requested to confirm the abort.

Neither humor or admonishment should be used in structuring prompt messages. The dialogue should be strictly factual and informative. Error messages should appear as close as possible in time and space to the user entry that caused the message. If a user repeats an entry error, the second error message should be revised to include a noticeable change so that the user may be certain that the computer has processed the attempted correction.

Prompting messages should be displayed in a standardized area of the display. Prompts and help instructions for system-controlled dialogue should be clear and explicit. The user should not be required to memorize lengthy sequences or refer to secondary written procedural references.

8.10 Defaults

Manufacturer's default settings and configurations should be provided in order to reduce user workload. Currently defined default values should be displayed automatically in their appropriate data fields with the initiation of a data entry transaction. The user should indicate acceptance of the default values. Upon user request, manufacturers should provide a convenient means by which the user may restore factory default settings.

Users should have the option of setting their own default values for alarms and configurations on the basis of personal experience. A device may retain and store one or more sets of user default settings. Activation of these settings should require deliberate action by the user.

8.11 Error Management/Data Protection

When users are required to make entries into a system, an easy means of correcting erroneous entries should be provided. The system should permit correction of individual errors without requiring reentry of correctly entered commands or data elements.

Homework Exercises

1. Do a web search on the author Jeff(rey) Cooper, and isolate the papers referring to mishaps. Locate and report on one of his human factors papers relevant to anesthesia.

2. Visit the ANSI web site, search for the number of standards relating to "color", "alarms", "human factors", and "labeling". Comment on your results.

3. Observe the layout of controls on your car, versus the layout of controls on a different brand. Where and why are there differences?

4. There has been a significant trend in using "internationally recognized" symbols rather than text to denote controls. Find and report on one example in your environment.

5. Discuss the differences in expectations for medical devices such as dialysis equipment to be used in the home versus in a clinic.

6. Discuss the differences in expectations for blood pressure determination in the home versus in the clinic.

7. Do a web search to locate ergonomic data. Why are designs generally aimed at the 5% female to 95% male ranges?

8. Do a web search for front panel web simulator software, report on your results. Find an example of a car dashboard layout.

9. Prototype a front panel layout for display of pulse oximeter data for joggers.

10. How would you redesign an operating room for a deaf anesthesiologist?

11. What branches of medicine are available for a blind physician? Why?

References

Association for the Advancement of Medical Instrumentation (AAMI), *Human Factors Engineering Guidelines and Preferred Practices for the Design of Medical Devices.* Arlington, VA: Association for the Advancement of Medical Instrumentation, 1993.

Backinger, C. and P. Kingsley, *Write It Right: Recommendations for Developing User Instruction Manuals for Medical Devices Used in Home Health Care.* Rockville, MD: U. S. Department of Health and Human Services, 1993.

Bogner, M. S., *Human Error in Medicine.* Hillsdale, NJ: Lawrence Erlbaum Associates, 1994.

Brown, C.M., *Human-computer Interface Design Guidelines.* Norwood, NJ: Ablex Publishing Company, 1989.

Cooper JB, Newbower RS, Kitz RJ. An analysis of major errors and equipment failures in anesthesia management: Considerations for prevention and detection. Anesthesiology 1984;60:34-42

Fries, Richard C., "Human Factors and System Reliability", in *Medical Device Technology*. Volume 3, Number 2, March, 1992.

Fries, Richard C., *Reliable Design of Medical Devices*. New York: Marcel Dekker, Inc., 1997.

Hartson, H. Rex, *Advances in Human-Computer Interaction*. Norwood, N J: Ablex Publishing Corporation, 1985.

Le Cocq, Andrew D., "Application of Human Factors Engineering in Medical Product Design", *Journal of Clinical Engineering*. Volume 12, Number 4, July-August, 1987.

Mathiowetz, V. et al, "Grip and Pinch Strength: Normative Data for Adults", in *Archives of Physical Medicine and Rehabilitation*. Volume 66, 1985.

MIL-HDBK-759, *Human factors Engineering Design for Army Material*. Washington, DC: Department of Defense, 1981.

MIL-STD-1472, *Human Engineering Design Criteria for Military Systems, Equipment and Facilities*. Washington, DC: Department of Defense, 1981.

Morgan, C.T., *Human Engineering Guide to Equipment Design*. New York: Academic Press, 1984.

Philip, J. H., "Human Factors Design of Medical Devices: The Current Challenge", *First Symposium on Human Factors in Medical Devices*, December 13-15, 1989. Plymouth Meeting, PA: ECRI, 1990.

Pressman, R. S., *Software Engineering*. New York: McGraw Hill, 1987.

Sawyer, Dick, "*Do It By Design, An Introduction to Human Factors in Medical Devices*", an FDA publication available on the web at: http://www.fda.gov/cdrh/humfac/doit.html

Weinger, Matthew B. and Carl E. Englund, "Ergonomic and Human Factors Affecting Anesthetic Vigilance and Monitoring Performance in the Operating Room Environment", *Anesthesiology*. Volume 73, Number 5, November, 1990.

Wiklund, Michael E., "How to Implement Usability Engineering," in *Medical Device and Diagnostic Industry.* Volume 15, Number 9, 1993.

Wiklund, Michael E., *Medical Device and Equipment Design - Usability Engineering and Ergonomics.* Buffalo Grove: Interpharm Press, Inc., 1995.

Woodson, W. E., *Human Factors Design Handbook.* New York: McGraw Hill, 1981.

Yourdon, E., *Modern Structured Analysis.* Englewood Cliffs, NJ: Yourdon Press, 1989.

Chapter 9

Industrial Design

"The future of the aircraft industry is still the responsibility of the engineer. Money alone never did and never will create anything."
Aviation Magazine (now *Aviation Week*)

Industrial design is the professional service of creating and developing concepts and specifications that optimize the function, value, and appearance of products and systems for the mutual benefit of both user and manufacturer. Industrial designers develop these concepts and specifications through collection, analysis and synthesis of data guided by the special requirements of the client or manufacturer. They are trained to prepare clear and concise recommendations through drawings, models and verbal descriptions. Industrial design services are often provided within the context of cooperative working relationships with other members of a development group. Typical groups include management, marketing, engineering and manufacturing specialists. The industrial designer expresses concepts that embody all relevant design criteria determined by the group.

The industrial designer's unique contribution places emphasis on those aspects of the product or system that relate most directly to human characteristics, needs and interests. This contribution requires specialized understanding of visual, tactile, safety and convenience criteria, with concern for the user. Education and experience in anticipating psychological, physiological and sociological factors that influence and are perceived by the user are essential industrial design resources. Industrial designers also maintain a practical concern for technical processes and requirements for manufacture; marketing opportunities and economic constraints; and distribution sales and servicing processes. They work to ensure that design recommendations use materials and technology effectively, and comply with all legal and regulatory requirements.

In addition to supplying concepts for products and systems, industrial designers are often retained for consultation on a variety of problems that have to do with a client's image. Such assignments include product and organization identity systems, development of communication systems, interior space planning and exhibit design, advertising devices and packaging and other related services. Their expertise is sought in a wide variety of administrative arenas to assist in developing industrial standards, regulatory guidelines and quality control procedures to improve manufacturing operations and products. Industrial designers, as professionals, are guided by their awareness of obligations to fulfill contractual responsibilities to clients, to protect the public safety and well-being, to respect the environment and to observe ethical business practice.

The term *industrial design* was coined early in the twentieth century to descrbe for mass-produced devices the creative role previously performed by an individual artisan. In keeping with the complexity of mass production, industrial designers work with other professions involved in conceiving, developing, and manufacturing products, including:

- marketing experts
- design engineers
- biomedical engineers
- human factors specialists
- manufacturing engineers
- service personnel.

Together with human factors specialists, industrial designers conduct usability studies to enusre that a product meets the user's needs, wants, and expectations.

They often rearrange internal components to make products more efficient to manufacture and easy to assemble, service, and recycle.

9.1 Set Usability Goals

Usability goals are comparable to other types of engineering goals in the sense that they are quantitative and provide a basis for acceptance testing. Goals may be objective or subjective. A sample objective goal might be: on average, users shall require 3 seconds to silence an alarm. This goal is an objective goal because the user's performance level can be determined simply by observation. For example, you can use a stop watch to determine task times. Other kinds of objective goals concentrate on the number of user errors and the rate of successful task completion.

A sample subjective goal is: on average, 75% of users shall rate the intuitiveness of the alarm system as 5 or better, where 1 = poor and 7 = excellent. This goal is subjective because it requires asking the user's opinion about their interaction with the given product. A rating sheet can be used to record their answers. Other kinds of subjective goals concentrate on mental processing and emotional response attributes, such as learning, frustration level, fear of making mistakes, etc.

Every usability goal is based on a usability attribute, e.g., task, speed or intuitiveness, includes a metric such as time or scale and sets a target performance level, such as 3 seconds or a rating of 5 or better.

Typically, up to 50 usability goals may be written, two-thirds of which are objective and one-third which are subjective. The target performance level on each goal is based on findings from preceding user studies, particularly the benchmark usability testing. If there is no basis for comparison, i.e., there are no comparable products, then engineering judgement must be used to set the initial goals and adjust them as necessary to assure they are realistic.

9.2 Design User Interface Concepts

Concurrent design is a productive method of developing a final user interface design. It enables the thorough exploration of several design concepts before converging on a final solution. In the course of exploring alternative designs, limited prototypes should be built of the most promising concepts and user feedback obtained on them. This gets users involved in the design process at its early stages and assures that the final design will be closely matched to user's expectations.

Note that the design process steps described below assume that the product includes both hardware and software elements. Some steps would be moot if the product has no software user interface.

9.2.1 Develop conceptual model

When users interact with a product, they develop a mental model of how it works. This mental model may be complete and accurate or just the opposite. Enabling the user to develop a complete and accurate mental model of how a product works is a challenge. The first step is developing so-called conceptual models of how to represent the product's functions. This exercise provides a terrific opportunity for design innovation. The conceptual model may be expressed as a bubble diagram, for example, that illustrates the major functions of the product and functional interrelationships as you would like the users to think of them. You can augment the bubble diagram with a narrative description of the conceptual model.

9.2.2 Develop user interface structure

Develop alternative user interface structures that complement the most promising 2-3 conceptual models. These structures can be expressed in the form of screen hierarchy maps that illustrate where product functions reside and how many steps it will take users to get to them. Such maps may take the form of a single element, a linear sequence, a tree structure (cyclic or acyclic) or a network. In addition to software screens, such maps should show which functions are allocated to dedicated hardware controls.

9.2.3 Define interaction style

In conjunction with the development of the user interface structures, alternative interaction styles should be defined. Possible styles include question and answer dialogs, command lines, menus and direct manipulation.

9.2.4 Develop screen templates

Determine an appropriate size display based on the user interface structure and interaction style, as well as other engineering considerations. Using computer-based drawing tools, draw the outline of a blank screen. Next, develop a limited number (perhaps 3-5) of basic layouts for the information that will appear on the various screens. Normally, it is best to align all elements, such as titles, windows, prompts, numerics according to a grid system.

9.2.5 Develop hardware layout

Apply established design principles in the development of hardware layouts that are compatible with the evolving software user interface solutions. Assure that the layouts reinforce the overall conceptual model.

9.2.6 Develop a screenplay

Apply established design principles in the development of a detailed screenplay. Do not bother to develop every possible screen at this time. Rather, develop only those screens that would enable users to perform frequently used, critical and particularly complex functions. Base the screen designs on the templates. Create new templates or eliminate existing templates as required while continuing to limit the total number of templates. Assure that the individual screens reinforce the overall conceptual model. You may choose to get user feedback on the screenplay (what some people call a paper prototype).

9.2.7 Develop a refined design

Developing a hardware layout and developing a screenplay describe prototyping and testing the user interface. These efforts will help determine the most promising design concept or suggest a hybrid of two or more concepts. The next step is to refine the preferred design. Several reiterations of the preceding steps may be necessary, including developing a refined conceptual model, developing a refined user interface structure and developing an updated set of screen templates. Then, a refined screenplay and hardware layout may be developed.

9.2.8 Develop a final design

Once again, steps 5 and 6 describe prototyping and testing the user interface. These efforts will help you determine any remaining usability problems with the refined design and opportunities for further improvement. It is likely that design changes at this point will be limited in nature. Most can be made directly to the prototype.

9.3 Model the User Interface

Build a prototype to evaluate the dynamics of the user interface. Early prototypes of competing concepts may be somewhat limited in terms of their visual realism and how many functions they perform. Normally, it is best to develop a prototype that 1) presents a fully functional top-level that allows users to browse their basic options, and 2) enables users to perform a few sample tasks, i.e., walkthrough a few scenarios. As much as possible, include tasks that relate to the established usability goals.

User interface prototypes may be developed using conventional programming languages or rapid prototyping languages, such as SuperCard, Altia Design, Visual Basic, Toolbook, and the like. The rapid prototyping languages are generally preferable because they allow for faster prototyping and they are easier to modify based on core project team and user feedback.

Early in the screenplay development process, it may make sense to prototype a small part of the user interface to assess design alternatives or to conduct limited studies, such as how frequently to flash a warning. Once detailed screenplays of competing concepts are available, build higher fidelity prototypes that facilitate usability testing. Once a refined design is developed, build a fully functional prototype that permits a verification usability test. Such prototypes can be refined based on final test results and serve as a specification.

9.4 Test the User Interface

There are several appropriate times to conduct a usability test, including:

- at the start of a development effort to develop benchmarks
- when you have paper-based or computer-based prototypes of competing design concepts
- when you have a prototype of your refined design
- when you want to develop marketing claims regarding the performance of the actual product.

While the rigor of the usability test may change, based on the timing of the test, the basic approach remains the same. You recruit prospective users to spend a concentrated period of time interacting with the prototype product. The users may undertake a self-exploration or perform directed tasks. During the course of such interactions, you note the test participants comments and document their performance. At intermittent stages, you may choose to have the test participant complete a questionnaire or rating/ranking exercise. Videotaping test proceedings is one way to give those unable to attend the test a first-hand sense of user-product interactions. Sometimes it is useful to create a 10-15 minute highlight tape that shows the most interesting moments of all test sessions.

During testing, collect the data necessary to determine if you are meeting the established usability goals. This effort will add continuity and objectivity to the usability engineering process.

9.5 Specify the User Interface

9.5.1 Style guide

The purpose of a style guide is to document the rules of the user interface design. By establishing such rules, you can check the evolving design to determine any inconsistencies. Also, it assures the consistency of future design changes. Style guides, usually 10-15 pages in length, normally include a description of the conceptual model, the design elements and elements of style.

9.5.2 Screen hierarchy map

The purpose of a screen hierarchy map is to provide an overview of the user interface structure. It places all screens that appear in the screenplay in context. It enables the flow of activity to be studied in order to determine if it reinforces the conceptual model. It also helps to determine how many steps users will need to take to accomplish a given task. Graphical elements of the screen hierarchy map should be cross-indexed to the screenplay.

9.5.3 Screenplay

The purpose of a screenplay is to document the appearance of all major screens on paper. Typically, screen images are taken directly from the computer-based prototype. Ideally, the screenplay should present screen images in their actual scale and resolution. Each screen should be cross-indexed to the screen hierarchy map.

9.5.4 Specification prototype

The purpose of the specification prototype is to model accurately the majority of user interface interactions. This provides the core project team with a common basis for understanding how the final product should work. It provides a basis for writing the user documentation. It may also be used to orient those involved in marketing, sales and training.

9.5.5 Hardware layouts

The hardware layout may be illustrated by the specification prototype. However, the hardware may not be located proximal to the software user interface. If this is the case, develop layout drawings to document the final hardware layout.

9.6 Additional Industrial Design Considerations

The design of medical devices should reflect industrial design features that increase the potential for successful performance of tasks and for satisfaction of design objectives.

9.6.1 Consistency and simplicity

Where common functions are involved, consistency is encouraged in controls, displays, markings, codings, and arrangement schemes for consoles and instrument panels.

Simplicity in all designs is encouraged. Equipment should be designed to be operated, maintained, and repaired in its operational environment by personnel with appropriate but minimal training. Unnecessary or cumbersome operations should be avoided when simpler, more efficient alternatives are available.

9.6.2 Safety

Medical device design should reflect system and personnel safety factors, including the elimination or minimization of the potential for human error during operation and maintenance under both routine and non-routine or emergency conditions. Machines should be designed to minimize consequence of human error. For example, where appropriate, a design should incorporate redundant, diverse elements arranged in a manner that increases overall reliability when failure can result in the inability to perform a critical function.

Any medical device failure should immediately be indicated to the operator and should not adversely affect safe operation of the device. Where failures can affect safe operation, simple means and procedures for averting adverse effects should be provided.

When the device failure is life threatening or could mask a life-threatening condition, an audible alarm and a visual display should be provided to indicate the device failure. Wherever possible, explicit notification of the source of failure should be provided to the user. Concise instructions on how to return to operation or how to invoke alternate backup methods should be provided.

9.6.3 Environmental/organizational considerations

The design of medical devices should consider the following:

- the levels of noise, vibration, humidity, and heat that will be generated by the device and the levels of noise, vibration, humidity, and heat to which the device and its operators and maintainers will be exposed in the anticipated operational environment
- the need for protecting operators and patients from electric shock, thermal, infectious, toxicologic, radiologic, electromagnetic, visual, and explosion risks, as well as from potential design hazards, such as sharp edges and corners, and the danger of the device falling on the patient or operator
- the adequacy of the physical, visual, auditory, and other communication links among personnel and between personnel and equipment
- the importance of minimizing psychophysiological stress and fatigue in the clinical environment in which the medical device will be used
- the impact on operator effectiveness of the arrangement of controls, displays and markings on consoles and panels the potential effects of natural or artificial illumination used in the operation, control, and maintenance of the device
- the need for rapid, safe, simple, and economical maintenance and repair
- the possible positions of the device in relation to the users as a function of the user's location and mobility
- the electromagnetic environment(s) in which the device is intended to be used.

9.6.4 Documentation

Documentation is a general term that includes operator manuals, instruction sheets, online help systems, and maintenance manuals. These materials may be accessed by many types of users. Therefore, the documentation should be written to meet the needs of all target populations.

Preparation of instructional documentation should begin as soon as possible during the specification phase. This assists device designers in identifying critical human factors engineering needs and in producing a consistent human interface. The device and its documentation should be developed together.

During the planning phase, a study should be made of the capabilities and information needs of the documentation users, including:

- the user's mental abilities
- the user's physical abilities
- the user's previous experience with similar devices
- the user's general understanding of the general principles of operation and potential hazards associated with the technology
- the special needs or restrictions of the environment.

As a minimum, the operator's manual should include detailed procedures for setup, normal operation, emergency operation, cleaning and operator troubleshooting.

The operator manual should be tested on models of the device. It is important that these test populations be truly representative of end-users and that they not have advance knowledge of the device.

Maintenance documentation should be tested on devices that resemble production units.

Documentation content should be presented in language free of vague and ambiguous terms. The simplest words and phrases that will convey the intended meaning should be used. Terminology within the publication should be consistent. Use of abbreviations should be kept to a minimum, but defined where they are used.

Information included in warnings and cautions should be chosen carefully and with consideration of the skills and training of intended users. It is especially important to inform users about unusual hazards and hazards specific to the device.

Human Factors Engineering design features should assure that the device functions consistently, simply, and safely, that the environment, system organization and documentation are analyzed and considered in the design, thus increasing the potential for successful performance of tasks and for satisfaction of design objectives.

9.6.5 Alarms and signals

The purpose of an alarm is to draw attention to the device when the operator's attention may be focused elsewhere. Alarms should not be startling but should elicit the desired action from the user. When appropriate, the alarm message should provide instructions for the corrective action that is required. In general, alarm design will be different for a device that is continuously attended by a trained operator, such as an anesthesia machine, than for a device that is unattended and operated by an untrained operator, such as a patient-controlled analgesia device. False alarms, loud and startling alarms, or alarms that recur unnecessarily can be a source of distraction for both an attendant and the patient and thus be a hindrance to good patient care.

Alarm characteristics are grouped in the following three categories:

1. High priority: a combination of audible and visual signals indicating that immediate operator response is required
2. Medium priority: a combination of audible and visual signals indicating that prompt operator response is required
3. Low priority: a visual signal, or a combination of audible and visual signals indicating that operator awareness is required.

A red flashing light should be used for a high priority alarm condition unless an alternative visible signal that indicates the alarm condition and its priority is employed. A red flashing light should not be used for any other purpose.

A yellow flashing light should be used for a medium priority alarm condition unless an alternative visible signal that indicates the alarm condition and it priority is employed. A yellow flashing light should not be used for any other purpose.

A steady yellow light should be used for a low priority alarm condition unless an alternative visible signal that indicates the alarm condition and its priority is employed.

Audible signals should be used to alert the operator to the status of the patient or the device when the device is out of the operator's line of sight. Audible signals used in conjunction with visual displays should be supplementary to the visual signals and should be used to alert and direct the user's attention to the appropriate visual display.

Design of equipment should take into account the background noise and other audible signals and alarms that will likely be present during the intended use of the device. The lowest volume control settings of the critical life support audible alarms should provide sufficient signal strength to preclude masking by anticipated ambient noise levels. Volume control settings for other signals should similarly preclude such masking. Ambient noise levels in hospital areas can range from 50 dB in a private room to 60 dB in intensive care units and emergency rooms, with peaks as high as 65 to 70 dB in operating rooms due to conversations, alarms, or the activation of other devices. The volume of monitoring signals normally should be lower than that of high priority or medium priority audible alarms provided on the same device. Audible signals should be located so as to assist the operator in identifying the device that is causing the alarm.

The use of voice alarms in medical applications should normally not be considered for the following reasons:

- voice alarms are easily masked by ambient noise and other voice messages

- voice messages may interfere with communications among personnel who are attempting to address the alarm condition
- the information conveyed by the voice alarm may reach individuals who should not be given specific information concerning the nature of the alarm
- the types of messages transmitted by voice tend to be very specific, possibly causing complication and confusion to the user
- in the situation where there are multiple alarms, multiple voice alarms would cause confusion
- different languages may be required to accommodate various markets.

The device's default alarm limits should be provided for critical alarms. These limits should be sufficiently wide to prevent nuisance alarms, and sufficiently narrow to alert the operator to a situation that would be dangerous in the average patient.

The device may retain and store one or more sets of alarm limits chosen by the user. When more than one set of user default alarm limits exists, the activation of user default alarm limits should require deliberate action by the user. When there is only one set of user default alarm limits, the device may be configured to activate this set of user default alarm limits automatically in place of the factory default alarm limits.

The setting of adjustable alarms should be indicated continuously or on user demand. It should be possible to review alarm limits quickly. During user setting of alarm limits, monitoring should continue and alarm conditions should elicit the appropriate alarms. Alarm limits may be set automatically or upon user action to reasonable ranges and/or percentages above and/or below existing values for monitored variables. Care should be used in the design of such automatic setting systems to help prevent nuisance alarms or variables that are changing within an acceptable range.

An audible high or medium priority signal may have a manually operated, temporary override mechanism that will silence it for a period of time, e.g., 120 seconds. After the silencing period, the alarm should begin sounding again if the alarm condition persists or if the condition was temporarily corrected but has now returned. New alarm conditions that develop during the silencing period should initiate audible and visual signals. If momentary silencing is provided, the silencing should be visually indicated.

An audible high or medium priority signal may be equipped with a means of permanent silencing, that may be appropriate when a continuous alarm is likely to degrade user performance of associated tasks to an unacceptable extent and in cases when users would otherwise be likely to disable the device altogether. If provided, such silencing should require that the user either confirm the intent to silence a critical life support alarm or take more than one step to turn the alarm off. Permanent silencing should be visually indicated and may be signalled by a periodic audible reminder. Permanent silencing of an alarm should not affect the visual representation of the alarm and should not disable the alarm.

Life support devices and devices that monitor a life-critical variable should have an audible alarm to indicate a loss of power or failure of the device. The characteristics of this alarm should be the same as those of the highest priority alarm that becomes inoperative. It may be necessary to use battery power for such an alarm.

9.6.11 Displays

Visual displays should provide the operator with a clear indication of equipment or system status under all conditions consistent with the intended use and maintenance of the system. The information displayed to a user should be sufficient to allow the user to perform the intended task, but should be limited to what is necessary to perform the task or to make decisions. Information necessary for performing different activities, such as equipment operation versus troubleshooting, should not appear in a single display unless the activities are related and require the same information to be used simultaneously. Information should be displayed only within the limits of precision required for the intended user activity or decision making and within the limits of accuracy of the measure.

Graphic displays should be used for the display of information when perception of the pattern of variation is important to proper interpretation. The choice of a particular graphic display type can have significant impact on user performance. The designer should consider carefully the tasks to be supported by the display and the conditions under which the user will view the device before selecting a display type.

Numeric digital displays should be used where quantitative accuracy of individual data items is important. They should not be used as the only display of information when perception of the variation pattern is important to proper interpretation or when rapid or slow digital display rates inhibit proper perception.

Displays may be coded by various features, such as color, size, location, shape, or flashing lights. Coding techniques should be used to help discriminate among individual displays and to identify functionally related displays, the relationship among displays, and critical information within a display.

Display formats should be consistent within a system. When appropriate for users, the same format should be used for input and output. Data entry formats should match the source document formats. Essential data, text, and formats should be under computer, not user, control. When data fields have a naturally occurring order, such as chronological or sequential, such order should be reflected in the format organization of the fields. Where some displayed data items are of great significance, or require immediate user response, those items should be grouped and displayed prominently. Separation of groups of information should be accomplished through the use of blanks, spacing, lines, color coding, or other similar means consistent with the application.

The content of displays within a system should be presented in a consistent, standardized manner. Information density should be held to a minimum in displays used for critical tasks. When a display contains too much data for presentation in a single frame, the data should be partitioned into separately displayable pages. The user should not have to rely on memory to interpret new data. Each data display should provide the needed context, including the recapitulation of prior data from prior displays, as necessary.

An appropriate pointing device, such as a mouse, trackball, or touch screen, should be used in conjunction with applications that are suited to direct manipulation, such as identifying landmarks on a scanned image or selecting graphical elements from a palette of options. The suitability of a given pointing device to user tasks should be assessed.

9.6.12 Interactive control

General design objectives include consistency of control action, minimized need for control actions, and minimized memory load on the user, with flexibility of interactive control to adapt to different user needs. As a general principle, the user should decide what needs doing and when to do it. The selection of dialogue formats should be based on anticipated task requirements and user skills.

System response times should be consistent with operational requirements. Required user response times should be compatible with required system response time. Required user response times should be within the limits imposed by the total user task load expected in the operational environment.

Control-display relationships should be straightforward and explicit, as well as compatible with the lowest anticipated skill levels of users. Control actions should be simple and direct, whereas potentially destructive control actions should require focused user attention and command validation/confirmation before they are performed. Steps should be taken to prevent accidental use of destructive controls, including possible erasures or memory dump.

Feedback responses to correct user input should consist of changes in the state or value of those elements of the displays that are being controlled. These responses should be provided in an expected and logical manner. An acknowledgement message should be employed in those cases where the more conventional mechanism is not appropriate. Where control input errors are detected by the system, error messages and error recovery procedures should be available.

Menu selection can be used for interactive controls. Menu selection of commands is useful for tasks that involve the selection of a limited number of options or that can be listed in a menu, or in cases when users may have relatively little training. A menu command system that involves several layers can be useful when a command set is so large that users are unable to commit all the commands to memory and a reasonable hierarchy of commands exists for the user.

Form-filling interactive control may be used when some flexibility in data to be entered is needed and when the users will have moderate training. A form-filling dialogue should not be used when the computer has to handle multiple types of forms and computer response is slow.

Fixed-function key interactive control may be used for tasks requiring a limited number of control inputs or in conjunction with other dialogue types.

Command language interactive control may be used for tasks involving a wide range of user inputs and when user familiarity with the system can take advantage of the flexibility and speed of the control technique.

Question and answer dialogues should be considered for routine data entry tasks when data items are known and their ordering can be constrained, when users have little or no training, and when the computer is expected to have moderate response speed.

Query language dialogue should be used for tasks emphasizing unpredictable information retrieval with trained user. Query languages should reflect a data structure or organization perceived by the users to be natural.

Graphic interaction as a dialogue may be used to provide graphic aids as a supplement to other types of interactive control. Graphic menus may be used that display icons to represent the control options. This may be particularly valuable when system users have different linguistic backgrounds.

9.6.13 Feedback

Feedback should be provided that presents status, information, confirmation, and verification throughout the interaction. When system functioning requires the user to standby, WAIT or similar type messages should be displayed until interaction is again possible. When the standby or delay may last a significant period of time, the user should be informed. When a control process or sequence is completed or aborted by the system, a positive indication should be presented to the user about the outcome of the process and the requirements for subsequent user action. If the system rejects a user input, feedback should be provided to indicate why the input was rejected and the required corrective action.

Feedback should be self-explanatory. Users should not be made to translate feedback messages by using a reference system or code sheets. Abbreviations should not be used unless necessary.

9.6.16 Error management/data protection

When users are required to make entries into a system, an easy means of correcting erroneous entries should be provided. The system should permit correction of individual errors without requiring reentry of correctly entered commands or data elements.

Homework Exercises

1. Compare the work done by persons concerned primarily with human factors (Chapter 8) to the work done by Industrial Designers (this chapter).

2. Perform a web search using the search term "Industrial Design". Summarize the results from your first 10 hits.

3. Visit the web site for the Industrial Design Society of America (idsa.org). Find and report on their definition of industrial design.

4. Visit the web site devicelink.com, go to one of the expos listed (such as MD&M West). Search for the listing for contract manufacturers. Of the first ten or so, how many would qualify as Industrial Designers (list and discuss).

5. Do a web search for front panel web simulator software, report on your results. Find an example of a medical device panel layout.

6. Prototype a front panel layout for display of exercise data for a weight watchers clinic.

7. Which of the 11 problems in Chapter 8 may also apply to this chapter, and why?

References

Association for the Advancement of Medical Instrumentation (AAMI), *Human Factors Engineering Guidelines and Preferred Practices for the Design of Medical Devices.* Arlington, VA: Association for the Advancement of Medical Instrumentation, 1993.

Bogner, M. S., *Human Error in Medicine.* Hillsdale, NJ: Lawrence Erlbaum Associates, 1994.

Brown, C.M., *Human-computer Interface Design Guidelines.* Norwood, NJ: Ablex Publishing Company, 1989.

Fries, Richard C., "Human Factors and System Reliability", in *Medical Device Technology.* Volume 3, Number 2, March, 1992.

MIL-STD-1472, *Human Engineering Design Criteria for Military Systems, Equipment and Facilities.* Washington, DC: Department of Defense, 1981.

Morgan, C.T., *Human Engineering Guide to Equipment Design.* New York: Academic Press, 1984.

Wiklund, Michael E., "How to Implement Usability Engineering," in *Medical Device and Diagnostic Industry.* Volume 15, Number 9, 1993.

Wiklund, Michael E., *Medical Device and Equipment Design - Usability Engineering and Ergonomics.* Buffalo Grove: Interpharm Press, Inc., 1995.

Chapter 10

Biomaterials and Materials Selection

"Researchers have discovered that chocolate produces some of the same reactions in the brain as marijuana...The researchers also discovered other similarities between the two, but can't remember what they are."
Matt Lauer, on NBC's "Today" show, August 22, 1996

Biomaterials may be defined as nonviable materials used in or as a medical device with the intention of performing a medically related function. Biomaterials have been in existence for a number of years and their use and number of applications has exploded in the past century.

Gold was one of the first known substances to be used in dentistry. Use of gold dates back about 2000 years. Glass eyes have a shorter history. The use of wooden (George Washington had a set) and later ivory dentures date to the Middle Ages. The advent of aseptic surgery in the 1860s necessarily predated the first successful use of metal bone plates in 1900 and joint replacements in the 1930s. Accidental implantation of plastic shards from shattered airplane turrets during World War Two, and the recognition that a major rejection episode did not occur, probably led to the initiation of today's market for biomaterials. Blood vessels were being replaced in the 1950s, heart valves were implanted in the 1960s, and the field has expanded radically since.[1]

Example uses of biomaterials include the following:

- Replacement of diseased parts: dialysis with semipermable membranes (Cuprophane, 1960s)
- Treatment aids: catheters
- Replacement of diseased part: dental amalgams
- Replacement of burned or dead part: artificial skin
- Cosmetic correction: breast implants
- Assistive in healing: sutures
- Diagnostic aids: rectoscope
- Functional correction: spinal rods (Harrington)
- Improve function: soft contacts
- Monitor, diagnose, and treatment: pacemaker with defibrillator.

This field is sufficiently broad in scope that there exists, since 1975, the Society for Biomaterials, which coordinates the interests of students, faculty, and industry via an international organization, a searchable web site, and national meetings.[2] Other web sites contain databases for dental materials (University of Michigan)[3] and general materials (MATWEB).[4]

Biological evaluation of biomaterial and medical devices using biomaterial is performed to determine the potential toxicity resulting from contact of the component materials of the device with the body. The device materials should not, either directly or through the release of their material constituents:

- produce adverse local or systemic effects
- be carcinogenic
- produce adverse reproductive and developmental effects.

Therefore, evaluation of any new device intended for human use requires data from systematic testing to ensure that the benefits provided by the final product will exceed any potential risks produced by device materials.

When selecting the appropriate tests for biological evaluation of a medical device, one must consider the chemical characteristics of device materials and the nature, degree, frequency and duration of its exposure to the body. In general, the tests include:

- acutes
- sub-chronic and chronic toxicity
- irritation to skin, eyes and mucosal surfaces
- sensitization
- hemocompatibility
- genotoxicity
- carcinogenicity
- effects on reproduction including developmental effects.

However, depending on varying characteristics and intended uses of devices as well as the nature of contact, these general tests may not be sufficient to demonstrate the safety of some specialized devices. Additional tests for specific target organ toxicity, such as neurotoxicity and immunotoxicity may be necessary for some devices. For example, a neurological device with direct contact with brain parenchyma and cerebrospinal fluid (CSF) may require an animal implant test to evaluate its effects on the brain parenchyma, susceptibility to seizure, and effects on the functional mechanism of choroid plexus and arachnoid villi to secrete and absorb (CSF). The specific clinical application and the materials used in the manufacture of the new device determine which tests are appropriate.

Some devices are made of materials that have been well characterized chemically and physically in the published literature and have a long history of safe use. For the purposes of demonstrating the substantial equivalence of such devices to other marketed products, it may not be necessary to conduct all the tests suggested in the FDA matrix of this guidance. FDA reviewers are advised to use their scientific judgment in determining which tests are required for the demonstration of substantial equivalence under section 510(k). In such situations, the manufacturer must document the use of a particular material in a legally marketed predicate device or a legally marketed device with comparable patient exposure.

10.1 The FDA and Biocompatibility

In 1986, FDA, Health and Welfare Canada, and Health and Social Services UK issued the Tripartite Biocompatibility Guidance for Medical Devices. This Guidance has been used by FDA reviewers, as well as by manufacturers of medical devices, in selecting appropriate tests to evaluate the adverse biological responses to medical devices. Since that time, the International Standards Organization (ISO), in an effort to harmonize biocompatibility testing, developed a standard for biological evaluation of medical devices (ISO 10993). The scope of this 12-part standard is to evaluate the effects of medical device materials on the body. The first part of this standard "Biological Evaluation of Medical Devices: Part 1: Evaluation and Testing", provides guidance for selecting the tests to evaluate the biological response to medical devices. Most of the other parts of the ISO standard deal with appropriate methods to conduct the biological tests suggested in Part 1 of the standard.

The ISO Standard, Part 1, uses an approach to test selection that is very similar to the currently used Tripartite Guidance, including the same seven principles. It also uses a tabular format (matrix) for laying out the test requirements based on the various factors discussed above. The matrix consist of two tables: Initial Evaluation Tests for Consideration (Table 10-1) and Supplementary Evaluation Tests for Consideration (Table 10-2). In addition, FDA is in the process of preparing toxicology profiles for specific devices. These profiles will assist in determining appropriate toxicology tests for these devices.

To harmonize biological response testing with the requirements of other countries, FDA will apply the ISO standard, Part 1, in the review process in lieu of the Tripartite Biocompatibility Guidance.

FDA notes that the ISO standard acknowledges certain kinds of discrepancies. It states "due to diversity of medical devices, it is recognized that not all tests identified in a category will be necessary and practical for any given device. It is indispensable for testing that each device shall be considered on its own merits: additional tests not indicated in the table may be necessary." In keeping with this inherent flexibility of the ISO standard, FDA has made several modifications to the testing required by ISO 10993-Part 1. These modifications are required for the category of surface devices permanently contacting mucosal membranes (e.g., IUDs). The ISO standard would not require acute, sub-chronic, chronic toxicity and implantation tests. Also, for externally communicating devices, tissue/bone/dentin with prolonged and permanent contact (e.g., dental cements, filling materials etc.), the ISO standard does not require irritation, systemic toxicity, acute, sub-chronic and chronic toxicity tests. Therefore, FDA has included these types of tests in the matrix. Although several

Device Categories			Biological Effect							
Body Contact X = ISO evaluation tests for consideration O = Additional tests which may be applicable		Contact Duration A: 24 hrs B: 24 h rs to 30 days C: >30 days	Cytotoxicity	Sensitization	Irritation	System Toxicity	Sub-chronic Tox	Genotoxicity	Implantation	Hemocompatibility
Surface devices	Skin	A	X	X	X	.	.	.	.	.
		B	X	X	X	.	.	.	.	.
		C	X	X	X	.	.	.	.	.
	Mucosal membrane	A	X	X	X	.	.	.	.	.
		B	X	X	X	O	O	.	O	.
		C	X	X	X	O	X	X	O	.
	Breached or compromised surfaces	A	X	X	X	O	.	.	.	.
		B	X	X	X	O	O	.	O	.
		C	X	X	X	O	X	X	O	.
External communicating devices	Blood path, indirect	A	X	X	X	X	.	.	.	X
		B	X	X	X	X	O	.	.	X
		C	X	X	O	X	X	X	O	X

Table 10-1 Initial Evaluation Tests for Consideration

Device Categories			Biological Effects							
Body Contact X = ISO evaluation tests for consideration O = Additional tests which may be applicable	Contact Duration A: 24 hrs B: 24 h rs to 30 days C: >30 days	Cytoxicity	Sensitization	Irritation	System Toxicity	Sub-chronic Tox	Genotoxicity	Implantation	Hemocompatibility	
	Tissue/bone/dentin communicating	A	X	X	X	O	.	.	.	.
		B	X	X	O	O	O	X	X	.
		C	X	X	O	O	O	X	X	.
	Circulating blood	A	X	X	X	X	.	O	.	X
		B	X	X	X	X	O	X	O	X
		C	X	X	X	X	X	X	O	X
Implant devices	Tissue/bone	A	X	X	X	0	.	.	.	.
		B	X	X	O	O	O	X	X	.
		C	X	X	O	O	O	X	X	.
	Blood	A	X	X	X	X	.	.	X	X
		B	X	X	X	X	O	X	X	X
		C	X	X	X	X	X	X	X	X

Table 10-1 Initial Evaluation Tests for Consideration (continued)

Device Categories						
Body Contact X = ISO evaluation tests for consideration O = Additional tests which may be applicable		Contact Duration A: 24 hrs B: 24 h rs to 30 days C: >30 days	Chronic Toxicity	Carcinogenicity	Reproductive Dev	Biodegradable
Surface devices	Skin	A	.	.	.	.
		B	.	.	.	.
		C	.	.	.	.
	Mucosal membrane	A	.	.	.	.
		B	.	.	.	.
		C	O	.	.	
	Breached or compromised surfaces	A	.	.	.	.
		B	.	.	.	.
		C	O	.	.	.
External communicating devices	Blood path, indirect	A	.	.	.	.
		B	.	.	.	.
		C	X	X	.	.

Table 10-2 Supplementary Evaluation Tests for Consideration

Device Categories						
Body Contact X = ISO evaluation tests for consideration O = Additional tests which may be applicable	Contact Duration A: 24 hrs B: 24 h rs to 30 days C: >30 days	Chronic Toxicity	Carcinogenicity	Reproductive Dev	Biodegradable	
	Tissue/bone/dentin communicating	A	.	.	.	.
		B	.	.	.	.
		C	O	X	.	.
	Circulating blood	A	.	.	.	.
		B	.	.	.	.
		C	X	X	.	.
Implant devices	Tissue/bone	A	.	.	.	.
		B	.	.	.	.
		C	X	X	.	.
	Blood	A	.	.	.	.
		B	.	.	.	.
		C	X	X	.	.

Table 10-2 Supplementary Evaluation Tests for Consideration (continued)

tests were added to the matrix, reviewers should note that some tests are commonly requested while other tests are to be considered and only asked for on a case-by-case basis. Thus, the modified matrix is only a framework for the selection of tests and not a checklist of every required test.

Reviewers should avoid proscriptive interpretation of the matrix. If a reviewer is uncertain about the applicability of a specific type of test for a specific device, the reviewer should consult toxicologists in ODE.

FDA expects that manufacturers will consider performing the additional tests for certain categories of devices suggested in the FDA-modified matrix. This does not mean that all the tests suggested in the modified matrix are essential and relevant for all devices. In addition, device manufacturers are advised to consider tests to detect chemical components of device materials, which may be pyrogenic. The FDA believes that ISO 10993, Part 1, and appropriate consideration of the additional tests suggested by knowledgeable individuals will generate adequate biological data to meet its requirements.

Manufacturers are advised to initiate discussions with the appropriate review division in the Office of Device Evaluation, CDRH, prior to the initiation of expensive, long-term testing of any new device materials to ensure that the proper testing will be conducted. We also recognize that an ISO standard is a document that undergoes periodic review and is subject to revision. ODE will notify manufacturers of any future revisions to the ISO standard referenced here that affect this document's requirements and expectations.

10.2 International Regulatory Efforts

ISO is in the process of publishing a series of standards on the biological evaluation of medical devices—ISO 10993. Many parts of this series have been accepted as international standards, while the rest are under development (see Table 10-3). The subject of the first part, ISO 10993-1, is the categorizing and performance of safety testing. Part two of the standard, ISO 10993-2, is concerned with animal welfare requirements; another section, ISO 10993-12, deals with sample preparation and reference materials. Most of the remaining parts of the standard treat the individual tests.

The EU has issued a council directive—93/42/EEC, 1993—concerning medical devices. All medical devices to be sold on the EU market must comply with this directive after June 14, 1998. The European Committee for Standardization (CEN) is currently in the process of adopting the ISO 10993 standard as the European standard. In 1986 the responsible authorities in the United Kingdom, United States, and Canada issued the Tripartite document, which was guidance on the selection of toxicological tests for medical device safety testing. This document has now been replaced by ISO 10993-1 as a first step in the process of international harmonization. In 1995 FDA chose to accept the ISO 10993-1 standard, with a modification of the matrix listing (see sidebar below). Japanese authorities have also issued a guideline for toxicological testing of medical devices. This document is available in an unofficial translation as Guidelines for Basic Biological Tests of Medical Materials and Devices. It resembles ISO 10993 in structure and content, but recommends modified tests and sample preparations.

The procedure for using the ISO 10993-1 standard is illustrated by the flowchart in Figure 10-1. The standard is applicable only for devices that are directly or indirectly in contact with the body or body fluids. If a device is to be subjected to the standard, the first step is to characterize the material. Such characterization need not always be followed by biological evaluation, because there may be sufficient historical data to verify that the device meets the requirements of the standard. If the material and/or the intended use of the device is different from any historical safe device, biological evaluation has to be performed. By following the standard, a suitable test program can be chosen depending on the type and duration of body contact. Within the EU, all new medical devices must carry the CE mark from June 14, 1998. This should ensure the availability of relevant documentation regarding biocompatibility and the lack of health problems associated with the use of a device. It is noteworthy that the approval of such documentation is not, as it was previously, accorded by the national health authorities, but rather by the so-called notified bodies, whose experts review the products and production facilities of medical device manufacturers.

10.3 Device Category and Choice of Test Program

The need to evaluate a medical device biologically depends on the material used in the device, the intended body contact, and the duration of that contact. A device designed for surface contact for a limited time is not as likely

Part	Title
1	Evaluation and Testing
2	Animal Welfare Requirements
3	Tests for Genotoxicity, Carcinogenicity, and Reproductive Toxicity
4	Selection of Tests for Interactions with Blood
5	Tests for Cytotoxicity – In Vitro Methods
6	Tests for Local Effects after Implantation
7	Ethylene Oxide Sterilization Residuals
8	Clinical Investigation of Medical Devices
9	Degradation of Materials Related to Biological Testing
10	Test for Irritation and Sensitization
11	Test for Systemic Toxicity
12	Sample Preparation and Reference Material
13	Identification and Quantification of Degradation Products from Polymers
14	Identification and Quantification of Degradation Products from Ceramics
15	Identification and Quantification of Degradation Products from Coated and Uncoated Metals and Alloys
16	Toxicokinetic Study Design for Degradation Products and Leachables
17	Glutaraldehyde and Formaldehyde Residues in Industrially Sterilized Medical Devices

Table 10-3 Listing of Individual Parts of ISO 10993

to be bioincompatible as a permanent-exposure implant device made of the same material. The ISO 10993-1 standard divides medical devices into three main categories: surface devices, externally communicating devices, and implant devices. Each category is further divided into subcategories according to the type of contact to which the patient is exposed (see Table 10-4).

The ISO test matrix should not be considered as a checklist for the different tests that have to be performed, but rather as a guide for qualified toxicologists who also take into consideration material information and historical data from similar devices. The certifying authorities in most countries (e.g., notified bodies, FDA, Japanese authorities) are generally cooperative when a company must decide on a test program for a device. It is therefore advisable to maintain close contact with the relevant authorities during the entire process. However, testing should not be performed simply to meet regulatory

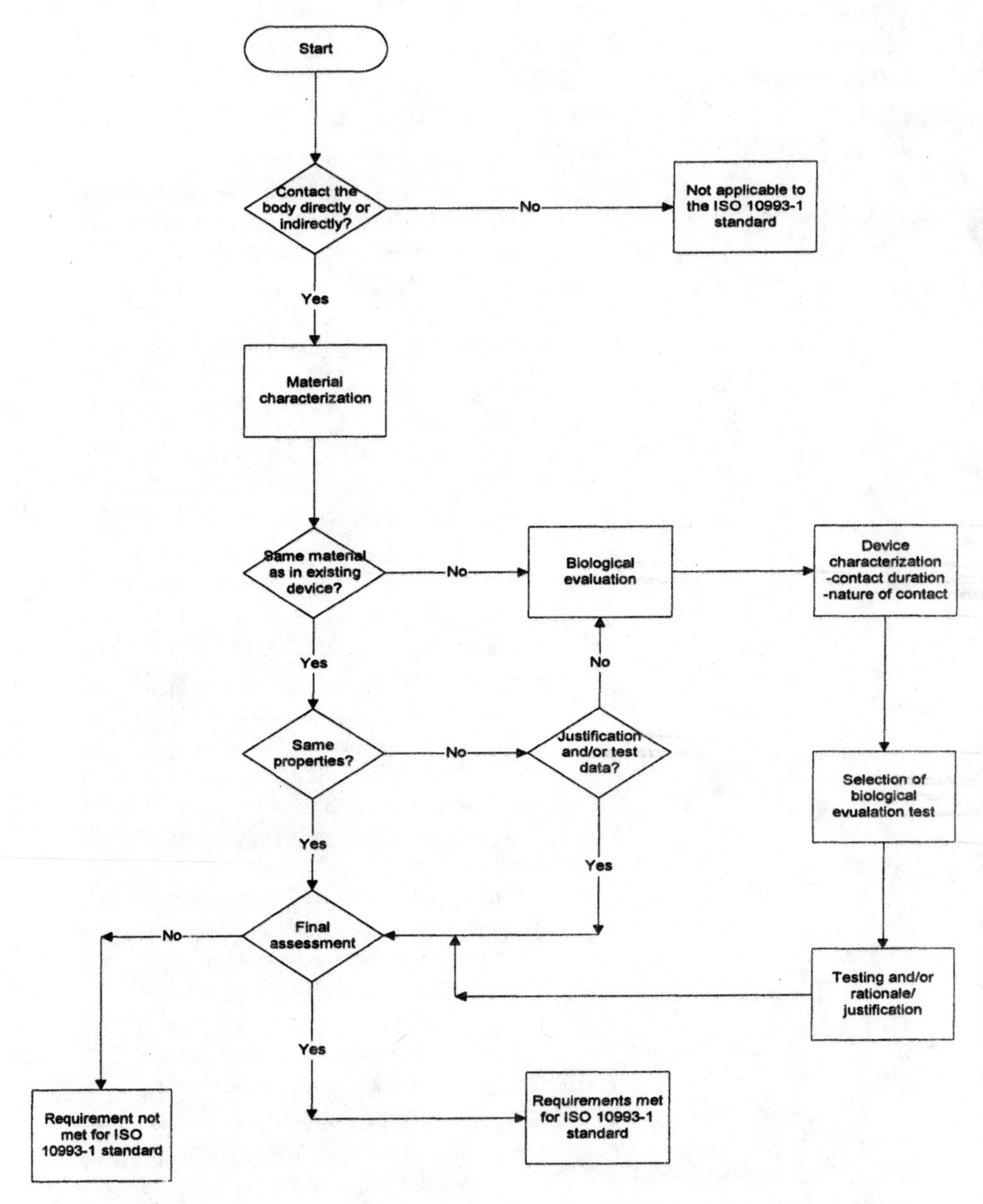

Figure 10-1 Steps in the biological evaluation of medical devices.

requirements. This is important not only to lessen the risk of over testing and excessive use of experimental animals, but also because a strict regulatory approach may mask potential negative health effects that might be identified via optional or nonroutine testing procedures.

The choice of test program for a device in a given category depends on the duration of the contact. Three different time spans are given: limited contact (<24 hours), prolonged contact (24 hours-30 days), and permanent contact (>30 days). ISO 10993-1 lists the tests that must be considered for each category.

As regards CE marking of existing products on the market or safety evaluation of medical devices already in clinical use, appropriate historical or clinical data should be employed whenever possible to avoid unnecessary testing.

10.4 Preparation of Extracts

ISO 10993-12 describes how samples for biological evaluation should be selected, prepared, and extracted. Other guidelines provide similar descriptions, which differ slightly in the specifics of the extraction procedures.

The device to be tested (the test article) should be a representative specimen of the mass-produced device. It should also be finished or treated (e.g., coated or sterilized) in the same way as the mass-produced device.

Because the toxic potential of materials and devices depends to a substantial degree on the leachability and toxicity of soluble components, extracts of the device are normally used in the tests. In some tests, however, an evaluation under normal-use conditions is mimicked by using the device or a piece of the device directly. Ideally, extraction media should constitute a series of media with decreasing polarity to ensure the extraction of components of widely different solubility properties. The most commonly used extraction media are physiological saline, vegetable oil, dimethylsulfoxide, and ethanol. Other extraction media such as polyethylene glycol or aqueous dilutions of ethanol may be selected in certain cases. For in vitro cytotoxicity testing, complete cell-culture medium is most often employed. The various guidelines also differ somewhat with respect to the temperature at which the extraction is conducted. Some leachable compounds may be chemically altered at high

Device Categories		Examples
Surface Devices	Skin	Electrodes, external prostheses, fixation tapes, compression bandages, monitors various types
	Mucous membrane	Contact lenses, urinary catheters, intravaginal and intraintestinal devices, endotracheal tubes, bronchoscopes, dental prostheses, orthodontic devices
	Breached or compromised surfaces	Ulcer, burn, and granulation tissue dressings or healing devices, occlusive patches
Externally Communicating Devices	Blood path indirect	Solution administration sets, extension sets, transfer sets, blood administration sets
	Tissue/bone/dentin communicating	Laparoscopes, arthroscopes, draining systems, dental cements, dental filling materials, skin staples
	Circulating blood	Intravascular catheters, temporary pacemaker electrodes, oxygenators, extracorporeal oxygenator tubing and accessories, dialyzers, dialysis tubing and accessories, hemoadsorbents and immunoadsorbents
	Tissue/bone implant devices	Orthopedic pins, plates, replacement joints, bone prostheses, cements and intraosseous devices, pacemakers, drug-supply devices, neuromuscular sensors and simulators, replacement tendons, breast implants, artificial larynxes, subperiosteal implants, ligation clips
	Blood	Pacemaker electrodes, artificial arteriovenous fistulae, heart valves, vascular grafts, internal drug-delivery catheters, ventricular-assist devices

Table 10-4 Device Categories and Examples According to ISO 10993-1

temperatures, and it is now generally recommended that extraction be conducted at 37°C—simulating body temperature—for 72 hours. This procedure will probably become increasingly accepted as the most appropriate extraction method. For in vitro cytotoxicity tests, extraction at 37°C for 24 hours is usually recommended, since certain constituents of the media are relatively labile.

The amount of leachable substances released to the extraction media is related to the surface area and thickness of the product to be extracted. Recommendations vary from 1.25 to 6 cm2 of product per milliliter of extraction medium, depending on the size and shape of the product, or from 0.1 to 0.2g of product per milliliter of extraction medium when a surface area cannot readily be estimated (e.g., for powders or granulates). In any case, the specific properties of the product must be taken into account in order to make usable extracts.

For cases in which a medical device comprises several components made from different materials, the ideal procedure from a toxicological point of view would be to test extracts of the components separately. However, in some situations this is not practical, and extracts of the whole device may be used instead.

10.5 Biological Control Tests

Biological control tests are not described in the ISO 10993 standard for biological evaluation of medical devices, since these particular tests are designed primarily for batch-control purposes. Such tests are also used during the product development phase to identify sources of contamination and to establish procedures that ensure the intended quality of the end product.

10.5.1 Microbiological control tests

Microbiological control tests are necessary to establish the microbiological status of an end product—factors such as sterility, absence of pathological bacteria, or limits for microbial counts. Furthermore, it is often necessary to monitor the microbiological load of raw materials and intermediary products, or to check the efficiency of production and sterilization processes. The tests are performed by rinsing the materials or products in physiological saline and assessing the rinsing medium for microbes, or by directly incubating the products in growth media.

10.5.2 Tests for endotoxins

Even sterile medical devices may contain cell-wall lipopolysaccharides originating from gram-negative bacteria. Such so-called endotoxins or pyrogens can cause an abrupt fever reaction after entering directly into the body from sources such as venous catheters, syringes, or implant components. Two different biological assays can be used to measure the presence of endotoxins: the rabbit pyrogen test and the Limulus test. In both cases, an eluate is prepared—normally by rinsing the surfaces of the product with water—and then tested for endotoxins. In the rabbit pyrogen test, the eluate is injected intravenously and the rectal temperature of the animal is measured after the injection. In the Limulus test, the eluate is incubated together with lysate from the blood of the horseshoe crab (Limulus polyphemus), which contains a substance that forms a gel in the presence of endotoxins.

10.5.3 Test for nonspecific toxicity

This test is designed to assess any nonspecific adverse effect that occurs following intravenous injection of a device eluate in mice. The test is often performed with the same eluate used for the pyrogen test. The mice are inspected regularly for any signs of ill health, which can indicate the presence of toxic substances leaching from the product.

10.6 Tests for Biological Evaluation

This section provides a brief description of the individual tests included in the ISO 10993/EN 30993 standard.

10.6.1 Cytotoxicity

The aim of in vitro cytotoxicity tests is to detect the potential ability of a device to induce sub lethal or lethal effects as observed at the cellular level. According to ISO 10993-1, the in vitro cytotoxicity assay is one of two tests--the other is the sensitization test described below--that must be considered in the evaluation of all device categories.

Three main types of cell-culture assays have been developed:

- the elution test
- the direct-contact test
- the agar diffusion test.

In the elution test, an extract (eluate) of the material is prepared and added in varied concentrations to the cell cultures. Growth inhibition is a widely used parameter, but others may also be used. In the direct-contact test, pieces of test material are placed directly on top of the cell layer, which is covered only by a layer of liquid cell-culture medium. Toxic substances leaching from the test material may depress the growth rate of the cells or damage them in various ways. In the agar diffusion test, a piece of test material is placed on an agar layer covering a confluent monolayer of cells. Toxic substances leaching from the material diffuse through the thin agar layer and kill or disrupt adjacent cells in the monolayer. As always, the physical and chemical properties of the test material should be considered before the choice of the test system is made.

There is usually a good qualitative correlation between results from cell-culture tests and studies performed in vivo with respect to cytotoxicity versus primary tissue effects. It is important to recognize, however, that although cell-culture toxicity is in general a good and sensitive indicator of primary tissue compatibility, exceptions may arise in cases where leaching substances cause tissue damage in vivo through more complex mechanisms. At present, the in vitro cytotoxicity assays should be used as screening tests and considered primarily as supplements to the various in vivo tests.

10.6.2 Sensitization

The sensitization test recognizes a potential sensitization reaction induced by a device, and is required by the ISO 10993-1 standard for all device categories. The sensitization reaction is also known as allergic contact dermatitis, which is an immunologically mediated cutaneous reaction. This is in contrast to irritant contact dermatitis (skin irritation)--a skin reaction caused by the primary and direct effect of a substance on the skin. In animals, the sensitization reactions manifest themselves as redness (erythema) and swelling (edema).

The preferred animal species for sensitization testing is the albino guinea pig. There is no reliable alternative in vitro test that can predict the sensitizing potential of a substance. The various available guinea pig methods have certain features in common: an induction (sensitization) phase, when the potential allergen is presented to the organism, followed by a rest period and a subsequent challenge phase to determine whether or not sensitization has occurred.

One of the most recognized and validated assays is the guinea pig maximization test (GPMT). A test design very similar to the GPMT is widely used for assessing the sensitizing potential of medical devices. After a challenge period, the skin reactions are graded on a ranking scale according to the degree of erythema and edema.

Predictive tests in guinea pigs are important tools in identifying the possible hazard to a population repeatedly exposed to a substance. Nevertheless, results from sensitization tests in guinea pigs have to be evaluated carefully. A positive test result in this assay may rate a substance as a stronger sensitizer than it appears to be during actual use. On the other hand, a negative result in such a sensitive assay ensures a considerable safety margin regarding the potential risk to humans.

10.6.3 Skin irritation

The ISO 10993-10 standard describes skin-irritation tests for both single and cumulative exposure to a device. The preferred animal species is the albino rabbit, whose highly sensitive, light skin makes it possible to detect even very slight skin irritation caused by a substance. Skin-irritation tests of medical devices are performed either with two extracts obtained with polar and nonpolar solvents or with the device itself.

In the single-exposure test, rabbits are treated for several hours only, whereas for the cumulative test the same procedure is repeated for several days. All extracts and extractants are applied to intact skin sites. Skin reaction is seen as redness or swelling and is graded according to a specified classification system.

Dermal irritation is the production of reversible changes in the skin following the application of a substance, whereas dermal corrosion is the production of irreversible tissue damage (scar formation) in the skin. Materials that leak corrosive substances are not likely candidates for medical device production.

10.6.4 Intracutaneous reactivity

The intracutaneous reactivity test is designed to assess the localized reaction of tissue to leachable substances. The test is required for consideration in nearly all the device categories in ISO 10993-1 (see Table III). Polar and nonpolar solvent extracts are administered as intracutaneous injections to rabbits. Undesirable intracutaneous reactivity includes redness or swelling.

10.6.5 Acute systemic toxicity

Acute systemic toxicity is the adverse effect occurring within a short time after administration of a single dose of a substance. ISO 10993-1 requires that the test for acute systemic toxicity be considered for all device categories that indicate blood contact. For this test, extracts of medical devices are usually administered intravenously or intraperitoneally in rabbits or mice.

Determining acute systemic toxicity is usually an initial step in the assessment and evaluation of the toxic characteristics of a substance. By providing information on health hazards likely to arise from short-term exposure, the acute systemic toxicity test can serve as a first step in the establishment of a dosage regimen in sub chronic and other studies, and can also supply initial data on the mode of toxic action of a substance. The test is similar to the nonspecific toxicity test. Normally, only one of these two procedures is included in a test battery.

10.6.6 Genotoxicity

Genetic toxicology tests are used to investigate materials for possible mutagenic effects--that is, damage to the body's genes or chromosomes. The tests are performed both in vitro and in vivo. ISO 10993- 1 requires the genotoxicity (mutagenicity) test to be considered for all device categories indicating permanent (>30 days) body contact (except for surface devices with skin contact only).

A mutation is a change in the formation content of the genetic material (DNA code) that is propagated through subsequent generations of cells. Mutations can be classified into two general types:

- gene mutations
- chromosomal mutations.

Gene mutations are changes in nucleotide sequences at one or several coding segments within a gene; chromosomal mutations are morphological alterations or aberrations in the gross structure of the chromosomes.

The simplest and most sensitive assays for detecting induced gene mutations are those using bacteria. Gene mutations can also be detected in cultured mammalian cells. Current in vivo assays for gene mutations are cumbersome and not widely used. The simplest and most sensitive assays for investigating chromosomal aberrations are those that use cultured mammalian cells. However, two well-established in vivo procedures are also available: chromosomal aberrations can be studied in bone marrow or peripheral blood cells of rodents dosed with a suspect chemical or extract either by counting micronuclei in maturing erythrocytes (micronucleus test) or by analyzing chromosomes in metaphase cells.

In addition to these mutagenicity tests, various assays can measure the induction of an overall genotoxic response--an indirect indicator of potential damage to the genetic material.

10.6.7 Implantation

Implantation tests are designed to assess any localized effects of a device designed to be used inside the human body. Implantation testing methods essentially attempt to imitate the intended use conditions of an implanted material. Although different tests use various animal species, the rabbit has become the species of choice, with implantation performed in the paravertebral muscle. Implantation can be either surgical or nonsurgical: the surgical method involves the creation of a pouch in the muscle into which the implant is placed, while the nonsurgical method uses a cannula and stylet to insert a cylinder-shaped implant. Through a macroscopic examination (which may be supplemented with microscopic analysis), the degree of tissue reaction in the paravertebral muscle is evaluated as a measure of biocompatibility.

10.6.8 Hemocompatibility

The purpose of hemocompatibility testing is to look for possible undesirable changes in the blood caused directly by a medical device or by chemicals leaching from a device. Undesirable effects of device materials on the blood may include hemolysis, thrombus formation, alterations in coagulation parameters, and immunological changes. According to the ISO 10993-4 (EN 30993-4) standard, devices that only come into very brief contact with circulating blood--for example, lancets, hypodermic needles, or capillary tubes--generally do not require blood/device interaction testing.

ISO 10993-4 describes hemocompatibility tests in five different categories:

- thrombosis
- coagulation
- platelets
- hematology
- immunology.

Most of the individual tests are not discussed in detail, but they may be performed either in vivo or, preferably, in vitro. There is still some uncertainty with respect to what is actually required by the regulatory authorities for the hemocompatibility test.

10.6.9 Subchronic and chronic toxicity

Subchronic toxicity is the potentially adverse effect that can occur as a result of the repeated daily dosing of a substance to experimental animals over a portion of their life span. In the assessment and evaluation of the toxic characteristics of a chemical, the determination of subchronic toxicity is carried out after initial information on toxicity has been obtained by acute testing, and provides data on possible health hazards likely to arise from repeated exposures over a limited time. Such testing can furnish information on target organs and the possibilities of toxin accumulation, and provide an estimate of a no-effect exposure level that can be used to select dose levels for chronic studies and establish safety criteria for human exposure.

In subchronic or chronic toxicity studies, one or two animal species are dosed daily, usually for a period of 3 to 6 months; the rat is the standard animal species of choice. The animals are given the test substance in increasing doses. The dose level of the low-dose group should be at the level of human exposure. When extracts of medical devices are employed, one dose level (the highest practically applicable volume) is often sufficient, since strong toxicity is generally not expected.

10.6.10 Carcinogenicity

The objective of long-term carcinogenicity studies is to observe test animals over a major portion of their life span to detect any development of neoplastic lesions (tumor induction) during or after exposure to various doses of a test substance. Carcinogenicity testing is normally conducted with oral dosing. For implants and medical devices, however, only extracts can be tested and they must be administered intravenously, necessitating certain modifications of the standard procedure. There are only a very few products for which this comprehensive test can be justified.

In carcinogenicity studies, mice or rats are dosed every day for 18 to 24 months. For medical device extracts, one dose level (again the highest practically applicable volume) is usually sufficient. At the completion of the dosing period, all surviving animals are sacrificed and their organs and tissues examined microscopically for the presence of tumors. An increased incidence of one or more category of tumors in the dosed group would indicate that the product tested has the potential to induce tumors and could be considered a possible carcinogen in humans.

10.7 Alternative Test Methods

As mentioned previously, a major goal in international toxicological testing is to reduce not only the use of in vivo studies but also the number of animals employed in these tests. A few of the in vivo procedures used today for testing medical devices may be of questionable worth for safety evaluation. However, the availability of accepted and validated in vitro assays is still limited. Substantial resources have been made available for validation of alternative in vitro assays in toxicology as replacements for animal tests, but it may take years before validated methods can be implemented, and any goal of replacing all in vivo studies with in vitro assays will probably never be met.

Recently, a working group under the auspices of the European Center for Validation of Alternative Methods (ECVAM) has recommended a few alternative methods that can be used for safer testing of medical devices. These include two in vitro tests as potential substitutes for the in vivo assays for skin and eye irritation. However, the implementation of validated protocols and internationally accepted guidelines for these tests is likely to be delayed into the next century.

10.8 Endnote

There have been some disasters involving biomaterials. These disasters have emphasized the need for diligence in testing of biomaterials. These include toxic shock syndrome, latex allergies, the use of talc on gloves, and perhaps reactions to silicon gel leakage from breast implants. Continuing diligence, especially when new substances are being tested, is mandated by law.

Homework Exercises

1. You are charged with developing the coating material for an implantable brain stimulator for reduction of tremor due to Parkinson's disease. You may begin with a web search to determine what materials are currently in use, if any. What materials will you consider and what tests will need to be run? Refer to the charts in this chapter.
2. You are interested in building an inexpensive EKG transmitter for implantation in mice. Do a literature (or web search) to determine a list of acceptable coatings. Which would you use if the experiment were to only last one day? Which if the work was to continue for a month? Why?
3. Do a literature search to determine the history of implant materials. What are some of the earliest signs that the human body accepted a foreign object?
4. How old is the history of implantation of materials into human teeth? Why was this done?

5. Do a web search using the term "biocompatibility testing"; categorize the first several hits as to their relevance to this chapter. Do a similar search using the term "animal care and use form."
6. Why are rabbits so often used for pyrogen testing? What is unique about rabbits?
7. The horseshoe crab is of value in compatibility testing. What is special about this animal?
8. "The use of earrings and other body piercing adornments has been linked to an increase in one of the hepatitis strains in the users." Do a web or literature search to deny or defend this statement.
9. In post-war Germany an operation was performed on amputees called a cineplasty, wherein a carbon-coated rod was passed through the muscle above the amputation. With time, the tunnel often grew skin on its surface and the subject could use his or her remaining muscle to move prostheses, such as a primitive grasper hand. Research this history and speculate on what might have ensued if there had been no long-term problems.
10. Research on of the four problems referenced in the endnote section. What was involved in the problem and what was the outcome?

References

[1] Ratner, B.D., et al., *Biomaterials Science*, Academic Press, 1996, pg. 11.
[2] The web site is www.biomaterials.org as of this writing.
[3] http://www.lib.umich.edu/dentlib/Dental_tables/intro.html
[4] http://www.matweb.com/main.htm

Biological Evaluation of Medical Devices, ISO 10993 Standard Series, Geneva, International Organization for Standardization, ongoing.

Bollen, Lise S. and Ove Svendsen, "Regulatory Guidelines for Biocompatibility Safety Testing," in *Medical Plastics and Biomaterials.* May, 1997.

Council Directive 93/42/EEC of 14 June 1993 Concerning Medical Devices, Official Journal of the European Communities, vol. 36, July, 1993.

Gad, S.C., *Safety Evaluation of Medical Devices*, Marcel Dekker, 1997.

Hill, D., Design Engineering of Biomaterials for Medical Devices, Wiley, 1998.

Toxicology Subgroup, Tripartite Subcommittee on Medical Devices, "Tripartite Biocompatibility Guidance for Medical Devices," Rockville, MD, FDA, Center for Devices and Radiological Health (CDRH), 1986.

Guidelines for Basic Biological Tests of Medical Materials and Devices. Unofficial translation of Japanese guideline ISBN 4-8408-0392-7.

Svendsen O, Garthoff B, Spielmann H, et al., Alternatives to the Animal Testing of Medical Devices (the Report and Recommendations of ECVAM Workshop 17 to be published in ATLA, in press, 1996).

Chapter 11

Safety Engineering: Devices and Processes

"Early and provident fear is the mother of safety."
Edmund Burke

The Accreditation Board for Engineering and Technology (ABET) requirements for design state that "Students must be prepared for engineering practice through the curriculum culminating in a major design experience based upon the knowledge and skills acquired in earlier coursework and incorporating engineering standards and realistic constraints that include most of the following considerations: economic; environmental; sustainability; manufacturability; ethical; health and safety; social; and political." [1] That biomedical engineering design work would involve health aspects is obvious, but should also include the several aspects involving safety and the potential for liability requires a discussion of the need for safety consideration in the design and redesign of medical devices, and in somewhat similar activities in process design. This chapter will first cover some aspects of safe design processes as relate to device design, then will conclude with a brief overview of redesign of medical processes with an eye toward safer practices in clinics.

The recently published National Academy Press publication "To Err is Human: Building a Safer Health System"[2] has provided several notable statistics, specifically "The human cost of medical errors is high. Based on the findings of one major study, medical errors kill some 44,000 people in U.S. hospitals each year. Another study puts the number much higher, at 98,000. Even using the lower estimate, more people die from medical mistakes each year than from highway accidents, breast cancer, or AIDS." This statistic permits comparing medical error deaths to the number of deaths due to other accidental causes, such as may be found from the National Safety Council website (www.nsc.org) , and to the number of deaths due to specific diseases. The safety council data estimates 150,445 total deaths due to injuries in 1998, a statistic on a par with the above. The magnitude of the numbers above should impress one as to the need for safety considerations, not just for public activities, but also for medical activities, such as is involved in the design of medical devices and systems. (Similar, but older statistics may be obtained in Reference 3).

11.1 Medical Case Example

Let us illustrate the above discussion with an example based upon an actual event. A young Down's syndrome patient with multiple heart defects died from an air embolism during a preoperative cardiac flow/oxygenation catheterization study. Evidence acquired from the hospital involved the following data and devices:

- The medical record for the patient
- Testimony regarding the procedure
- Complete records of blood pressure and ekg as various sites were checked for pressures and sampled for oxygen saturation levels, blood pressure was sampled periodically using the system below
- The catheterization system, which included a three port connection system (manifold) for blood pressure determination, saline infusion and blood sampling/injection via a syringe
- A typical saline bag and connector assembly
- An opaque pressurization jacket used to pressurize the saline bag to ensure saline flow when the saline port was opened.

There are two items to be determined at this point. It is a given that the patient died of an air embolus. How did this occur and what could have been done to prevent this are two of the questions to be asked. Let us ask the second first, discussing some of the general procedures that must be used to analyze safe devices and procedures.

11.2 Safety in Design

Good design practices should consider means by which a given design may cause harm, and should – via guide sentences, structure, or checklists, assist the designer in determination of improvements to the system under study. Let us illustrate this with another example: Drink machines have been known to tip over and kill or maim persons shaking them when irate over non-delivery of drinks (a few deaths per year in the U.S.). How can this be prevented?

A quick checklist can be found that helps one begin the solution to this problem; this checklist can read as the following[3]:

- Eliminate by design
- Guard against
- Warn the user
- Train the user
- Mandate the use of personal protective equipment
- Other.

As the drink machine manufacturer, what solutions are possible here? Mandating that the user wear protective equipment is not likely, nor is training the user. One might warn the user to not tilt the drink machine in order to get a drink, but it is not likely that you would win a case involving the death of a user of your machine. Guarding against the machine tilting would seem to be a better approach; strapping the machine to a nearby wall should enable this outcome. A far better approach would be to eliminate the problem by design by placing the weight of the unsold drinks at the base of the machine, rather than at the top (which enables gravity feed of the drinks and thus a cheaper design).

The above checklist is simply an outline; in practice each of the subheadings can have various gradations. For example, the warning of the user can be visual or audible, color coded, flashing, etc.

Implied in the above discussion are a few other concepts that are mandatory to understand if one is to analyze unsafe designs. One is the term hazard, which may be defined as a source of potential harm or a situation with a potential for harm. Another is risk, which is a combination of the probability of occurrence of harm and the severity of that harm. If you as the manufacturer of the machine above decide to not redesign anything, you are apparently assuming that your risk of financial harm due to a lawsuit is less than your cost to prevent the problem in the first place. Good design practices will include hazard analysis and risk assessment at every stage of the design, with an ultimate goal of risk reduction. As safe design is mandated for medical devices, this practice must be documented as a device is developed. As the variety of users in the medical environment is so varied in terms of education and responsibilities and other tasks, good design must involve a fairly comprehensive list of items.

Let us once again use the drink machine example above to look at this process of safe design. A typical approach to an analysis could include the following steps:

- Identify users (for example, drink installer, general public).
- Identify hazards each users may be subjected to, this hazard list is associated with a checklist such as mechanical hazards, chemical, health, etc. (Mechanical problems would be paramount here.)
- Begin the risk assessment, using a guide sentence such as "when doing the (task) the harm may be (harm)." One of the guide sentences here would be – "When shaking the machine it could tip and crush the user."
- Identify the severity of the harm (catastrophic, serious, slight, minimal), the exposure to harm (frequent, occasional, remote, none), and the probability of harm (probable, possible, unlikely, negligible) and therefore the risk level (High, moderate, or low). A high risk level implies the outcome of severe to moderate injury or death, moderate implies moderate to low probability of harm, low implies moderate to mild injury. The risk of death from an unsercured drink machine falling on one is high, the exposure is remote (it does happen!), the probability of it occurring with an untethered machine is high.

- The complete analysis would then involve the identification of methods to reduce the risk (such as guarding), the revised exposure and risk data, and the personnel in charge of this activity.

Special attention should be given to situations where the device may be misused in order to "cover all bases" in an analysis. Additionally, especially in the case of devices used in a clinical environment, special consideration should be given to not only the primary users of the device, but also to casual users (cleaning crew) and special needs patients (elderly, very young, very ill, AIDs, at-risk, etc.). Human factors analyses should also be considered, especially in light of situations where there might be high stress on the part of the user (see Chapter 8).

11.3 Medical Case Example – Revisited

Let us revisit the case mentioned above regarding the death of a young Down's syndrome child with multiple heart defects. What considerations should there be in this case – regarding instrumentation, risk, and fault? Below are a few of the points to consider when looking at this case:

- The patient was described as young. A far smaller amount of air can cause death from air embolism in young patients as compared to adults – children are "at risk" for this problem compared to adults.
- Down's syndrome children often have heart problems; this particular patient was described as having multiple heart defects. Heart shunts predispose patients to risks from air emboli; this patient had shunts (the reason for the study and determination of oxygenation levels).
- The diagnosis was that the patient died of an air embolus. Where did the air come from?

The solution to this case (as a legal case) lies in determining how the air got into the patient. How can this be used to redesign the process or the mentioned devices to ensure that this does not happen again? The answer lies in application of good safety engineering principles.

The particular hazard being addressed in this discussion is one of several that accompany this type of diagnostic workup, but let us address only this one concern (the air). The hazard to be investigated is a dramatic decrease in the ability of the heart to pump blood due to the inadvertent introduction of air into the patient. How could air get into the patient? A few of the ways include:

- Air entering the patient through the catheter insertion point in the groin
- Air entering the patient via a medication line
- Accidental opening of the blood pressure sensor port, suction of air into the patient
- Flushing of the blood pressure sensor port with air, rather than saline
- Accidental infusion of air from the surgeon's sampling syringe, rather than sampling of blood at this site
- Infusion of air from the saline drip bag.

Five of these were eliminated very quickly based upon the medical records in the case. The patient was supine, thus the risk of #1 was minimal. Even if air had been inserted at this point, the likelihood of damage was minimal. Medication lines were patent, there was no evidence of air in them. Suction of air into the patient due to an opened pressure sensor line was unlikely, the pressures recorded in the patient at all sites were positive with respect to atmospheric, with only a few milliseconds per beat occasionally becoming sub atmospheric (insufficient time to cause air to enter). #4 is not likely, had it occurred only a syringe full of air could have been injected (10 ml or so), it is not likely that the air could have made it to the patient. #5 is unlikely also, again the dose of air would have been 10 ml maximum (this has happened). Implicated – air from the infusion bag, due to the pressurizing jacket – entered the patient. For the particular bags in use, there is about 35 ml of air, an amount adequate to cause death in a young at-risk patient. The pressurization bag ensured that the air was indeed pumped to the patient, a simulation of the situation showed that this could occur in less than 5 seconds at the measured pressures involved. Too quick if one was otherwise involved with measuring data from the patient!

Why is there air in the infusion bag? To ensure that – when drugs are injected into the bag – that mixing can occur by shaking the bag. What would have been a safe design for this situation? Simply elect to NOT use a pressurization jacket.

11.4 Process Improvement

Most hospitals have a safety process in place that looks for methods to improve the processes of health care delivery. This group may operate with the name of quality improvement, quality assurance, patient safety committee, or the like. Some of the processes involved in their work involve the types of analyses just discussed, some of their work involves flowcharting (see Chapter 2), some involves the use of cause-and-effect diagrams. Figure 11.1 illustrates the use of this concept. This particular diagram was generated to look at the process for "bad infusion outcomes" to assist in identifying the potential cause of this outcome.[4] Of interest is the fact that, while the administration was asking for additional in-service training for personnel doing infusions, this particular chart was of value in identifying the real cause of the problem, a change in the supplied concentration of the drug in question. Note the causes: People, Policies, Patients, and Equipment, and how they relate to the outcome.

11.5 Miscellaneous Issues

Major design problems in some devices and drugs have resulted from drug interactions and materials failures. The need for both animal and human testing for drug interactions and possible materials testing for implanted materials serves as a beginning point for discussions of these topics. Much of this testing is mandated by the FDA in terms of required test protocols. Specifically, the drug thalidomide and some of the early experiences with heart valves deserve mention in discussions on historical problems, many of which are covered in the references cited here.[5,6,7] A discussion of patent medicines and quack medical devices, with their inherent risks to human safety are addressed in the following references.[8,9]

11.6 Other Process Issues

Many of the mistakes made in the hospital environment are due to communication issues. Redesign of hospital systems should pay special attention to the interfaces between people, with an emphasis on correct communication. To this end, computerization of drug and medication dosing should be stressed, avoiding all oral transfers of information if at all possible. Double-checking of doses and allergies to medicines can help alleviate many medication errors.

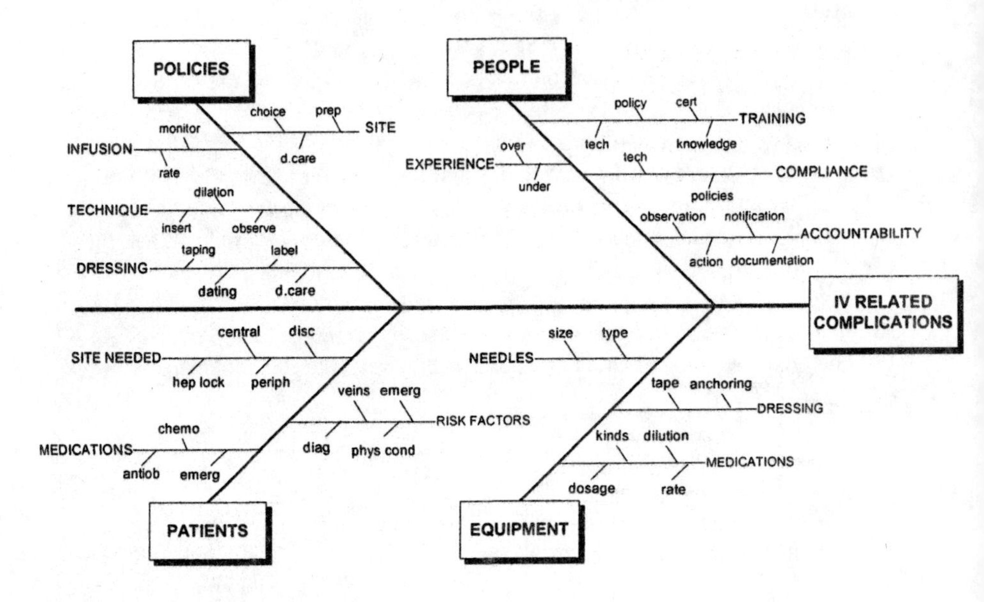

Figure 11.1 Cause-and-effect diagram, IV complications.

A long overdue policy on the part of the FDA is the ending of sound-alike and look-alike medication names by fiat.

11.7 Summary

Designing with safety in mind is mandatory. Appropriate design for safe and effective devices and processes may cost more in the initial design, but should pay continuing benefits in the long run.

Homework Exercises

1. Visit a site such as www.designsafe.com, download the demo version of the software. Perform an analysis of a your design project or one of your instructor's choosing.
2. Visit the FDA MAUDE site, do a search for any device that caused a death in the past two months. Perform a safety analysis on this device.
3. Visit the FDA MAUDE site, do a search for any device that caused an accidental injury in the past few months. Discuss the harm caused and the possible correction of this problem.
4. There are several variations on safety analyses. Define and discuss FMEA and its applications to medicine.
5. Do a search for the term "anticipatory failure determination" and report on the value of this type of software.
6. Develop a cause and effect diagram for the air embolus case discussed in this chapter.
7. Search for information on thalidomide, discuss what went wrong with the use of this drug. Find and discuss at least one other drug example.
8. Some of the early heart valves had mechanical problems. Discuss how this is not a likely event today.
9. Search for information on the failure rate of implant pumps for the alleviation of male erectile dysfunction. What design problems occurred in these devices?
10. Major accidents sometimes cause a rethinking of basic procedures. Investigate the major accident at Bhopal and some of the recommendations that arose from this event.
11. Find and describe the specific wording that requires safety in medical devices, both for the FDA and for CE marking.
12. What is the value of ASA and surgical risk classification schemes?
13. Read and report on one relevant chapter from Geddes (Medical Device Accidents) or Casey (Set Phasers on Stun). (See References 7 and 8).
14. Do a search and report on the term "Inherently Safer Design".
15. Discuss the necessary components of a system to guarantee a proper patient-blood transfusion match.

References

[1] From the ABET website, www.abet.org.
[2] "To Err is Human; Building a Safer Health System," National Academy Press, 2000.
[3] From the program *designsafe,* from Designsafe Engineering.
[4] Provided by Dr. Doris Quinn, Nashville, TN: Vanderbilt Quality Assurance Department.
[5] Witkin, Karen B. 1997, *Clinical Evaluation of Medical Devices: Principles and Case Studies*, Humana Press.
[6] Casey, S., 1993, *Set Phasers on Stun and other True Tales of Design, Technology, and Human Error*, Santa Barbara, CA, Aegean Publishing Company.
[7] Geddes, Leslie, 1998, *Medical Device Accidents With Illustrative Cases*, New York, CRC Press.
[8] http://www.cyberus.ca/~sjordan/pmmain.htm
[9] http://www.mtn.org/quack

Chapter 12

Prototyping and Testing

"Experience is a hard teacher. She gives the test first and the lessons afterward."
Anonymous

Prototyping and testing of hardware and/or software based systems are the logical activities to be performed during the product development cycle once a well-developed idea for a product has been established. Prototyping allows the idea to become a reality that can be seen, touched, and maneuvered to determine if the idea meets the needs of the potential customer. Testing then allows the developer to determine if the design meets the requirements of the product specification and whether it is robust enough to withstand the stresses and ordinary use and misuse by the customer.

12.1 Prototyping

Once the idea for a new design has been established, the next step in the development process is the production of a prototype. Prototypes are developed for the system, including both hardware and software. For hardware, a prototype may be defined:

An easily modified and extensible model of a system, including location of individual hardware components.

The hardware model is usually made from material such as wood, foam, cardboard or other suitable material. The purpose of the hardware prototype is a model of the potential system that can be taken to customer sites for reaction to the design. Customer feedback includes:

- Is the size of the system correct for the application?
- Are the components placed properly for ease of use?
- Is the display (if applicable) placed for ease of use?

Dependent on the project, and the size of the project, the hardware model may be preceded by a series of simulation models, where the initial layout and design of the panels may be done at little cost using one of several available software prototyping tools that have made the market in the past several years. Some of the packages will animate events, other packages can and do emulate two and three-dimensional dynamics. Such software has been used to do initial dashboard layouts, cockpit layouts, and medical instrument panel design.[1]

If software is part of the final product, constructing a prototype of the software is an essential part of the development process. A software prototype may be defined:

An easily modified and extensible model (representation, simulation or demonstration) of a planned software system, likely including its interface and input/output functionality.

Unlike the hardware prototype, which is a non-functioning example of the device, the software prototype is a functioning example of the final product that a potential customer could actually operate and determine if the product satisfies their needs. Thus, the software prototyping acts as a means of risk reduction, as the developer determines early in the process whether the software system will satisfy the customer's needs.

In addition to customer feedback, the software prototype serves to provide information to the software development team, especially in the area of timing constraints. If the prototype is an accurate functional representation of the relevant features of the product, then measurements made on the prototype should give the developers a good idea as to whether the timing constraints can be achieved.

Software tools also exist to allow testing of changes in processes prior to actual implementation of changes. Such tools require that reasonable assumptions be made about the effects of modifications of a process event changed. Such tools have been used for processes involving chemical plants, manufacturing processes, and clinic flows.[2]

12.1.1 Types of prototypes

There are several types of prototypes that may be classified as follows:

- LOW-FIDELITY: a set of drawings (e.g., storyboard) that provide a static, non-computerized, non-working mock-up of user interface for the planned system
- HIGH-FIDELITY: a set of screens that provide a dynamic, computerized, working model of the planned system
- EXPLORATORY: a throw-away prototype used to clarify project goals, to identify requirements, to examine alternative designs, or to investigate a large and complex system
- EXPERIMENTAL: a prototype used to validate system specifications
- OPERATIONAL: an iterative prototype that is progressively refined until it becomes the final system
- HORIZONTAL: a prototype that models many features but with little detail; a horizontal slice of a system's structure chart from the top down to a specific depth most useful in the early stages of design
- VERTICAL: a prototype that models few features but with much detail; a vertical slice of a system's structure chart from top to bottom most useful in the later stages of design
- DIAGONAL: a prototype that is horizontal down to a particular level, then vertical below that point

- GLOBAL: a prototype of the entire system; an expanded horizontal prototype that models a greater number of features and covers multiple levels of the system's structure chart
- LOCAL: a prototype of a single usability-critical system component; a vertical prototype that is focused on one feature.

12.1.2 The prototype process

The prototype process consists of four steps that follow in logical sequence, although the second step is an iterative one and may account for the majority of the prototyping time:

- Build a low-fidelity prototype to clarify initial requirements.
- Iterate (re-specify, re-design, re-evaluate) until the team, both users and developers, agree that the fidelity and completeness of the evolving prototype are sufficiently high.
- Freeze these specifications.
- Finish building the product exactly as documented in the frozen specifications.

12.2 Testing

Testing may be defined as subjecting a device to conditions that indicate its weaknesses, behavior characteristics, and modes of failure. It is a continuous operation throughout the development cycle that provides pertinent information to the development team. Testing may be performed for three basic reasons: basic information, verification, and validation.

Basic information testing may include vendor evaluation, vendor comparison, and component limitability. Verification is the process of evaluating the products of a given phase to ensure correctness and consistency with respect to the products and standards provided as input to that phase.

Validation includes proving the subsystems and system meet the requirements of the Product Specification.

Testing is an essential part of any engineering development program. If the development risks are high, the test program becomes a major component of the overall development effort. To provide the basis for a properly integrated development test program, the design specification should cover all criteria to be tested including function, environment, reliability, and safety. The test program should be drawn up to cover assurance of all these design criteria.

The ultimate goal of testing is assuring that the customer is satisfied. It is the customer who pays the bills, and if we are to be successful in business, we have to solve their problems. We aim for quality, but quality isn't just an abstract ideal. We are developing systems to be used, and used successfully, not to be admired on the shelf. If quality is to be a meaningful and useful goal in the real world, it must include the customer.

12.2.1 Testing defined

Definitions matter, although consensus as to what testing really is is less important than being able to use these definitions to focus our attention on the things that should happen when we are testing. Historically, testing has been defined in several ways:

- establishing confidence that a device does what it is supposed to do
- the process of operating a device with the intent of finding errors
- detecting specification errors and deviations from the specification
- verifying that a system satisfies its specified requirements or identifying differences between expected and actual results
- the process of operating a device or component under specified conditions, observing or recording the results, and making an evaluation of some aspect of the system or component.

All these definitions are useful, but in different ways. Some focus on what is done while testing, others focus on more general objectives like assessing quality and customer satisfaction, while others focus on goals like expected results. If customer satisfaction is a goal, this satisfaction, or what would constitute it, should be expressed in the requirements. Identifying differences between expected and actual results is valuable because it focuses on the fact that when we are testing, we need to be able to anticipate what is supposed to happen. It is then possible to determine what actually does happen and compare the two.

If a test is to find every conceivable fault or weakness in the system or component, then a good test is one that has a good probability of detecting an as yet undiscovered error, and a successful test is one that detects an as yet undiscovered error. The focus on showing the presence of errors is the basic attitude of a good test.

Testing is a positive and creative effort of destruction. It takes imagination, persistence and a strong sense of mission to systematically locate the weaknesses in a complex structure and to demonstrate its failures. This is one reason why it is so hard to test our own work. There is a natural real sense in which we don't want to find errors in our own material.

Errors are in the work product, not in the person who made the mistake. With the "test to destroy" attitude, we are not attacking an individual in an organization or team of developers, but rather are looking for errors in those developers' work products.

Everyone on the development team needs to understand that tests add value to the product by discovering errors and getting them on the table as early as possible - to save the developers from building products based on error-ridden sources, to ensure the marketing people can deliver what the customer wants, and to assure management gets the bottom line on the quality and finance they are looking for.

12.2.2 Parsing test requirements

No matter what type of test is conducted, there are certain requirements that must be proven as a result of the test. Before testing begins, it is helpful to place all requirements into a database where they may be sorted on a variety of attributes, such as responsible subsystem. The purpose of the database is to assure all requirements are addressed in the test protocol as well as providing a convenient tracking system for the requirements. Where the number of requirements is small, manual collation of the requirements is effective. Where the number of requirements is large, the use of a software program to parse requirements is most helpful.

Once the requirements are listed, they can be used to develop the various test protocols necessary for testing. In addition, the list of requirements can be made more useful by turning them into a checklist, as seen in Figure 22-1, by adding space for additional information, such as reference to the location of a particular requirement, location of the test protocol, location of the test results, the initials of the person performing and completing the test, and the date of test completion. This checklist is also invaluable in tracking all requirements to satisfy Quality Assurance and Regulatory departments as well as FDA and ISO auditors.

12.2.3 Test protocol

It has been said that testing without a plan is not testing at all, but an experiment. Therefore, it is essential that each test performed be detailed in a test protocol which includes:

- the name of the device under test
- the type of test being performed
- the purpose of the test
- a definition of potential failures during the test
- any special requirements
- the number of units on test
- the length of the test in hours or cycles
- a detailed procedure for running the test or reference to a procedure in another document, such as a standard
- the parameters to be recorded.

12.2.4 Determining sample size and test length

Once you determine the type of test to be performed, you need to decide on the test sample size and the length of time necessary to accomplish your testing goal. Sample size and test time are dependent upon the MTBF goal, originally defined in the Product Specification and on the confidence level at which the test will be conducted.

The formula for determining the sample size and test time is derived from the following equation:

$$\text{MTBF goal} = (\text{sample size})(\text{test time})\,(2)/X^2_{\alpha;2r+2} \qquad 12.1$$

The equation thus becomes:

$$(\text{sample size})(\text{test time}) = \text{MTBF goal}\,(X^2_{\alpha;2r+2})/2 \qquad 12.2$$

To complete the equation, we must first understand the Chi Square chart, included in Appendix 1. To use this chart, first find the risk factor that the chart is based upon. The risk factor is derived from the confidence level:

$$\text{Confidence level} = 1 - \alpha$$

where α is the risk factor.

Thus, a confidence level of 90% yields a risk factor of 10%, while a confidence level of 95% yields a risk factor of 5%. Using the 90% confidence level, $\alpha = 0.10$ in equation 12.2.

The "r" in equation 12.2 is the number of failures. When calculating sample size and test time, it is assumed there will be no failures. This results in the minimal test time. Thus $v=(2r+2) = 2(0)+2$ or 2 and equation 12.2 becomes

$$(\text{sample size})(\text{test time}) = (\text{MTBF goal})(X^2_{0.10;2})/2$$

Looking at the Chi Square chart in Appendix 1, go across the top row of the chart and find 0.10, or *. Go down that column to the line for $v = 2$. There you will find the number 4.605, or 4.61. Put this into the equation:

$$(\text{sample size})(\text{test time}) = \text{MTBF goal}\,(4.61)/2 \qquad 12.3$$

Inserting the MTBF goal into the equation and solving it yields the unit test time or (sample size)(test time). Recall that design goals typically call for MTBF to be reported in events per million hours of use, this implies a significant time to test if only a few units are to be tested. Field use data may be needed if bench testing cannot be completed in a reasonable length of time.

12.3 Types of Testing

Testing may be of various types, dependent upon the particular result desired. Various test types include:

- **Verification**: procedures that attempt to determine that the product of each phase of the development process is an implementation of a previous phase, i.e., it satisfies it. Each verification activity is a phase of the testing life cycle. The testing objective in each verification activity is to detect as many errors as possible. The testing team should leverage its efforts by participating in any inspections and walkthroughs conducted by development and by initiating verification, especially at the early stages of development.
- **Validation**: validation is the process of evaluating a system or component during or at the end of the development process to determine whether it satisfies specified requirements.
- **Black Box**: the easiest way to understand black box testing is to visualize a black box with a set of inputs coming into it and a set of outputs coming out of it. The black box test is performed without any knowledge of the internal structure. The black box test verifies that the end-user requirements are met from the end-user's point of view. Black box testing is a data driven testing scheme. The tester views the device or program as a black box, i.e., the tester is not concerned about the internal behavior and structure. The tester is only interested in finding circumstances in which the device or program does not behave according to its specification. Black box testing that is used to detect errors leads to exhaustive input testing, as every possible input condition is a test case.
- **White box**: white box testing is the opposite of black box testing. It is performed by personnel who are

knowledgeable of the internal structure and are testing from the developer's point of view. White box testing is a logic driven testing scheme. The tester examines the internal structure of the device or program and derives test data from an examination of the internal structure. White box testing is concerned with the degree to which test cases exercise or cover the structure of the device or program. The ultimate white box test is an exhaustive path test.

- **Hardware Testing**: hardware testing includes various types of tests depending on the intended use of the device. Testing which occurs during almost every product development cycle includes:

    - vendor evaluation
    - component variation
    - environmental testing
    - safety evaluation
    - shipping tests
    - standards evaluation
    - product use/misuse
    - reliability demonstration.

  Often, hardware testing, especially that associated with the calculation of reliability parameters is performed twice during the development process. The first occurs immediately after the design phase and evaluates the robustness and reliability of the design. The second occurs after production of customer units begins. This testing evaluates the robustness and reliability of the manufacturing process.

- **Software Testing**: software testing consists of several levels of evaluation. Initially, module testing occurs, where the individual modules of the software program are evaluated and stress tested. This testing consists of verifying the design and implementation of the specification at the smallest component of the program. Testing involves running each module independently to assure it works, and then inserting errors, possibly through the use of an emulator. The test is basically an interface between the programmer and the software environment. Integration testing occurs after each of the modules have been successfully tested. The various modules are then integrated with each other and tested to assure they work together. System testing consists of merging the software with the hardware to assure both will work as a system. Testing involves verifying the external software interfaces, assuring the system requirements are met, and assuring the system, as a whole, is operational. Acceptance testing is the final review of all the requirements specified for the system and assuring both hardware and software address them.

- **Functional Testing**: Functional testing (Table 12-1) is designed to verify that all the functional requirements have been satisfied. This type of testing verifies that given all the expected inputs then all of the expected outputs are produced. This type of testing is termed success oriented testing because the tests are expected to produce successful results.

  Testing of the functional capabilities involves the exercising of the operational modes and the events that allow a transition between the various software operational states. These tests are performed to verify that proper mode transitions are executed and proper outputs are generated given the correct inputs. These tests also verify that the software generates the expected output given the expected user input. A communication test tool should be utilized to test the proper operation of the remote communications protocol and functionality of the communications software located in the product under test.

  Timing tests should be performed for system critical functions relating to the system critical time and the operational window. Battery tests should be performed whenever a software change to the software that monitors the battery levels has been made. In addition, if new functionality is pushing the product to the absolute performance edge, then battery tests should also be

Test Type	Example
Functional Modes	Transitions between operational modes Correct inputs generate correct outputs Inputs and outputs include switches, tones, messages and alarms
Remote Communications	Connect and disconnect tests Valid commands and inquiries tests Handling of invalid commands and inquiries Tests for all baud rates supported Corrupted frames tests Error handling in general and the interface to the error handler Control Mode testing with emphasis on safety Monitor Mode testing with emphasis on fidelity of values reported
Timing	Active failure tests are completed within the system critical time Passive failure tests are completed within the operational window
Battery	Ramp up and ramp down of voltages Test the various levels of warnings, alarms, and errors

Table 12.1 Examples of Functional Testing

performed because of its potential effect on any power down software routines.

- **Robustness Testing**: robustness testing (Table 12-2) is designed to determine how the software performs given unexpected inputs. Robustness testing determines whether the software recovers from an unexpected input, locks the system in an indeterminate state or continues to operate in a manner which is unpredictable. This type of testing is termed failure oriented because the test inputs are designed to cause the product to fail given foreseeable and reasonably unforeseeable misuse of the product.

Robustness testing is performed in order to determine software responses at the boundary limits of the product or test and manufacturing equipment and the test cases should include negative values.
As a part of robustness testing, algorithms are tested for overflow and underflow. the user interface is tested by entering unexpected values and sequences. Routines, tasks, or processes that are time constrained are altered to introduce reasonable delays in order to determine the reaction of the product or equipment. Communication software is given unexpected commands and data that is then transmitted to the remote communications handler. Robustness testing should include rapid data input rates, such as might occur when a book is placed on an input keyboard.

- **Stress Testing**: stress testing (Table 12-3) is designed to ascertain how the product reacts to a condition in which the amount or rate of data exceeds the amount or rate expected. Stress tests can help determine the margin of safety that exists in the product or equipment.
Stress tests are performed which exercise the equipment continuously over varying periods of time and operating parameters if latent errors exist in the software. Generally, these tests consist of overnight runs and weekend runs that gain the optimum benefit of the allotted test time. Global buffers and data structures are tested under loaded and overflow conditions in order to determine the response of the software. Remote communications load tests should be performed which verify the remote communications interface transfer rate at the maximum transfer rate under worst case and maximum load conditions. Worst case scenario tests verify the product or equipment operating capability under the projected worst case scenario. The worst case scenario for products generally includes highest execution rate and event overload for event driven systems. These tests should be limited to reasonable environmental tests which do not include temperature and vibration testing.

Test Type	Example
Boundary	Over and under specified limits Numerical values which determine logic flow based on a maximum or minimum value Negative numerical values
Overflow and Underflow	Values too large for all algorithms Values too small for all algorithms
User Interface	Enter unexpected values Enter unexpected sequences
Execution Time Line Processing	Routines which have execution time limits are altered to introduce delays Tasks which have execution time limits are altered to introduce delays Routines with execution constraints due to parametric calculations are altered
Data Transmission	Unexpected commands are transmitted to the remote communications handler Unexpected data are transmitted to the remote communications handler

Table 12-2 Examples of Robustness Testing

- **Safety testing**: Safety testing (Table 12-4) is designed to verify that the product performs in a safe manner and that a complete assessment of the safety design has been accomplished. Fail-safe tests should be performed specifically to verify the fail-safe provisions of the software design. These tests cover the error conditions only and do not address warnings or alarms which are more appropriately tested under the functional tests. Limited, non-destructive fault insertion tests should be

Test Type	Example
Duration	Over night runs Weekend runs Others types of software burn-in tests
Buffer Overload	Global buffers tested under loaded and overlfow conditions Global data structures tested under loaded and overflow conditions
Remote Communications	Verify the transfer at the maximum transfer rate Verify the transfer at the maximum transfer rate under maximum load conditions
Worst Case Scenario	Verify the product and test and manufacturing equipments operating capability under projected worst case Highest execution rate Event overload for event driven system

Table 12-3 Example of Stress Testing

performed by the software verification and validation engineers. Products require an analysis of the error handling routines as well as data corruption tests to ensure an acceptable level of safety. The analysis must include a review of the products active failure tests so that they are completed within the system critical time and within the product defined operational window. A number of safety aspects that must also be addressed are the protection of critical parameters and events that lead to a loss of safety critical indicators. Safety testing of the product must utilize the hazards analysis in relation to failures. In addition, validation safety tests and internal product safety self tests that were performed on past products should be compiled, executed, and compared against the new product under test in order to arrive at a consistent and growing list of mandatory safety tests.

- **Regression Testing**: regression testing (Table 12-4) is performed whenever a software change or a hardware change that affects the software has occurred. Regression testing verifies that the change produces the desired effect on the altered component and that no other component that relies on the altered component is adversely affected. Regression testing is performed on products and test and manufacturing equipment that have made a change to an established, validated baseline. Regression testing begins by comparing the new software to the existing baseline with a version difference tool and the generation of a cross reference listing to assess the changes and to ensure that no unintended side effects are introduced. From this, an assessment of the amount of changes and their criticality is made, the level of effort that is required to perform the regression is estimated and the risk is assessed. The alterations are tested and a compiled list of core tests are executed in order to establish that no new unintended changes have been introduced. Special attention must be made to the safety implications.

Homework Exercises

1. Perform a web search with the search term being "prototyping tool". Briefly list the variety of tools found. Download and run one of the demos that can be found (such as at http://www.altia.com/demos/demos.html). Comment on the results.
2. Perform a web search using the term "process simulation". Briefly list the variety of tools found. Download and run a demo if found, comment on your results.
3. A variety of companies advertise that they will build prototypes for a fee. Find a series of companies that will do this.
4. Stereolithography is used for prototyping. Find a company that performs this activity. Find the cost of a stereolithography machine, suggest a use for it in a design course.

Test Type	Example
Fail-Safe	Verify that fail safe provisions of the software design Test error conditions and handling Test data corruption
Active Failure	Tests completion within system critical time ROM testing via CRC computation and comparison to a stored value RAM testing for stuck bits in data and address paths RAM testing for address decoding problems LED indicators voltage tests Processor and controller tests
Passive Failure	Watchdog timer test Watchdog disable tests Hardware RAM tests CRC generator Battery Test Audio generators and speaker tests EEPROM tests
Safety	Critical parameters and their duplicates Events that lead to a loss of audio indicators Events that lead to a loss of visual indicators Events that lead to tactile errors, such as a key press Error handling for corrupted vectors and structures Error handling for corrupted sanity checks Sufficiency of periodic versus aperiodic tests
From Hazard Analysis	Single point failures Normal power up, run-time and power down safety tests

Table 12-4 Examples of Safety Testing

Sequence Step	Activity
1	Compare the new software to the existing baseline
2	Generate a cross reference listing to assess changes and to ensure no unintended side effects
3	Assess the amount of changes and the criticality
4	Determine the level of effort required and assess the risk
5	Test the new functions and the debug fixes
6	Execute a predetermined set of core tests to confirm no new unintended changes
7	Devote special attention to the safety implications

Table 12-5 Regression Testing Sequence

5. Calculate the test time for a device that has an estimated MTBF of 10 per million hours if you have only ten units to test. List your assumptions and comment on your results.

References

[1] Easily found with web searches using the term "prototyping tool", packages such as Altia Simulation Graphics, Interface Consultant, and Working Model3-D may be located, among others.
[2] Web search using the term "process simulation", many tools such as Design II for Windows and Stella can be found.

Fries, Richard C., *Reliability Assurance for Medical Devices, Equipment and Software*. Buffalo Grove, IL: Interpharm Press, 1991.

Fries, Richard C., *Reliable Design of Medical Devices.* New York: Marcel Dekker, Inc., 1997.

Kit, Edward, *Software Testing in the Real World - Improving the Process.* Reading, MA: Addison-Wesley Publishing Company, 1995.

Laplante, Phillip, *Real-Time Systems Design and Analysis - An Engineer's Handbook.* New York: The Institute of Electrical and Electronic Engineers, Inc., 1993.

Myers, Glenford J., *The Art of Software Testing.* New York: John Wiley & Sons, 1979.

Neufelder, Ann Marie, *Ensuring Software Reliability.* New York: Marcel Dekker, Inc., 1993.

Schach, Stephen R., *Classical and Object-Oriented Software Engineering.* New York: WCB/McGraw-Hill, 1999.

Chapter 13

Quality Control and Improvement, Reliability, and Liability

"Why is there never enough time to develop a product correctly, but always enough time to do it over?"
Anonymous

The term reliability is a term that has been used extensively, but is often misunderstood. Reliability has been described by some as a group of statisticians spewing endless streams of data. Others have described it as testing a device "ad nauseam". Reliability is neither of these.

Reliability is a characteristic that describes how good a device or process really is. Physicians and medical processes will be dealt with briefly in section 13.9.8, the major thrust of this chapter will apply to devices – electronic, mechanical, software based, and systems. In that context, reliability is a measure of the dependability of the device. It is a characteristic that must be planned for, designed and manufactured into a device. The inclusion of reliability in manufacturing is important, because no matter how reliably a device is designed, it will not be a success unless it is manufactured and serviced reliably. Thus, reliability is the state of mind which all personnel associated with a product must be in. It is a philosophy that dictates how good a device will be.

13.1 Reliability versus Unreliability

If reliability is a measure of how good a device is, unreliability is a measure of the potential for the failure of a device. It is the result of the lack of planning for design and manufacturing activities. It is a philosophy that states the manufacturer does not care how good their device will be. The consequences of such a philosophy include:

- high cost
- wasted time
- customer inconvenience
- poor customer reputation.

Because reliability is preferable to unreliability, processes should be instituted to avoid the causes of unreliability, including:

- improper design
- improper materials
- manufacturing errors
- assembly and inspection errors
- improper testing
- improper packaging and shipping
- user abuse
- misapplication.

To illustrate the above, consider that the company Home Depot (9/99) recalled more that 10,000 stepladders (they were the distributor, not the manufacturer). The steps on the ladders were too short and some were improperly attached, failure of the ladder was possible. Consider the loss to the manufacturer, and to Home Depot for this defect.

13.2 Quality versus Reliability

The terms "quality" and "reliability" are sometimes used interchangeably, although they are quite different. The difference grew out of the need for a time-based concept of quality. This distinction of time marks the difference between the traditional quality control concept and the modern approach to reliability.

The traditional concept of quality does not include the notion of a time base. The term *quality* is defined in ISO 8402 as:

> *the totality of features or characteristics of a product or service that bear on its ability to satisfy stated or implied needs.*

The definition refers to this totality at a particular instant of time. Thus, we may speak of the quality of a component at incoming, the quality of a subassembly in manufacturing test, or the quality of a device at set-up.

In terms of this definition, a medical device is assessed against a specification or set of attributes. Having passed the assessment, the device is delivered to a customer, accompanied by a warranty, so that the customer is relieved of the cost implications of early failures. The customer, upon accepting the device, realizes that it might fail at some future time, hopefully far into the future. This approach provides no measure of the quality of the device outside the warranty period. It assumes this is the customer's responsibility and not the company's.

Reliability, on the other hand, is quality over a specific time period, such as the five year expected life of a device or an eight-hour operation. It has been described as the science of estimating, controlling and managing the probability of failure over time. (As such, this also implies that warranty costs must be factored into sales costs.)

If the medical device is assessed against a specification or set of attributes, but was additionally designed for a Mean Time Between Failures of 5 years prior to being sent to the customer, reliability is being designed into the product (A Mean Time Between Failure of 5 years means 63% of the units in the field would have failed once within the five year period). A company must realize that, if they want to be successful and build a satisfied customer base, the responsibility for the quality of the device outside the warranty period belongs to them.

13.3 The Definition of Reliability

This idea of quality over a period of time is reflected in the more formal definition of reliability:

the probability, at a desired confidence level, that a device will perform a required function, without failure, under stated conditions, for a specified period of time.

This definition contains four key requirements:

- To perform a required function, the function must have been established through such activities as customer and/or market surveys. Thus, reliability requires the device to be fully specified prior to design.
- To perform without failure, the normal operation of the device must be defined, in order to establish what a failure is. This activity also includes anticipating the misuse to which the device could be subjected and designing around it.
- To perform under stated conditions, the environment in which the device will operate must be specified. This includes typical temperature and humidity ranges, methods of shipping, shock and vibration experienced in normal usage and interference from associated equipment or to other equipment.
- To operate for a specified period of time, the life expectancy of the device must be defined as well as the typical daily usage.

In summary, reliability assumes that preliminary thought processes have been completed and that the device and its environment have been thoroughly defined. These conditions make the task of the designer easier and less costly in time and effort. It assumes that failure-free or failure- tolerant design principles are used. It assumes manufacturing processes are designed so that they will not reduce the reliability of the device.

Reliability, like any science, depends upon other technical areas as a base for its functionality. These include:

- Basic mathematics and statistics
- Current regulatory standards
- Design principles
- Software Quality Assurance
- System interface principles

- Human factors
- Cost/benefit analysis
- Common sense.

13.4 History of Reliability

Reliability originated during World War II, when the Germans first introduced the concept to improve the operation of their V-1 and V-2 rockets. Prior to this time, most equipment was mechanical in nature and failures could usually be isolated to a simple part. Products were expected to be reliable and safety margins in stress-strength, wear or fatigue conditions were employed to assure it. Then, as electronics began to grow, so did reliability.

From 1945 to 1950, various military studies were conducted in the United States on equipment repair, maintenance costs and failure of electronic equipment. As a result of these studies, the Department of Defense established an ad hoc committee on reliability in 1950. This committee became a permanent group in 1952, known as the Advisory Group on the Reliability of Electronic Equipment (AGREE). In 1957, this group published a report that led directly to a specification on the reliability of military electronic equipment.

In the early 1960s, the field of reliability experienced growth and widespread application in the aerospace industry, especially following the failure of Vanguard TV3 and several satellites. During this time engineers also began to realize that to really improve reliability, one must eliminate the source of failures. This led to the first Physics of Failure Symposium in 1962. This was followed by a period of growth in other highly technical areas, such as computers.

Today many industries and government agencies employ specialists in the area of reliability. Reliability is moving in the direction of more realistic recognition of causes and effects of failures, from the system to the component level. These companies have come to realize that poor reliability is costly, leads to poor customer reputation and the subsequent loss of market share. Industries that are regulated must also comply with reliability requirements established by the regulating agencies.

13.5 Types of Reliability

Reliability is composed of three primary subdivisions, each with their own particular attributes:

- Electronic reliability
- Mechanical reliability
- Software reliability.

13.5.1 Electronic reliability

Electronic reliability (Figure 13-1) is a function of the age of a component or assembly. The failure rate is defined in terms of the number of malfunctions occurring during a period of time. As is evident from the figure, the graph is divided into three distinct time periods:

- Infant mortality
- Useful life
- Wearout.

13.5.1.1 Infant mortality

Infant mortality is the beginning of the life of an electronic component or assembly. This period is characterized by an initial high failure rate, which decreases rapidly and then stabilizes. These failures are caused by gross, built-in flaws due to faulty workmanship, bad processes, manufacturing deviations from the design intent or transportation damage.
Examples of early failures include:

- Poor welds or seals
- Poor solder joints
- Contamination on surfaces or in materials
- Voids, cracks, or thin spots on insulation or protective coatings.

Many of these failures can be prevented by improving the control over the manufacturing process, by screening components or by burn-in procedures. improvements in design or materials are necessary for these manufacturing deviations.

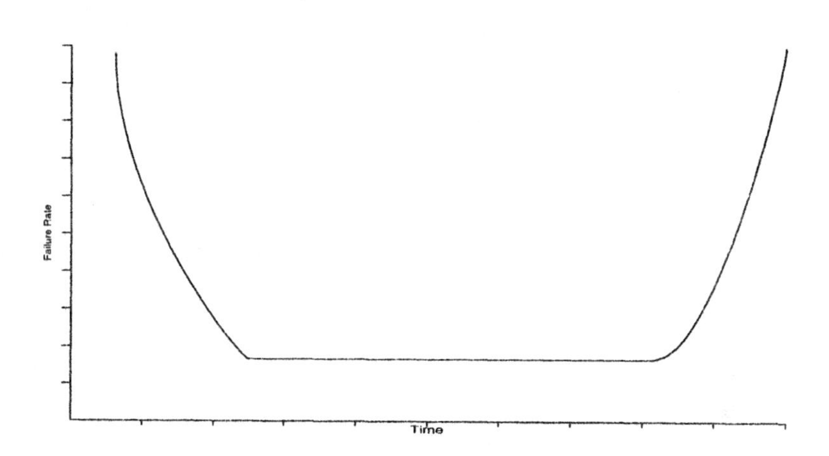

Figure 13-1 Electronic reliability curve. (From Fries, 1997.)

13.5.1.2 Useful life

The useful life period of a component or assembly is the largest segment of the life cycle and is characterized by a constant failure rate. During this period, the failure rate reaches its lowest level and remains relatively constant. Failures occurring during this period are either stress related or occur by chance. These are the most difficult to repeat or analyze.

13.5.1.3 Wearout

The final period in the life cycle occurs when the failure rate begins to increase rapidly. Wearout failures are due primarily to deterioration of the design strength of the components or assemblies, as a consequence of operation and/or exposure to environmental fluctuations. Such deterioration may result from:

- Corrosion or oxidation
- Insulation breakdown or leakage
- Ionic migration of metals on surfaces or in vacuum

- Frictional wear or fatigue
- Shrinkage and cracking in plastics.

Replacing components prior to reaching the wearout period through a preventive maintenance program can prevent wearout failures.

13.5.2 Mechanical reliability

Mechanical reliability (Figure 13-2) differs considerably from electronic reliability in its reaction to the aging of a component or assembly. Mechanical components or assemblies begin their life cycle at a failure rate of zero and experience a rapidly increasing failure rate. This curve approximates the wearout portion of the electronics life curve.

Mechanical failures are due primarily to deterioration of the design strength of the component or assembly. Such deterioration may result from:

- Frictional wear
- Shrinkage and/or cracking in plastics
- Fatigue
- Surface erosion
- Corrosion
- Creep
- Material strength deterioration.

Optimization of mechanical reliability occurs with timely elimination of components or assemblies through preventive maintenance, before the failure rate reaches unacceptably high levels.

13.5.3 Software reliability

The *IEEE Standard Glossary of Software Engineering Terminology* gives the following definition of reliability:

The ability of a system or component to perform its required functions, under stated conditions for a specified period of time.

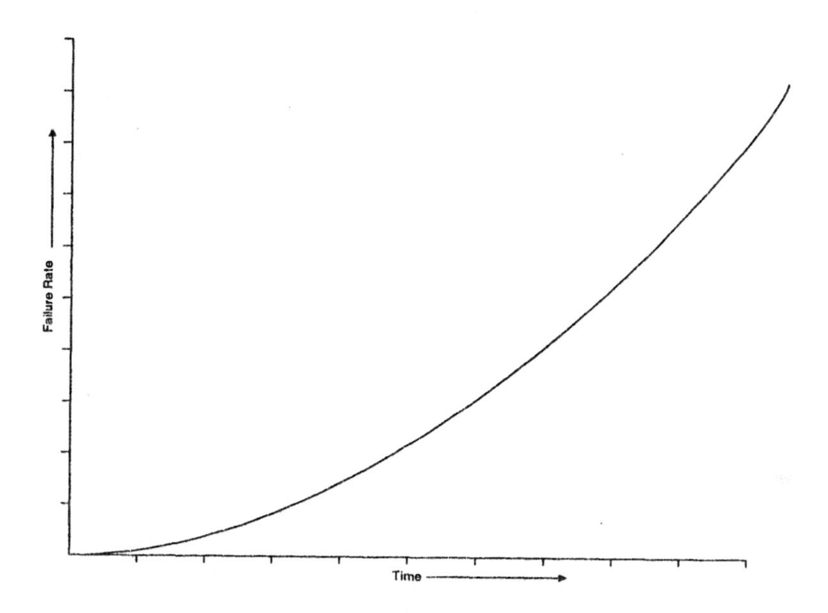

Figure 13-2 Mechanical reliability curve. (From Fries, 1997.)

In the case of medical device software, that definition should be expanded to include the concepts of safety and efficacy as follows:

The ability of a system or component to perform its required functions in a safe and effective manner, under stated conditions, for a specified period of time.

The main point of this definition is that reliability, safety, and efficacy are inseparable requirements for medical device software.

In order to apply this definition, the software developer must know exactly what the "required functions" of the particular medical device are. Sometimes such functional definitions are obvious, but in general they are not. Such knowledge requires the existence of a formal software specification.

In addition, the software developer must know the "stated conditions." This means the environment in which the software is to operate must be fully defined. This may include whether the software will be operated during a stressful situation, the lighting and noise levels in the area of operation, and the technical knowledge of the user.

"For a specified period of time" indicates the reliability is being measured for a specific period of time, known as a mission time. This may be the length of a surgical case, the warranty period for the device, or the total operational life of the device.

Software reliability differs considerably from both electronic and mechanical reliability in that software is not subject to the physical constraints of electronic and mechanical components. Software reliability consists of the process of preventing failures through structured design and detecting and removing errors in the coding. Once all "bugs" are removed, the program will operate without failure forever (Figure 13-3). However, practically, the software reliability curve may be as shown in Figure 13-4, with early failures as the software is first used and a long period of constant failures, as bugs are fixed.

Software failures are due primarily to:

- Specification errors
- Design errors
- Typographical errors
- Omission of symbols.

13.6 Device Reliability

The life cycle of any medical device may be represented by a graph known as the Reliability Bathtub Curve (Figure 13-5). It is a graph of failure rate versus the age of the device.

The graph is identical to that for electronics described above. As with the electronics life curve, there are three distinct time periods:

- Infant mortality
- Useful life
- Wearout.

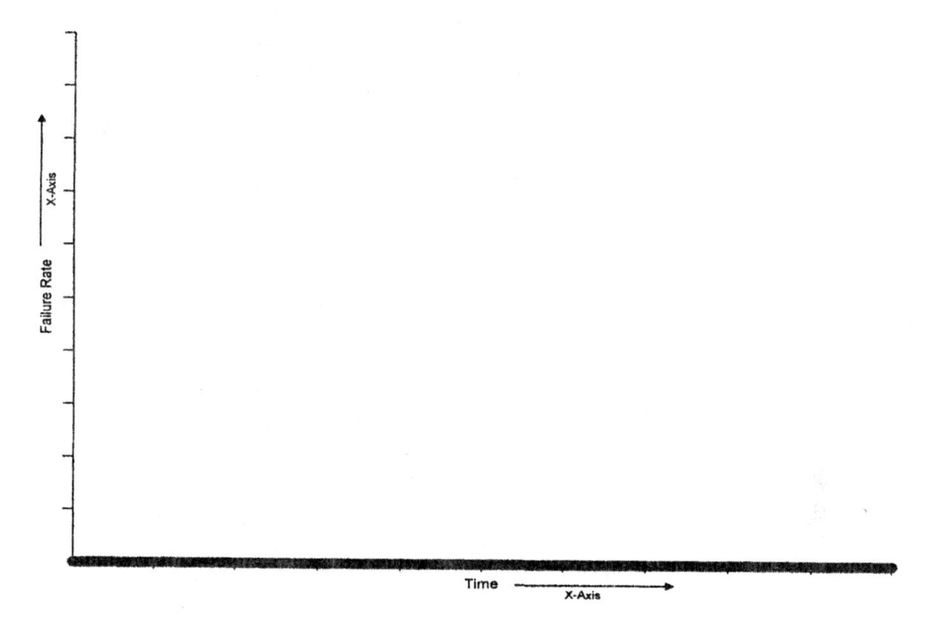

Figure 13-3 Ideal software reliability curve. (From Fries, 1997.)

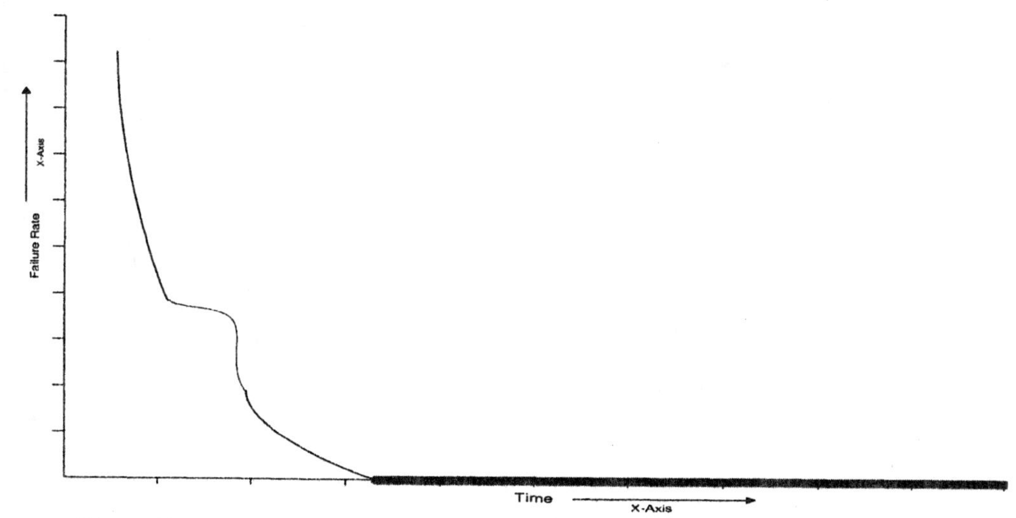

Figure 13-4 Practical software reliability curve. (From Fries, 1997.)

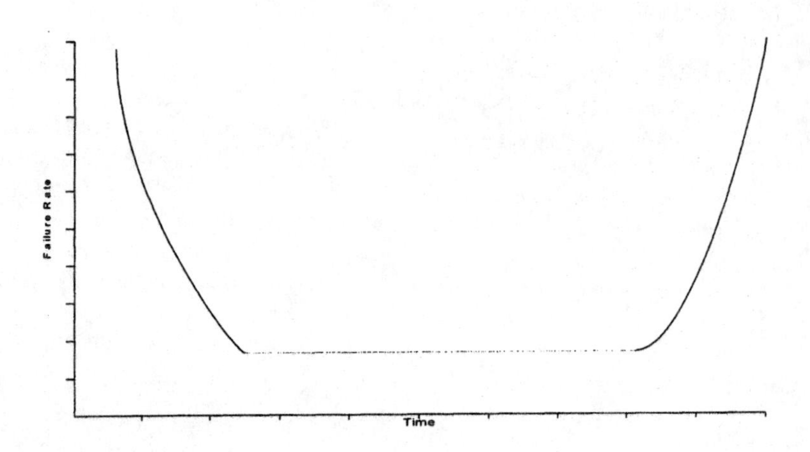

Figure 13-5 Reliability bathtub curve. (From Fries, 1997.)

The discussion of the three life periods contained in the section on electronic reliability applies to device reliability as well.

13.7 Optimizing Reliability

Reliability optimization involves consideration of each of the life cycle periods. Major factors that influence and degrade a system's operational reliability must be addressed during design in order to control and maximize system reliability. Thus, early failures may be eliminated by a systematic process of controlled screening and burn-in of components, assemblies and the device. Stress related failures are minimized by providing adequate design margins for each component and the device. Wearout failures may be eliminated by conducting timely preventive maintenance on the device, with appropriate replacement of effected components.

13.8 Reliability's Effect on Medical Devices

Subjecting a medical device to a reliability program provides a structured approach to the product development process. It provides techniques that improve the quality of the device over a period of time as well as reduce development and redevelopment time and cost. It yields statistical data that quantifies the success, or lack of success, of the development process and predicts future performance. It also assures regulatory requirements are satisfied and gives confidence that regulatory inspections will produce no major discrepancies.

The use of the various reliability techniques results in decreased warranty costs and the resultant increase in customer acceptance. This naturally leads to an enhanced customer perception of the manufacturer and the resultant increase in market share. Reliability techniques also reduce the risk of liability by assuring safety has been the primary concern during the design and development process. By reducing up-front costs, limiting liability risks and increasing future profits, reliability is essential to the success of any company.

Most importantly, the inclusion of reliability gives development personnel a feeling of confidence that they have optimized the design to produce a device that is safe and effective for its intended use and will remain that way for a long period of time. This confidence will foster success in future products.

13.9 Product Liability

Law can be defined as the collection of rules and regulations by which society is governed. The law regulates social conduct in a formal binding way while it reflects society's needs, attitudes, and principles. Law is a dynamic concept that lives, grows, and changes. It can be described as a composite of court decisions, regulations, and sanctioned procedures, by which laws are applied and disputes adjudicated.

The three most common theories of liability for which a manufacturer may be held liable for personal injury caused by its product are negligence, strict liability, and breach of warranty. These are referred to as common-law causes of action, which are distinct from causes of action based on federal or state statutory law. Although within the last decade federal legislative action that would create a uniform federal product liability law has been proposed and debated, no such law exists today. Thus, such litigation is governed by the laws of each state.

These three doctrines are called "theories of recovery" because an injured person cannot recover damages against a defendant unless he alleges and proves, through use of one or more of these theories, that the defendant owed him a legal duty and that the defendant breached that duty, thereby causing the plaintiff's injuries. Although each is conceptually distinct, similarities exist between them. Indeed, two or more theories are asserted in many product defect suits.

13.9.1 Negligence

Since much of medical malpractice litigation relies on negligence theory, it is important to clearly establish the elements of that cause of action. Negligence may be defined as conduct which falls below the standard established by law for the protection of others against unreasonable risk of harm. There are four major elements of the negligence action:

- that a person or business owes a duty of care to another
- that the applicable standard for carrying out the duty be breached
- that as proximate cause of the breach of duty a compensable injury results
- that there be compensable damages or injury to the plaintiff.

The burden is on the plaintiff to establish each and every element of the negligence action.

The basic idea of negligence law is that one should have to pay for injuries that he or she causes when acting below the standard of care of a reasonable, prudent person participating in the activity in question. This standard of conduct relates to a belief that centers on potential victims: that people have a right to be protected from unreasonable risks of harm. A fundamental aspect of the negligence standard of care resides in the concept of foreseeability.

A plaintiff in a product liability action grounded in negligence, then, must establish a breach of the manufacturer's or seller's duty to exercise reasonable care in the manufacture and preparation of a product. The manufacturer in particular must be certain that the product is free of any potentially dangerous defect that might become dangerous upon the happening of a reasonably anticipated emergency. The obligation to exercise reasonable care has been expanded to include reasonable care in the inspection or testing of the product, the design of the product, or the giving of warnings concerning the use of the product.

A manufacturer must exercise reasonable care even though he is but a link in the production chain that results in a finished product. For example, a manufacturer of a product which is designed to be a component part of another manufactured product is bound by the standard of reasonable care. Similarly, a manufacturer of a finished product which incorporates component parts fabricated elsewhere has the same legal obligation.

A seller of a product, on the other hand, is normally held to a less stringent standard of care than a manufacturer. The lesser standard is also applied to distributors, wholesalers, or other middlemen in the marketing chain. This rule pertains because a seller or middleman is viewed as simply a channel through which the product reaches the consumer.

In general, the duty owed at any particular time varies with the degree of risk involved in a product. The concept of reasonable care is not static, but changes with the circumstances of the individual case. The care must be commensurate with the risk of harm involved. Thus, manufacturers or sellers of certain hazardous products must exercise a greater degree of care in their operations than manufacturers or sellers of other less dangerous products.

13.9.2 Strict liability

Unlike the negligence suit, in which the focus is on the defendant's conduct, in a strict liability suit, the focus is on the product itself. The formulation of strict liability states that one who sells any product in a defective condition unreasonably dangerous to the user or consumer or to his property is subject to liability for physical harm thereby caused to the ultimate user or consumer or to his property if the seller is engaged in the business of selling such a product, and it is expected to and does reach the user or consumer without substantial change to the condition in which it is sold. Therefore, the critical focus in a strict liability case is on whether the product is defective and unreasonably dangerous. A common standard applied in medical device cases to reach that determination is the risk/benefit analysis - that is, whether the benefits of the device outweigh the risks attendant with its use.

The result of strict liability is that manufacturers, distributors, and retailers are liable for the injuries caused by defects in their products, even though the defect may not be shown to be the result of any negligence in the design or manufacture of the product. Moreover, under strict liability, the manufacturer cannot assert any of the various defenses available to him in a warranty action.

Strict liability means that a manufacturer may be held liable even though he has exercised all possible care in the preparation and sale of this product. The sole necessity for manufacturer liability is the existence of a defect in the product and a causal connection between this defect and the injury which resulted from the use of the product.

13.9.3 Breach of warranty

A warranty action is contractual rather than tortious in nature. Its basis lies in the representations, either express or implied, which a manufacturer or a seller makes about its product.

A third cause of action that may be asserted by a plaintiff is breach of warranty. There are three types of breaches of warranty that may be alleged:

- breach of the implied warranty of merchantability ("King's Pacemakers", for example)
- breach of the implied warranty of fitness for a particular purpose (use of the term pacemaker, for example)
- breach of an express warranty ("cures 100%," for example).

13.9.3.1 Implied warranties

Some warranties accompany the sale of an article without any express conduct on the part of the seller. These implied warranties are labeled the warranties of merchantability and of fitness for a particular purpose.

A warranty that goods shall be merchantable is implied in a contract for their sale, if the seller is a merchant who commonly deals with such goods. At a minimum, merchantable goods must:

- pass without objection in the trade under the contract description
- be fit for the ordinary purposes for which they are used
- be within the variations permitted by the sales agreement, of even kind, quality, and quantity within each unit and among all units involved
- be adequately contained, packaged, and labeled as the sales agreement may require
- conform to the promises or affirmations of fact made on the container or label.

The implied warranty of fitness for a particular purpose arises when a buyer makes known to the seller the particular purpose for which the goods are to be used, and the buyer, relying on the seller's skill or judgement, receives goods which are warranted to be sufficient for that purpose.

13.9.3.2 Exclusion of warranties

The law has always recognized that sellers may explicitly limit their liability upon a contract of sale by including disclaimers of any warranties under the contract. The Uniform Commercial Code embodies this principle and provides that any disclaimer, exclusion, or modification is permissible under certain guidelines. However, a disclaimer is not valid if it deceives the buyer.

These warranty causes of action do not offer any advantages for the injured plaintiff that cannot be obtained by resort to negligence and strict liability claims and, in fact, pose greater hurdles to recovery. Thus, although a breach of warranty claim is often pled in the plaintiff's complaint, it is seldom relied on at trial as the basis for recovery.

13.9.4 Defects

The term "defect" is used to describe generically the kinds and definitions of things that courts find to be actionably wrong with products when they leave the seller's hands. In the decisions, however, the courts sometimes distinguish between defectiveness and unreasonable danger. Other considerations in determining defectiveness are:

- consumer expectations
- presumed seller knowledge
- risk-benefit balancing
- state of the art
- unavoidably unsafe products.

A common and perhaps the prevailing definition of product unsatisfactoriness is that of "unreasonable danger." This has been defined as the article sold must be dangerous to an extent beyond that which would be contemplated by the ordinary consumer who purchases it, with the ordinary knowledge common to the community as to its characteristics.

Another test of defectiveness sometimes used is that of presumed seller knowledge: would the seller be negligent in placing a product on the market if he had knowledge of its harmful or dangerous condition? This definition contains a standard of strict liability, as well as one of defectiveness, since it assumes the seller's knowledge of a product's condition even though there may be no such knowledge or reason to know.

Sometimes a risk-benefit analysis is used to determine defectiveness, particularly in design cases. The issue is phrased in terms of whether the cost of making a safer product is greater or less than the risk or danger from the product in its present condition. If the cost of making the change is greater than the risk created by not making the change, then the benefit or utility of keeping the product as is outweighs the risk and the product is not defective. If on the other hand, the cost is less than the risk then the benefit or utility of not making the change is outweighed by the risk and the product in its unchanged condition is defective.

Risk-benefit or risk-burden balancing involves questions concerning state of the art, since the burden of eliminating a danger may be greater than the risk of that danger if the danger cannot be eliminated. State of the art is similar to the unavoidably unsafe defense where absence of the knowledge or ability to eliminate a danger is assumed for purposes of determining if a product is unavoidably unsafe. "State of the art" is defined as the state of scientific and technological knowledge available to the manufacturer at the time the product was placed in the market.

Determining defectiveness is one of the more difficult problems in products liability, particularly in design litigation. There are three types of product defects:

- manufacturing or production defects
- design defects
- defective warnings or instructions.

The issue implicates questions of the proper scope of the strict liability doctrine, and the overlapping definitions of physical and conceptual views of defectiveness.

Manufacturing defects can rarely be established on the basis of direct evidence. Rather, a plaintiff who alleges the existence of a manufacturing defect in the product must usually resort to the use of circumstantial evidence in order to prove that the product was defective. Such evidence may take the form of occurrence of other similar injuries resulting from use of the product, complaints received about the performance of the product, defectiveness of other units of the product, faulty methods of production, testing or analysis of the product, elimination of other causes of the accident, and comparison with similar products.

A manufacturer has a duty to design his product so as to prevent any foreseeable risk of harm to the user or patient. A product which is defectively designed can be distinguished from a product containing a manufacturing defect. While the latter involves some aberration or negligence in the manufacturing process, the former encompasses improper planning in connection with the preparation of the product. Failure to exercise reasonable care in the design of a product is negligence. A product which is designed in a way which makes it unreasonably dangerous will subject the manufacturer to strict liability. A design defect, in contrast to a manufacturing defect, is the result of the manufacturer's conscious decision to design the product in a certain manner.

Product liability cases alleging unsafe design may be divided into three basic categories:

- cases involving concealed dangers
- cases involving a failure to provide appropriate safety features
- cases involving construction materials of inadequate strength.

A product has a concealed danger when its design fails to disclose a danger inherent in the product which is not obvious to the ordinary user.

Some writers treat warning defects as a type of design defect. One reason for doing this is that a warning inadequacy, like a design inadequacy, is usually a characteristic of a whole line of products, while a production or manufacturing flaw is usually random and atypical of the product.

13.9.5 Failure to warn of dangers

An increasingly large portion of product liability litigation concerns the manufacturer's or seller's duty to warn of actual or potential dangers involved in the use of the product. Although the duty to warn may arise under all three theories of product liability, as mentioned above, most warnings cases rely on negligence principles as the basis for the decision. The general rule is that a manufacturer or seller who has knowledge of the dangerous character of the product has a duty to warn users of this danger. Thus, failure to warn where a reasonable man would do so is negligence.

13.9.6 Plaintiff's conduct

A manufacturer or seller may defend a product liability action by demonstrating that the plaintiff either engaged in negligent conduct that was a contributing factor to his injury, or used a product when it was obvious that a danger existed and thereby assumed the risk of his injury. Another type of misconduct which may defeat recovery is when the plaintiff misuses the product by utilizing it in a manner not anticipated by the manufacturer. The applicability of these defenses in any given product suit is dependent upon the theory or theories of recovery which are asserted by the plaintiff.

13.9.7 Defendant's conduct

Compliance with certain standards by a manufacturer may provide that party with a complete defense if the product leaves the manufacturer's or seller's possession or control and when it is a substantial or proximate cause of the plaintiff's injury. Exceptions to this rule include alterations or modifications made with the manufacturer's or seller's consent, or according to manufacturer's/seller's instructions.

13.9.8 Defendant-related issues

When a medical device proves to be defective, potential liability is created for many parties who may have been associated with the device. Of all the parties involved, the injured patient is least able to bear the financial consequences. To place the financial obligation upon the proper parties, the courts must consider the entire history of the product involved, often from the time the design concept was spawned until the instant the injury occurred. The first parties encountered in this process are the designers, manufacturers, distributors, and sellers of the product. Secondarily, and often of highest import to a case, is when the device failure has been well documented in the FDA MAUDE database. If similar injuries have been reported over a period of time, and no corrective action has been taken, the assumption of fault on the part of the manufacturer is easily justified.

Physicians and hospitals are also subject to liability through medical malpractice actions for their negligence, whether or not a defective product is involved. Where such a product is involved, the doctor or hospital may be liable for:

- negligent misuse of the product
- negligent selection of the product
- failure to inspect or test the product
- using the product with knowledge of its defect.

Negligent behavior on the part of the physician or other members of the health care team also can be a basis for a lawsuit. Medical errors, such as mistranscription of drug type or dose, misadministration of dose, etc. have been grounds for suits. The parallel for implied warranty is implied credentials; a physician who advertises for a specialty must be credentialed in that specialty (such as surgery or anesthesiology). The records of the Joint Commission on the Accreditation of Health Care Organizations is open to the public, one of their responsibilities is the inspection of credentials in residency programs.

The health care industry has generally accepted the need for quality assurance. The current climate in the United States, with the publication of *To Err is Human, Building a Safer Health System* and the estimated 40-90,000 deaths per year via medical errors, has prompted an upgrade in efforts to improve safety and therefore reliability in the health care system. To this end, new funding initiatives are being put in place to study and reduce medical errors.

13.9.9 Manufacturer's and physician's responsibilities

Manufacturers of medical devices have a duty with regard to manufacture, design, warnings, and labeling. A manufacturer is required to exercise that degree of care that a reasonable, prudent manufacturer would use under the same or similar conditions. A manufacturer's failure to comply with the standard in the industry, including failing to warn or give adequate instructions, may result in a finding of liability against the manufacturer.

With regard to medical devices, a manufacturer must take reasonable steps to warn physicians of dangers of which it is aware or reasonably should be aware where the danger would not be obvious to the ordinary competent physician dispensing a particular device. The responsibility for the prudent use of the medical device is with a physician. A surgeon who undertakes to perform a surgical procedure has the responsibility to act reasonably.

It is therefore required of the manufacturer to make a full disclosure of all known side effects and problems with a particular medical device by use of appropriate warnings given to physicians. The physician is to act as the learned intermediary between the manufacturer and the patient and transmit appropriate information to the patient. The manufacturer, however, must provide the physician with the information in order that he can pass it on to the patient.

In addition, the manufacturer's warnings must indicate the scope of potential danger from the use of a medical device and the risks of its use. This is particularly important where there is "off label use" (the practice of using a product approved for one application in a different application) by a physician.

The manufacturer's warnings must detail the scope of potential danger from the use of a medical device, including the risks of misuse. The warnings must alert a reasonably competent physician to the dangers of not using a product as instructed. It would seem then the manufacturer may be held liable for failing to disclose the range of possible consequences of the use of a medical device if it has knowledge that the particular device is being used "off label."

The duty of a manufacturer and physician for use of a medical device will be based upon the state of knowledge at the time of the use. The physician therefore has a responsibility to be aware of the manufacturer's warnings as he considers the patient's condition. This dual responsibility is especially relevant in deciding what particular medical device to use. Physician judgement and an analysis of the standard of care in the community should predominate the court's analysis in determining liability for possible misuses of the device.

A concern arises if the surgeon has received instruction as to the specific device from a manufacturer outside an investigative device exemption (IDE) clinical trail approved by the FDA. In such circumstances, plaintiffs will maintain that the manufacturer and physician conspired to promote a product that is unsafe for "off label use."

13.10 Conclusion

Products liability will undoubtedly continue to be a controversial field of law, because it cuts across so many fundamental issues of our society. It will also remain a stimulating field of study and practice, since it combines a healthy mixture of the practical and theoretical. The subject will certainly continue to change, both by statutory and by common law modification.

Products liability implicates many of the basic values of our society. It is a test of the ability of private industry to accommodate competitiveness and safety. It tests the fairness and the workability of the tort system of recovery, and of the jury system as a method of resolving disputes.

Homework Exercises

1. Sketch and properly label the reliability curve for a software package. Describe the different sections.
2. List and briefly describe the legal grounds for liability due to medical device malfunction.
3. Define the following terms in one sentence (each): reliability, failure, quality, warranty period, risk.
4. A new class of sensors is currently being developed - biosensors. Do a web search on this term, copy a brief definition for this term. What type of reliability curve do you predict for this type of device? Why?
5. A young lady has injured her lower back while using a "Thigh Master". How would you prove that her injury was due to the device? What grounds would you sue under?
6. What devices follow a "bathtub" failure curve? Give one example. How would a good QI (quality improvement) program change this curve?
7. A patient is scalded by a warming humidifier used in surgery. As a lawyer for the patient, which claims would you file prior to the taking of initial testimony?
8. George P. Turpentine has a stand on the corner that sells "Wonder Fizz", a drink that he claims is good for head problems, back problems, hip problems, muscle aches, insomnia. He'll even go on to tell that it will make you grow 2 inches and you'll have smarter children as a result of its wonderful effects. How might George be liable under the three main principals of legal liability (*negligence, strict liability, breach of warranty*)? Do a web search to determine the difference between quality improvement and quality assessment.
9. Search the MAUDE database for a medical device accident during the week of your birthday in the past year. Print out the report. Discuss the likely lawsuit that may have arisen and the grounds for the lawsuit.
10. Do a web search using the term "medical negligence". Print out the headers for the first 20 hits; classify the results and comment on them.

References

Boardman, Thomas A. and Thomas Dipasquale, "Product Liability Implications of Regulatory Compliance or Non-Compliance," in *The Medical Device Industry - Science, Technology, and Regulation in a Competitive Environment.* New York: Marcel Dekker, Inc., 1990.

Boumil, Marcia Mobilia and Clifford E. Elias, *The Law of Medical Liability in a Nutshell.* St. Paul, MN: West Publishing Co., 1995.

Buchholz, Scott D., "Defending Pedicle Screw Litigation," in *For the Defense.* Volume 38, Number 3, March, 1996.

Dhillon, B. S., *Reliability Engineering in Systems Design and Operation.* New York: Van Nostrand Reinhold Company, 1983.

Fries, Richard C., *Reliability Assurance for Medical Devices, Equipment and Software.* Buffalo Grove, IL: Interpharm Press, Inc., 1991.

Fries, Richard C., *Reliable Design of Medical Devices.* New York: Marcel Dekker, Inc., 1997.

Gingerich, Duane, *Medical Product Liability: A Comprehensive Guide and Sourcebook.* New York: F & S Press, 1981.

Goldberg, M. F. and J. Vaccaro, editors. *Physics of Failure in Electronics.* Spartan Books, Inc., 1963.

IEEE Std. 610.12, *Standard Glossary of Software Engineering Terminology.* New York: Institute of Electrical and Electronics Engineers, 1990.

ISO 8402, *Quality Vocabulary.* Switzerland: International Organization for Standardization, 1986.

Kanoti, George A. "Ethics, Medicine, and the Law," in *Legal Aspects of Medicine.* New York: Springer-Verlag, 1989.

Kececioglu, Dimitri, *Reliability Engineering Handbook.* Englewood Cliffs, NJ: PTR Prentice Hall Inc, 1991.

Langer, E. and J. Meltroft, editors. *Reliability in Electrical and Electronic Components and Systems*. North Holland Publishing Company, 1982.

Lloyd, D. K. and M. Lipow, *Reliability Management, Methods and Mathematics*. 2nd Edition, Milwaukee, Wisconsin: The American Society for Quality Control, 1984.

MIL-STD-721C, *Definition of Terms for Reliability and Maintainability*. Washington, DC: Department of Defense, 1981.

Niehoff, Ken, "Designing Reliable Software." *Medical Device and Diagnostic Industry*, Volume 16, Number 9, September 1994

O'Connor, P. D. T. *Practical Reliability Engineering*. 2nd Edition, New York: John Wiley and Sons, 1985.

Phillips, Jerry J., *Products Liability in a Nutshell*. 4th edition, St. Paul, MN: West Publishing Co., 1993.

Reliability Analysis Center. *Reliability Design Handbook*. Chicago: ITT Research Institute, 1975.

Sandberg, J. B. "Reliability For Profit...Not Just Regulation", in *Quality Progress*, August 1987.

Shapo, Marshall S., *Products Liability and the Search for Justice*. Durham, NC: Carolina Academic Press, 1993.

Chapter 14

The Food and Drug Administration

"Leaders get out in front and stay there by raising the standards by which they judge themselves - and by which they are willing to be judged."
Fredrick Smith

FDA literature dates its significant prehistory as including the appointment of a director of the Department of Agriculture by President Lincoln in 1862, and the later 1883 request for petitions to pass laws prohibiting adulteration and misbranding of foods and drugs. Many patent medicines at the time relied more on alcohol content for relief than on any useful ingredients (Lydia Pinkham's Vegetable Compound was 15 to 20% alcohol). Others cured rheumatism, sprains, boils, headache, etc, others purified the blood, etc.

The publication of *The Jungle*, in 1906, by Upton Sinclair is said to be one of the primary driving forces in the initiation of the FDA. Sinclair wrote a thinly disguised damnation of the meat packing industry. The minor quote (from chapter 10) to follow may serve to illuminate why the public became aroused: "*...with the hot weather there descended upon Packingtown a veritable Egyptian plague of flies; there could be no describing this--the houses would be black with them. There was no escaping; you might provide all your doors and* *windows with screens, but their buzzing outside would be like the swarming of bees, and whenever you opened the door they would rush in as if a storm of wind were driving them."* The Food and Drug Administration was formed in 1906, it banned (and therefore regulated) interstate commerce in adulterated and or misbranded food, drink, and drugs.

It took the deaths in 1938 of 107 individuals, primarily children, due to the ingestion of "Elixir of Sulfanilamide", a toxic combination of diethylene glycol and sulfa for the FDA to be given the power to act on the behalf of the public under the 1938 Federal Food, Drug, and Cosmetic Act. The drug enforcement requirements will be discussed in depth in Chapter 16, sections 6 and 7. The FDA was given the power to enforce labeling of food, extended the power of the FDA to cosmetics and therapeutic devices, and added the ability to use injunctions to the previous powers of seizures and prosecutions.

14.1 Recent History of Device Regulation

Regulation of medical devices is intended to protect consumer's health and safety by attempting to ensure that marketed products are effective and safe. Prior to 1976, the FDA had limited authority over medical devices under the Food, Drug, and Cosmetic Act of 1938. Beginning in 1968, Congress established a radiation control program to authorize the establishment of standards for electronic products, including medical and dental radiology equipment. From the early 1960s to 1975, concern over devices increased and six US Presidential messages were given to encourage medical device legislation.

In 1969, the Department of Health, Education, and Welfare appointed a special committee (the Cooper Committee) to review the scientific literature associated with medical devices. The Committee estimated that over a 10-year period, 10,000 injuries were associated with medical devices, of which 731 resulted in death. The majority of problems were associated with three device types: artificial heart valves, cardiac pacemakers, and intrauterine contraceptive devices. There activities culminated in passage of the Medical Devices Amendments of 1976.

Devices marketed after 1976 are subject to full regulation unless they are found substantially equivalent to a device already on the market in 1976. By the end of 1981, only about 300 of the 17,000 products submitted for clearance to the FDA after 1976 had been found not substantially equivalent.

In the years following World War II, the FDA focused much of the attention on drugs and cosmetics. Over-the-counter drugs became regulated in 1961. In 1962, the FDA began requesting safety and efficacy data on new drugs and cosmetics.

By the mid-1960s, it became clear that the provisions of the FFD&C Act were not adequate to regulate the complex medical devices of the times to assure both patient and user safety. Thus, in 1969, the Cooper Committee was formed to examine the problems associated with medical devices and to develop concepts for new regulations.

In 1976, with input from the Cooper Committee, the FDA created the Medical Device Amendments to the FFD&C Act, which were subsequently signed into law. The purpose of the amendments was to assure that medical devices were safe, effective and properly labeled for their intended use. To accomplish this mandate, the amendments provided the FDA with the authority to regulate devices during most phases of their development, testing, production, distribution and use. This marked the first time the FDA clearly distinguished between devices and drugs. Regulatory requirements were derived from this 1976 law.

In 1978, with the authority granted the FDA by the amendments, the Good Manufacturing Practices (GMP) were promulgated. The GMP represents a quality assurance program intended to control the manufacturing, packaging, storage, distribution and installation of medical devices. This regulation was intended to allow only safe and effective devices to reach the market place. It is this regulation that has the greatest effect on the medical device industry. It allows the FDA to inspect a company's operations and take action on any noted deficiencies, including prohibition of device shipment.

Recent regulations specific to medical devices are the Medical Device Reporting (MDR) regulation of 1984, the Device Reconditioner/Rebuilder (DRR) regulation of 1988, and the Safe Medical Devices Act of 1992.

Currently, the FDA has powers in the following areas: Food, Drugs, Medical Devices, Biologics, Animal Feed and Drugs, Cosmetics, and Radiation Emitting Devices. We will concentrate on medical devices for the remainder of this chapter.

14.2 Device Classification

According to the FDA definition, a medical device is:

"an instrument, apparatus, implement, machine, contrivance, implant, in vitro reagent, or other similar or related article, including a component part, or accessory which is:

- recognized in the official National Formulary, or the United States Pharmacopoeia, or any supplement to them,
- intended for use in the diagnosis of disease or other conditions, or in the cure, mitigation, treatment, or prevention of disease, in man or other animals, or
- intended to affect the structure or any function of the body of man or other animals, and which does not achieve any of it's primary intended purposes through chemical action within or on the body of man or other animals and which is not dependent upon being metabolized for the achievement of any of its primary intended purposes."

From 1962, when Congress passed the last major drug law revision, and first attempted to include devices, until 1976 when device laws were finally written, there were almost constant congressional hearings. Testimony was presented by medical and surgical specialty groups, industry, basic biomedical sciences, and various government agencies, including all the FDA. All of the viewpoints and arguments that we hear today were proposed, and considered in public discussion. Nearly two dozen bills were rejected as either inadequate or inappropriate.

The Cooper Committee concluded that the many inherent and important differences between drugs and devices necessitated a regulatory plan specifically adapted to devices. They recognized that some degree of risk is inherent in the development of many devices, so that all hazards cannot be eliminated, that there is often little or no prior experience on which to base judgments about safety and effectiveness, that devices undergo performance improvement modifications during the course of clinical trials, and that results also depend upon the skill of the user.

They therefore rejected the drug-based approach and created a new and different system for evaluating devices. All devices were placed into classes based upon the degree of risk posed by each individual device and its use. The Pre-Market Notification Process (510(k)) and the Pre-Market Approval Application (PMAA) became the regulatory pathways for device approval. The Investigational Device Exemption (IDE) became the mechanism to establish safety and efficacy in clinical studies for PMAAs.

14.2.1 Class I devices

Class I devices were defined as not life sustaining, their failure poses no risk to life, and there is no need for performance standards. Basic standards, however, such as premarket notification (510(k)), registration, device listing, good manufacturing practices (GMP), and proper record keeping are all required. Nonetheless, the FDA has exempted many of the simpler Class I devices from some or all of these requirements. For example, tongue depressors and stethoscopes are both Class I devices, both are exempt from GMP, tongue depressors are exempt from 510(k) filing, whereas stethoscopes are not. Examples may be found on the FDA website of multiple devices and their classifications, the FDA is willing to advise beforehand on the device classification to be sought. Note, however, that any classification applies only to the petitioned for use of the device. Thus, a lung sound stethoscope may not also be called (without FDA approval) a heart sounds stethoscope.

14.2.2 Class II devices

Class II devices were also defined in 1976 as not life sustaining. However, they must not only comply with the basic standards for Class I devices, but must meet specific controls or performance standards. For example, sphygmomanometers, although not essential for life, must meet standards of accuracy and reproducibility.

Premarket notification is documentation submitted by a manufacturer that notifies the FDA that a device is about to be marketed. It assists the agency in making a determination about whether a device is "substantially equivalent" to a previously marketed predecessor device. As provided for in section 510(k) of the Food, Drug, and Cosmetic Act, the FDA can clear a device for marketing on the basis of premarket notification that the device is substantially equivalent to a pre-1976 predecessor device. The decision is based on premarket notification information that is provided by the manufacturer and includes the intended use, physical composition, and specifications of the device. Additional data usually submitted include in vitro and in vivo toxicity studies.

The premarket notification or 510(k) process was designed to give manufacturers the opportunity to obtain rapid market approval of these noncritical devices by providing evidence that their device is "substantially equivalent" to a device that is already marketed. The device must have the same intended use and the same or equally safe and effective technological characteristics as a predicate device.

Class II devices are usually exempt from the need to prove safety and efficacy. The FDA, however, may require additional clinical or laboratory studies. On occasion these may be as rigorous as for an IDE in support of a PMA, although this is rare. The FDA responds with an "order of concurrence" or nonconcurrence with the manufacturer's equivalency claims.

The Safe Medical Device Act of 1990 and the Amendments of 1992 attempted to take advantage of what had been learned since 1976 to give both the FDA and manufacturers greater leeway by permitting down-classification of many devices, including some life supporting and life sustaining devices previously in Class III, provided that reasonable assurance of safety and effectiveness can be obtained by application of "Special Controls" such as performance standards, post market surveillance, guidelines and patient and device registries.

14.2.3 Class III devices

Class III Devices were defined in 1976 as either sustaining or supporting life so that their failure is life threatening. For example, heart valves, pacemakers and PCTA balloon catheters are all Class III devices. Class III devices almost always require a PMAA, a long and complicated task fraught with many pitfalls that has caused the greatest confusion and dissatisfaction for both industry and the FDA.

The new regulations permit the FDA to use data contained in four prior PMAs for a specific device, that demonstrate safety and effectiveness, to approve future PMA applications by establishing performance standards or actual reclassification. Composition and manufacturing methods which companies wish to keep as proprietary secrets are excluded. Advisory Medical panel review is now elective.

However, for PMAAs that continue to be required, all of the basic requirements for Class I and II devices must be provided, plus failure mode analysis, animal tests, toxicology studies and then finally human clinical studies, directed to establish safety and efficacy under an IDE.

It is necessary that preparation of the PMA must actually begin years before it will be submitted. It is only after the company has the results of all of the laboratory testing, pre-clinical animal testing, failure mode analysis and manufacturing standards on their final design, that their proof of safety and efficacy can begin, in the form of a clinical study under an IDE.

At this point the manufacturer must not only have settled on a specific, fixed design for his device, but with his marketing and clinical consultants must also have decided on what the indications, contraindications, and warnings for use will be. The Clinical Study must be carefully designed to support these claims.

Section 520(g) of the Federal Food, Drug, and Cosmetic Act, as amended, authorizes the FDA to grant an IDE to a researcher using a device in studies undertaken to develop safety and effectiveness data for that device when such studies involve human subjects. An approved IDE application permits a device that would otherwise be subject to marketing clearance to be shipped lawfully for the purpose of conducting a clinical study. An approved IDE also exempts a device from certain sections of the Act. All new significant risk devices not granted substantial equivalence under the 510(k) section of the Act must pursue clinical testing under an IDE.

An Institutional Review Board (IRB) is a group of physicians and lay people at a hospital who must approve clinical research projects prior to their initiation. The IRB is discussed in detail in Section 6.6.1.

14.3 Registration and Listing

Under section 510 of the Act, every person engaged in the manufacture, preparation, propagation, compounding or processing of a device shall register their name, place of business and such establishment. This includes manufacturers of devices and components, repackers, relabelers, as well as initial distributors of imported devices. Those not required to register include manufacturers of raw materials, licensed practitioners, manufacturers of devices for use solely in research or teaching, warehousers, manufacturers of veterinary devices, and those who only dispense devices, such as pharmacies.

Upon registration, the FDA issues a device registration number. A change in the ownership or corporate structure of the firm, the location, or person designated as the official correspondent must be communicated to the FDA device registration and listing branch within 30 days. Registration must be done when first beginning to manufacture medical devices and must be updated yearly.

Section 510 of the Act also requires all manufacturers to list the medical devices they market. Listing must be done when first beginning to manufacture a product and must be updated every 6 months. Listing includes not only informing the FDA of products manufactured, but also providing the agency with copies of labeling and advertising.

Foreign firms that market products in the United States are permitted but not required to register, and are required to list. Foreign devices that are not listed are not permitted to enter the country.

Registration and listing provides the FDA with information about the identity of manufacturers and the products they make. This information enables the agency to schedule inspections of facilities and also to follow up on problems. When the FDA learns about a safety defect in a particular type of device, it can use the listing information to notify all manufacturers of those devices about that defect.

14.4 The 510(k) Process

14.4.1 Determining substantial equivalency

A new device is substantially equivalent if, in comparison to a legally marketed predicate device, it has the same intended use and 1) has the same technological characteristics as the predicate device or 2) has different technological characteristics and submitted information that does not raise different questions of safety and efficacy, and demonstrates that the device is as safe and effective as the legally marketed predicate device. Figure 14-1 is an overview of the substantial equivalence decision-making process.

14.4.2 Preparing a 510(k)

14.4.2.1 Types of 510(k)s

There are several types of 510(k) submissions that require different formats for addressing the requirements. These include:

- Submissions for Identical Devices
- Submissions for Equivalent but Not Identical Devices
- Submissions for Complex Devices or for Major Differences in Technological Characteristics
- Submissions for Software-Controlled Devices.

The 510(k) for simple changes, or for identical devices should be kept simple and straightforward. The submission should refer to one or more predicate devices, it should contain samples of labeling, it should have a brief statement of equivalence, and it may be useful to include a chart listing similarities and differences.

The group of equivalent but not identical devices includes combination devices where the characteristics or functions of more than one predicate device are relied on to support a substantially equivalent determination. This type of 510(k) should contain all of the information listed above as well as sufficient data to demonstrate why the differing characteristics or functions do not affect safety or effectiveness. Submission of some functional data may be necessary. It should not be necessary, however, to include clinical data; bench or pre-clinical testing results should be sufficient. Preparing a comparative chart showing differences and similarities with predicate devices can be particularly helpful to the success of this type of application.

Submissions for complex devices or for major differences in technological characteristics is the most difficult type of submission, since it begins to approach the point at which the FDA will need to consider whether a 510(k) is sufficient of whether a PMAA must be submitted. The key is to

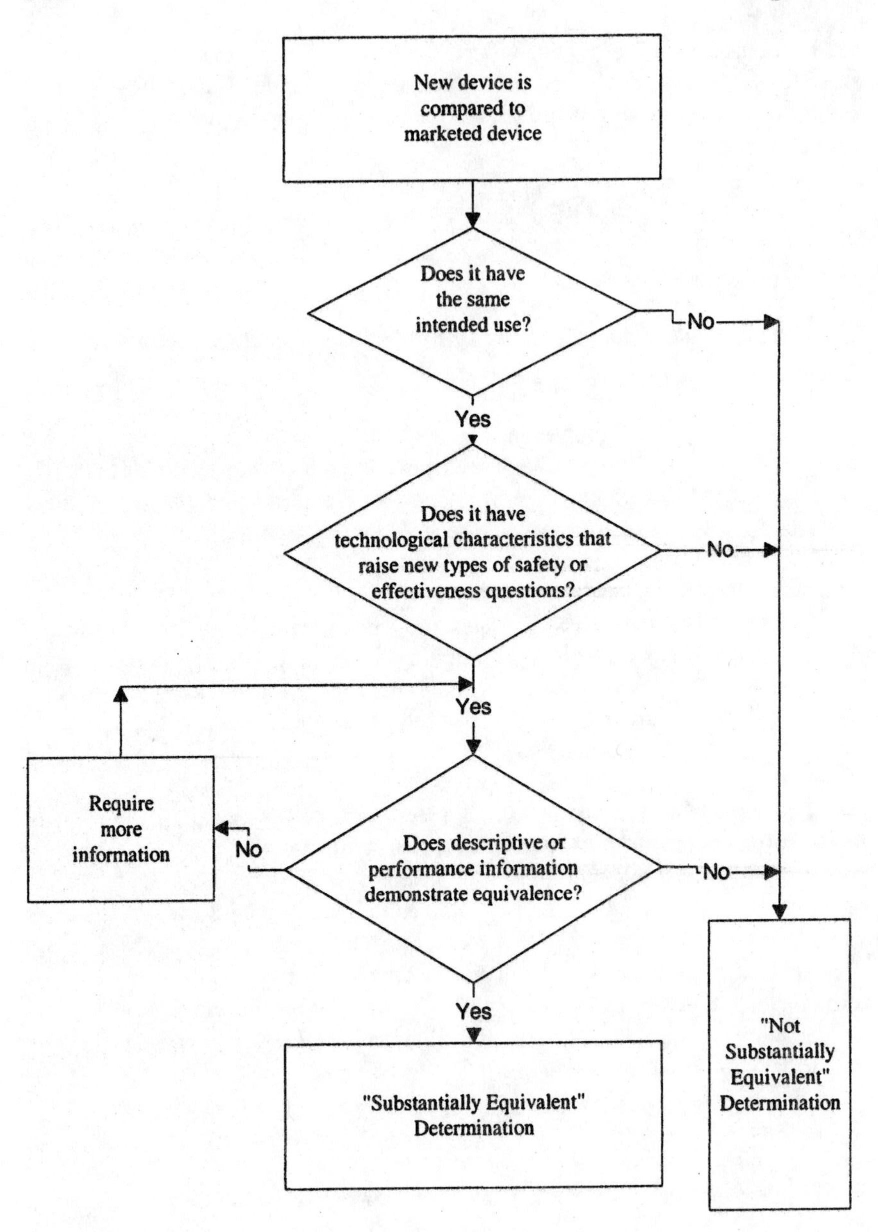

Figure 14-1 The substantial equivalence process. (From Fries, 1997.)

demonstrate that the new features or the new uses do not diminish safety or effectiveness and that there are no significant new risks posed by the device. In addition to the types of information described above, this type of submission will almost always require submission of some data, possibly including clinical data.

As a general rule, it often is a good idea to meet with FDA to explain why the product is substantially equivalent, to discuss the data that will be submitted in support of a claim of substantial equivalence, and to learn the FDA's concerns and questions so that these may be addressed in the submission. The FDA's guidance documents can be of greatest use in preparing this type of submission.

The term software includes programs and or data that pertain to the operation of a computer-controlled system, whether they are contained on floppy disks, hard disks, magnetic tapes, laser disks, or embedded in the hardware of a device. The depth of review by the FDA is determined by the "level of concern" for the device and the role that the software plays in the functioning of the device. Levels of concern are listed as minor, moderate, and major and are tied very closely with risk analysis.

In reviewing such submissions, the FDA maintains that end-product testing may not be sufficient to establish that the device is substantially equivalent to the predicate devices. Therefore, a firm's software development process and/or documentation should be examined for reasonable assurance of safety and effectiveness of the software-controlled functions, including incorporated safeguards. 510(k)s that are heavily software dependent will receive greater FDA scrutiny, and the questions posed must be satisfactorily addressed.

14.4.2.2 The 510(k) format

The actual 510(k) submission will vary in complexity and length according to the type of device or product change for which substantial equivalency is sought. A submission shall be in sufficient detail to provide an understanding of the basis for a determination of substantial equivalence. All submissions shall contain the following information:

- The submitter's name, address, telephone number, a contact person, and the date the submission was prepared

- The name of the device, including the trade or proprietary name, if applicable, the common or usual name, and the classification name
- An identification of the predicate or legally marketed device or devices to which substantial equivalence is being claimed
- A description of the device that is the subject of the submission, including an explanation of how the device functions, the basic scientific concepts that form the basis for the device, and the significant physical and performance characteristics of the device such as device design, materials used, and physical properties
- A statement of the intended use of the device, including a general description of the diseases or conditions the device will diagnose, treat, prevent, cure, or mitigate, including a description, where appropriate, of the patient population for which the device is intended. If the indication statements are different from those of the predicate or legally marketed device identified above, the submission shall contain an explanation as to why the differences are not critical to the intended therapeutic, diagnostic, prosthetic, or surgical use of the device and why the differences do not affect the safety or effectiveness of the device when used as labeled
- A statement of how the technological characteristics (design, material, chemical composition, or energy source) of the device compare to those of the predicate or legally marketed device identified above.

510(k) summaries for those premarket notification submissions in which a determination of substantial equivalence is based on an assessment of performance data shall contain the following information in addition to that listed above:

- A brief discussion of the nonclinical tests and their results submitted in the premarket notification.

- A brief discussion of the clinical tests submitted, referenced, or relied on in the premarket notification submission for a determination of substantial equivalence.

This discussion shall include, where applicable, a description of the subjects upon whom the device was tested, a discussion of the safety and/or effectiveness data obtained with specific reference to adverse effects and complications, and any other information from the clinical testing relevant to a determination of substantial equivalence.

- The conclusions drawn from the nonclinical and clinical tests that demonstrate that the device is safe, effective, and performs as well as or better than the legally marketed device identified above.

The summary should be in a separate section of the submission beginning on a new page and ending on a page not shared with any other section of the premarket notification submission, and should be clearly identified as a "501(k) summary."

A 510 (k) statement submitted as part of a premarket notification shall state as follows:

I certify that (name of person required to submit the premarket notification) will make available all information included in this premarket notification on safety and effectiveness that supports a finding of substantial equivalence within 30 days of request by any person. The information I agree to make available does not include confidential patient identifiers.

This statement should be made in a separate section of the premarket notification submission and should be clearly identified as a 510(k) statement.

A Class III certification submitted as part of a premarket notification shall state as follows:

I certify that a reasonable search of all information known or otherwise available to (name of premarket notification submitter) about the types and causes of reported safety and/or effectiveness problems for the (type of device) has been conducted. I further certify that the types of problems to which the (type of device) is susceptible and their potential causes are listed in the attached Class III summary, and that this Class III summary is complete and accurate.

This statement should be clearly identified as a Class III certification and should be made in the section of the premarket notification submission that includes the Class III summary.

A 510(k) should be accompanied by a brief cover letter that clearly identifies the submission as a 510(k) premarket notification. To facilitate prompt routing of the submission to the correct reviewing division within FDA, the letter can mention the generic category of the product and its intended use.

When the FDA receives a 510(k) premarket notification, it is reviewed according to a checklist to assure its completeness. A sample 510(k) checklist is shown in Figure 14-2.

14.5 PMA Application

Premarket Approval (PMA) is an approval application for a Class III medical device, including all information submitted with or incorporated by reference. The purpose of the regulation is to establish an efficient and thorough device review process to facilitate the approval of PMAs for devices that have been shown to be safe and effective for their intended use and that otherwise meet the statutory criteria for approval, while ensuring the disapproval of PMAs for devices that have not been shown to be safe and effective or that do not otherwise meet the statutory criteria for approval.

14.5.1 The PMA process

The first step in the PMAA process is the filing of the investigational device exemption (IDE) application for significant risk devices. The IDE is reviewed by the FDA and once accepted, the sponsor can proceed with clinical trials.

14.5.2 Contents of a PMAA

Section 814.20 of 21 CFR defines what must be included in an application, including:

- name and address
- application procedures and table of contents summary
- complete device description
- reference to performance standards
- nonclinical and clinical investigations
- justification for single investigator
- bibliography
- sample of device
- proposed labeling
- environmental assessment
- other information.

The summary should include indications for use, a device description, a description of alternative practices and procedures, a brief description of the marketing history, and a summary of studies. This summary should be of sufficient detail to enable the reader to gain a general understanding of the application. The PMAA must also include the applicant's foreign and domestic marketing history as well as any marketing history of a third party marketing the same product.

The description of the device should include a complete description of the device, including pictorial presentations. Each of the functional components or ingredients should be described, as well as the properties of the device relevant to the diagnosis, treatment, prevention, cure, or mitigation of a disease or condition. The principles of the device's operation should also be explained. Information regarding the methods used in, and the facilities and controls used for the manufacture, processing, packing, storage, and installation of the device should be explained in sufficient detail so that a person generally familiar with current good manufacturing practices can make a knowledgeable judgment about the quality control used in the manufacture of the device.

To clarify which performance standards must be addressed, applicants may ask members of the appropriate reviewing division of the Office of Device Evaluation (ODE) or consult FDA's list of relevant voluntary standards or the Medical Device Standards Activities Report.

Critical Elements		
1	Is the product a device?	Yes☐ No☐
2	Is the device exempt from 510(k) by regulation or policy?	Yes☐ No☐
3	Is device subject to review by CDRH (Center for Devices and Radiological Health)?	Yes☐ No☐
4	Are you aware that this device has been the subject of a previous NSE (Not Substantially Equivalent) decision?	Yes☐ No☐
	If yes, does this new 510(k) address the NSE issue(s) (e.g., performance data)?	
5	Are you aware of the submitter being the subject of and integrity investigation? If yes, consult the ODE (Office of Device Evaluation) Integrity Officer.	Yes☐ No☐
6	(ii). Has the ODE Integrity Officer given permission to proceed with the review? (Blue Book Memo #I91-2 and Federal Register 90N-0332, September 10, 1990).	Yes☐ No☐
7	Does the submission contain the information required under Sections 510(k) , 513(f) and 513(i) of the Federal, Food, Drug and Cosmetic Act (Act) and Subpart E of Part 807 in Title 21 of the Code of Federal Regulations?	Yes☐ No☐
8	Device trade or proprietary name?	Yes☐ No☐
9	Device common or usual name or classification name?	Yes☐ No☐
10	Establishment registration number (only applies if establishment is registered)?	Yes☐ No☐
11	Class into which the device is classified under (21 CFR Parts 862 to 892)?	Yes☐ No☐
12	Classification panel?	Yes☐ No☐
13	Action taken to comply with Section 514 of the Act?	Yes☐ No☐
14	Proposed labels, labeling and advertisements (if available) that describe the device, its intended use, and directions for use (Blue Book Memo #G91-1)?	Yes☐ No☐
15	A 510(k) summary of safety and effectiveness or a 510(k) statement that safety and effectiveness information will be made available to any person upon request?	Yes☐ No☐
16	For Class III devices only, a Class III certification and a Class III summary?	Yes☐ No☐
17	Photographs of the device?	Yes☐ No☐
18	Engineering drawings for the device with dimensions and tolerances?	Yes☐ No☐
19	The marketed device(s) to which equivalence is being claimed including labeling and description of the device?	Yes☐ No☐
20	Statement of similarities and/or differences with marketed device(s)?	Yes☐ No☐
21	Data to show consequences and effects of a modified device(s)?	Yes☐ No☐
22	Additional Information that is necessary under 21 CFR 807.87(h)?	Yes☐ No☐
23	Submitter's name and address?	Yes☐ No☐
24	Contact person, telephone number and fax number?	Yes☐ No☐

	Critical Elements	
25	Representative/Consultant if applicable?	Yes☐ No☐
26	Table of Contents with pagination?	Yes☐ No☐
27	Address of manufacturing facility/facilities and, if appropriate, sterilization site(s)?	Yes☐ No☐
28	Additional Information that may be necessary under 21 CFR 807.87(h)?	Yes☐ No☐
29	Comparison table of the new device to the marketed device(s)?	Yes☐ No☐
30	Action taken to comply with voluntary standards?	Yes☐ No☐
31	Performance data:	Yes☐ No☐
	marketed device?	Yes☐ No☐
	bench testing?	Yes☐ No☐
	animal testing?	Yes☐ No☐
	clinical data?	Yes☐ No☐
	new device?	Yes☐ No☐
	bench testing?	Yes☐ No☐
	animal testing?	Yes☐ No☐
	clinical data?	Yes☐ No☐
32	Sterilization information?	Yes☐ No☐
33	Software information?	Yes☐ No☐
34	Hardware information?	Yes☐ No☐
35	If this 510(k) is for a kit, has the kit certification statement been provided?	Yes☐ No☐
36	Is this device subject to issues that have been addressed in specific guidance document(s)?	Yes☐ No☐
	If yes, continue review with checklist from any appropriate guidance documents.	
	If no, is 510(k) sufficiently complete to allow substantive review?	
37	Truthfulness certification?	Yes☐ No☐
38	Other (as required)?	Yes☐ No☐

Figure 14-2 Sample FDA 510(k) checklist. (From Fries, 1997.)

14.6 Investigational Device Exemptions

The purpose of the Investigational Device Exemption (IDE) regulation is to encourage the discovery and development of useful devices intended for human use while protecting the public health. It provides the procedures for the conduct of clinical investigations of devices. An approved IDE permits a device to be shipped lawfully for the purpose of conducting investigations of the device without complying with a performance standard or having marketing clearance.

14.6.1 Institutional review boards (IRBs)

Any human research is covered by Federal regulation will not be funded unless it has been reviewed by an IRB. The fundamental purpose of an IRB is to ensure that research activities are conducted in an ethical and legal manner. Specifically, IRBs are expected to ensure that each of the basic elements of informed consent, as defined by regulation, are included in the document presented to the research participant for signature or verbal approval.

The deliberations of the IRB must determine that:

- the risks to subjects is equitable
- the selection of subjects is equitable
- informed consent will be sought from each prospective subject or their legally authorized representative
- informed consent will be appropriately documented
- where appropriate, the research plan makes adequate provision for monitoring the data collected to assure the safety of the subjects
- where appropriate, there are adequate provisions to protect the privacy of subjects and to maintain the confidentiality of data.

It is axiomatic that the IRB should ensure that the risks of participation in a research study should be minimized. The IRB must determine that this objective is to be achieved by ensuring that investigators use procedures that are consistent with sound research design and that do not necessarily expose subjects to excessive risk. In addition, the IRB needs to assure that the investigators, whenever appropriate, minimize risk and discomfort to the research participants by using, where possible, procedures already performed on the subjects as part of routine diagnosis or treatment.

The Institutional Review Board is any board, committee, or other group formally designated by an institution to review, to approve the initiation of, and to conduct periodic review of biomedical research involving human subjects. The primary purpose of such review is to assure the protection of the rights and welfare of human subjects.

An IRB must comply with all applicable requirements of the IRB regulation and the IDE regulation in reviewing and approving device investigations involving human testing. An IRB has the authority to review and approve, require modification, or disapprove an investigation. If no IRB exists or if FDA finds an IRB's review to be inadequate, a sponsor may submit an application directly to FDA.

An investigator is responsible for:

- ensuring that the investigation is conducted according to the signed agreement, the investigational plan, and applicable FDA regulations
- protecting the rights, safety, and welfare of subjects
- control of the devices under investigation.

An investigator is also responsible for obtaining informed consent and maintaining and making reports.

14.6.2 IDE format

There is no preprinted form for an IDE application, but the following information must be included in an IDE application for a significant risk device investigation. Generally, an IDE application should contain the following:

- name and address of sponsor
- a complete report of prior investigations
- a description of the methods, facilities, and controls used for the manufacture, processing, packing, storage, and installation of the device
- an example of the agreements to be signed by the investigators and a list of the names and addresses of all investigators
- certification that all investigators have signed the agreement, that the list of investigators includes all investigators participating in the study, and that new investigators will sign the agreement before being added to the study
- a list of the names, addresses, and chairpersons of all IRBs that have or will be asked to review the investigation and a certification of IRB action concerning the investigation

- the name and address of any institution (other than those above) where a part of the investigation may be conducted
- the amount, if any, charged for the device and an explanation of why sale does not constitute commercialization
- a claim for categorical exclusion or an environmental assessment
- copies of all labeling for device
- copies of all informed consent forms and all related information materials provided to subjects
- any other relevant information that FDA requests for review of the IDE application.

14.7 Good Laboratory Practices

In 1978, FDA adopted Good Laboratory Practices (GLP) rules and implemented a laboratory audit and inspection procedure covering every regulated entity which conducts nonclinical laboratory studies for product safety and effectiveness. The GLPs were amended in 1984.

The GLP standard addresses all areas of laboratory operations including requirements for a Quality Assurance Unit to conduct periodic internal inspections and keep records for audit and reporting purposes, Standard Operating Procedures (SOPs) for all aspects of each study and for all phases of laboratory maintenance, a formal mechanism for evaluation and approval of study protocols and their amendments, and reports of data in sufficient detail to support conclusions drawn from them. The FDA inspection program includes GLP compliance, and a data audit to verify that information submitted to the agency accurately reflects the raw data.

14.8 Good Manufacturing Practices

FDA is authorized, under section 520(f) of the Act, to promulgate regulations detailing compliance with current Good Manufacturing Practices (GMP) and include the methods used in, and the facilities and controls used for, the manufacture, packing, storage and installation of a device. The GMP regulations were established as manufacturing safeguards to ensure the production of a safe and effective device and include all of the essential elements of a quality assurance program. Because manufacturers cannot test every device, the GMPs were established as a minimum standard of manufacturing to ensure that each device produced would be safe. If a product is not manufactured according to GMPs, even if it is later shown not to be a health risk, it is in violation of the Act and subject to FDA enforcement action.

The general objectives of the GMPs, not specific manufacturing methods, are found in Part 820 of the Code of Federal Regulations. The GMPs apply to the manufacture of every medical device. The proposed new GMP regulations, scheduled to be released in 1996, gives FDA the authority to examine the design area of the product development cycle for the first time. The regulation also parallels very closely the ISO 9000 set of standards.

14.9 Human Factors

In April, 1996, the FDA issued a draft primer on the use of Human Factors in medical device design. The purpose of the document was to improve the safety of medical devices by minimizing the likelihood of user error by systematic, careful design of the user interface, i.e., the hardware and software features that define the interaction between the users and the equipment. The document contains background information about human factors as a discipline, descriptions and illustrations of device problems, and a discussion of human factors methods. It also contains recommendations for manufacturers and health facilities.

As the source for this document, the FDA extensively used the guideline *Human Factors Engineering Guidelines and Preferred Practices for the Design of Medical Devices* published by the Association for the Advancement of Medical Instrumentation as well as interfacing with Human Factors consultants. It is expected that Human Factors requirements will become part of the product submission as well as the GMP inspection. Human Factors Engineering is discussed in detail in Chapter 8.

14.10 Design Control

With the anticipated publication of the new GMP regulations, the FDA will have the authority to cover design controls in their inspections. In preparation for this, the FDA issued a draft guidance document in March, 1996 entitled *Design Control Guidance for Medical Device Manufacturers.* The purpose of the document was to provide readers with an understanding of what is meant by "control" in the context of the requirements. By providing an understanding of what constitutes control of a design process, readers could determine how to apply the concepts in a way that was both consistent with the requirements and best suited for their particular situation.

Three underlying concepts served as a foundation for the development of this guidance:

- the nature of the application of design controls for any device should be proportional to both the complexity of and the risks associated with that device
- the design process is a multifunctional one that involves other departments beside design and development if it is to work properly, thus involving senior management as an active participant in the process
- the product life cycle concept serves throughout the document as the framework for introducing and describing the design control activities and techniques.

Design control concepts are applicable to process development as well as product development. The extent is dependent upon the nature of the product and processes used to manufacture the product. The safety and performance of a new product is also dependent on an intimate relationship between product design robustness and process capability.

The document covers the areas of:

- risk management
- design and development planning
- organizational and technical interfaces
- design input
- design output
- design review
- design verification
- design validation

- design changes
- design transfer.

14.11 The FDA and Software

The subject of software in and as a medical device has become an important topic for the FDA. This interest began in 1985 when software in a radiation treatment therapy device is alleged to have resulted in a lethal overdose. The FDA then analyzed recalls by fiscal year to determine how many were caused by software problems. In fiscal year 1985, for example, 20% of all neurology device recalls were attributable to software problems, while 8% of cardiovascular problems had the same cause. This type of analysis, along with the results of various corporate inspections, led the FDA to conclude that some type of regulation was required.

Since there are many type of software in use in the medical arena, the problem of the best way to regulate it has become an issue for the FDA. Discussions have centered around what type of software is a medical device, the type of regulation required for such software, and what could be inspected under current regulations. Agency concerns fall into three major categories: medical device software, software used in manufacturing, and software information systems used for clinical decision making.

For medical device software, FDA is responsible for assuring that the device utilizing the software is safe and effective. It only takes a few alleged serious injuries or deaths to sensitize the Agency to a particular product or generic component that deserves attention. The Agency's review of medical device reporting (MDR) incidents and analysis of product recalls has convinced the Agency that software is a factor contributing to practical problems within devices.

When software is used during manufacturing, FDA is concerned with whether or not the software controlling a tool or automatic tester is performing as expected. The FDA's perceptions are rooted in experiences with GMP inspections of pharmaceutical manufacturers, where computers are heavily depended upon for control of manufacturing processes. Although there are few incidents of device or manufacturing problems traceable to flaws in manufacturing software, GMP inspections have focused intensively on validation of software programs used in industry for control of manufacturing operations.

With regard to stand-alone software used to aid clinical decision making, the FDA is concerned with hypothetical problems rather than extensive records of adverse incidents. While most commercially available health care information systems replace manual systems that had a far higher potential for errors, FDA believes that regulations should apply to the kinds of systems that may influence clinical treatment or diagnoses. FDA has observed academic work of "expert systems" used by medical professionals and is concerned that such systems may be commercialized without sufficient controls.

A draft of a software policy was issued in September, 1987. The policy was a general statement of FDA thinking, including the definition of a medical device, establishment of a three class system for regulation of software, and a list of exemptions from the regulations. The draft is very general and leaves much room for personal interpretation. The draft does not address GMP issues nor the status of software as an inspectable commodity. The draft was revised in 1989, but did little to clear up the above issues. To date, a final policy has not been published.

The FDA has published guidelines for developing quality software, the requirements for product approval submissions (510k) and the inspection of software controlled test fixtures as a part of GMP inspections. They have also conducted training courses for their inspectors and submission reviewers on the subject of software and computer basics.

14.12 Software Classification

When a computer product is a component, part, or accessory of a product recognized as a medical device in its own right, the computer component is regulated according to the requirements for the parent device unless the component of the device is separately classified. Computer products that are medical devices and not components, parts or accessories of other products that are themselves medical devices are subject to one of three degrees of regulatory control depending on their characteristics. These products are regulated with the least degree of control necessary to provide reasonable assurance of safety and effectiveness. Computer products that are substantially equivalent to a device previously classified will be regulated to the same degree as the equivalent device. Those devices that are not substantially equivalent to a preamendment device or that are substantially equivalent to a Class III device are regulated as Class III devices.

Software classification, as listed in the FDA draft policy of 1987, follows a similar pattern to devices. Medical software is divided into three classes with regulatory requirements specific to each:

Class I software is subject to the Act's general controls relating to such matters as misbranding, registration of manufacturers, record keeping, and good manufacturing practices. An example of Class I software would be a program that calculates the composition of infant formula.

Class II software is that for which general controls are insufficient to provide reasonable assurance of safety and effectiveness and for which performance standards can provide assurance. This is exemplified by a computer program designed to produce radiation therapy treatment plans.

Class III software is that for which insufficient information exists to assure that general controls and performance standards will provide reasonable assurance of safety and effectiveness. Generally, these devices are represented to be life-sustaining or life-supporting and may be intended for a use that is of substantial importance in preventing impairment to health. They may be implanted in the body or present a potential unreasonable risk of illness or injury. A program that measures glucose levels and calculates and dispenses insulin based upon those calculations without physician intervention would be a Class III device.

14.13 The FDA Inspection

The FDA's power to inspect originates in Section 704 of the Federal Food, Drug, and Cosmetic Act. This provision allow FDA officials to inspect any factory, warehouse, or establishment in which devices are manufactured, processed, packed or held, for introduction into interstate commerce of after such introduction. In addition to the "establishments" specification, FDA is permitted to enter any vehicle used to transport or hold regulated products for export or in interstate commerce. The inspection power is specifically extended to medical device manufacturers by Sections 519 and 520 of the Federal Food, Drug, and Cosmetic Act.

Every FDA inspector is authorized by law to inspect all equipment that is used in the manufacturing process. Furthermore, investigators may examine finished and unfinished devices and device components, containers, labeling for regulated products, and all documents that are required to be kept by the regulations, such as device master records and device history records.

Despite the broad inspectional authority over restricted devices, the statute provides that regardless of the device's unrestricted status, certain information is excluded from FDA's inspectional gambit. The kind of information to which FDA does not have access includes financial data, sales data, and pricing data. The new GMPs due for release in 1996 give the FDA authority to inspect the design area and the qualifications of personnel in all aspects of the product development process.

14.14 Advice on Dealing with the FDA

Several recommendations can be made regarding how to deal with the FDA and its regulatory process. None of these bits of advice are dramatic or new, but in the course of observing a firm's interaction with the agency, it is amazing how many times the failure to think of these steps can result in significant difficulties.

Know your district office. This may not be an easy thing to accomplish, since, understandably, there is a great reluctance to walk into a regulatory agency and indicate you are there to get acquainted. As opportunities arise, however, they should not be overlooked. Situations such as responding to a notice of an investigator's observations at the conclusion of an inspection or a notice of adverse findings letter are excellent opportunities to hand deliver a reply instead of simply mailing it. The verbal discussion with the reply may make the content much more meaningful and will allow both sides to learn more about the intent and seriousness with which the subject is being approached.

Prepare for inspections. When the FDA investigator walks into your manufacturing facility or corporate offices, there should be a procedure established that everyone is familiar with as to who is called, who escorts the investigator through the facility, who is available to make copies of records requested, etc. A corollary to this suggestion is to be prepared to deal with adverse inspectional findings or other communications from the agency that indicate the FDA has found violations, a serious health hazard, or other information that requires high-level company knowledge and decision making.

Take seriously 483's and letters. Many regulatory actions are processed with no apparent indication that a firm seriously considered the violations noted by the agency.

Keep up with current events and procedures of the FDA. This will minimize the changes or surprise interpretations that could have an effect on a firm's operations and will allow for advance planning for new FDA requirements. The Agency publishes much of its new program information in bulletins and other broad distribution documents, but much more can be learned from obtaining copies of FDA Compliance Policy Guides and Compliance Programs.

Let the FDA know of your firm's opinions on issues, whether they are in the development state at the Agency or are policies or programs established and in operation. The Agency does recognize that the firms it regulates are the true experts in device manufacturing and distribution, and their views are important. The Agency also recognizes that the regulation of manufacturers in not the only bottom line - solving public health problems is equally or more important, and there are generally many ways to solve those problems.

14.15 Manufacturer and User Facility Device Experience Database

It is important to recognize that the FDA maintains a database for medical device "user experiences", most of which have some death, injury, or malfunction event label attached to it. Data entered include: Brand name, type of device, generic and brand name of device, catalog number, model, and family, PMA and 510k data, manufacturer information including contact, report source, event type (death, injury, malfunction, other), device age, operator, patient outcome, a brief memorandum regarding the circumstances, etc. Due to the freedom of information act, this information is available to everyone that can do a web search., thus a manufacturer that consistently has detrimental information reported in this database is liable for follow-up inspections by the FDA as well as is at a risk in lawsuits relating to these devices.

Homework Exercises

1. The meat industry is, despite efforts since 1906, still a major concern for some individuals. Find and discuss any recently reported hamburger spoilage problem.

2. Feedback mechanisms are of value in electronic and mechanical control systems. Why are they not useful for material flows, such as foodstuffs.
3. Perform a web search for patent medicines, document two interesting examples.
4. Why did the FDA not have intrastate control in 1906?
5. Find, using the FDA website, any warning letter of interest to you and report on it.
6. Use the MAUDE database to do a search for device=bed, outcome=death, for any recent year. Report on your results.
7. Select a medical device used by one of your acquaintances, do a MAUDE search to determine if there have been any negative outcomes in the past five years.
8. Perform a web search for quack medical devices. Report on one.
9. Much recent television advertising exaggerates claims for nonmedical drugs or devices (such as "Viagro" and muscle stimulators). Find and report on an example, discuss how "truth" is being "bent." What would it take to get the FDA involved?

References

Banta, H. David, "The Regulation of Medical Devices," in *Preventive Medicine.* Volume 19, Number 6, November, 1990.

Basile, Edward, "Overview of Current FDA Requirements for Medical Devices," in *The Medical Device Industry: Science, Technology, and Regulation in a Competitive Environment.* New York: Marcel Dekker, Inc., 1990.

Basile, Edward M. and Alexis J. Prease, "Compiling a Successful PMA Application," in *The Medical Device Industry: Science, Technology, and Regulation in a Competitive Environment.* New York: Marcel Dekker, Inc., 1990.

Bureau of Medical Devices, Office of Small Manufacturers Assistance, *Regulatory Requirements for Marketing a Device.* Washington, DC: U.S. Department of Health and Human Services, 1982.

Center for Devices and Radiological Health, *Devic Good Manufacturing Practices Manual.* Washington, DC: U.S. Department of Health and Human Services, 1987.

Food and Drug Administration, *Federal Food, Drug and Cosmetic Act, as Amended January, 1979.* Washington, DC: U.S. Government Printing Office, 1979.

Food and Drug Administration, *Guide to the Inspection of Computerized Systems in Drug Processing.* Washington, DC: Food and Drug Administration, 1983.

Food and Drug Administration, *FDA Policy for the Regulation of Computer Products.* Washington, DC: Federal Register, 1987.

Food and Drug Administration, *Software Development Activities.* Washington, DC: Food and Drug Administration, 1987.

Food and Drug Administration, *Medical Devices GMP Guidance for FDA Inspectors.* Washington, DC: Food and Drug Administration, 1987.

Food and Drug Administration, *Reviewer Guidance for Computer-Controlled Medical Devices.* Washington, DC: Food and Drug Administration, 1988.

Food and Drug Administration, *Investigational Device Exemptions Manual.* Rockville MD: Center for Devices and Radiological Health, 1992.

Food and Drug Administration, *Premarket Notification 510(k): Regulatory Requirements for Medical Devices.* Rockville MD: Center for Devices and Radiological Health, 1992.

Food and Drug Administration, *Premarket Approval (PMA) Manual.* Rockville MD: Center for Devices and Radiological Health, 1993.

Food and Drug Administration, *Design Control Guidance for Medical Device Manufacturers.* Draft. Rockville, MD: Center for Devices and Radiological Health, 1996.

Food and Drug Administration, *Do It By Design: An Introduction to Human Factors in Medical Devices*. Draft. Rockville, MD: Center for Devices and Radiological Health, 1996.

Fries, Richard C. et al, "Software Regulation" in *The Medical Device Industry: Science, Technology, and Regulation in a Competitive Environment*. New York: Marcel Dekker, Inc., 1990.

Ginzburg, Harold M., "Protection of Research Subjects in Clinical Research," in *Legal Aspects of Medicine*. New York: Springer-Verlag, 1989.

Gundaker, Walter E., "FDA's Regulatory Program for Medical Devices and Diagnostics," in *The Medical Device Industry: Science, Technology, and Regulation in a Competitive Environment*. New York: Marcel Dekker, Inc., 1990.

Holstein, Howard M., "How to Submit a Successful 510(k)," in *The Medical Device Industry: Science, Technology, and Regulation in a Competitive Environment*. New York: Marcel Dekker, Inc., 1990.

Jorgens III, J. and C. W. Burch, "FDA Regulation of Computerized Medical Devices," *Byte*. Volume 7, 1982.

Jorgens III, J., "Computer Hardware and Software as Medical Devices," *Medical Device and Diagnostic Industry*. May, 1983.

Jorgens III, J. and R. Schneider, "Regulation of Medical Software by the FDA," *Software in Health Care*. April-May, 1985.

Kahan, J. S., "Regulation of Computer Hardware and Software as Medical Devices," *Canadian Computer Law Reporter*. Volume 6, Number 3, January, 1987.

Munsey, Rodney R. and Howard M. Holstein, "FDA/GMP/MDR Inspections: Obligations and Rights," in *The Medical Device Industry: Science, Technology, and Regulation in a Competitive Environment*. New York: Marcel Dekker, Inc., 1990.

Office of Technology Assessment, Federal Policies and the Medical Devices Industry. Washington, DC: U.S. Government Printing Office, 1984.

Sheretz, Robert J. and Stephen A. Streed, "Medical Devices - Significant Risk vs Nonsignificant Risk," in *Journal of the American Medical Association*, Volume 272, Number 12, September 28, 1994.

Trull, Frankie L. and Barbara A. Rich, "The Animal Testing Issue," in *The Medical Device Industry: Science, Technology, and Regulation in a Competitive Environment*. New York: Marcel Dekker, Inc., 1990.

U. S. Congress, House Committee on Interstate and Foreign Commerce. Medical Devices. Hearings before the Subcommittee on Public Health and the Environment. Octover 23-24, 1973. Serial Numbers 93-61 Washington DC: U.S. Government Printing Office, 1973.

Wholey, Mark H. and Jordan D. Hailer, "An Introduction to the Food and Drug Administration and How It Evaluates New Devices: Establishing Safety and Efficacy," in *CardioVascular and Interventional Radiology*. Volume 18, Number 2, March/April 1995

Chapter 15

Licensing, Patents, Copyrights, and Trade Secrets

"Ultimately property rights and personal rights are the same thing"
Calvin Coolidge

"The march of invention has clothed mankind with powers of which a century ago the boldest imagination could not have dreamt"
Henry George

Intellectual property is a generic term used to describe the products of the human intellect that have economic value. Intellectual property is "property" because a body of laws has been created over the last 200 years that gives owners of such works legal rights similar in some respects to those given to owners of real estate or tangible personal property. Intellectual property may be owned, bought, and sold the same as other type of property.

There are four separate bodies of law that may be used to protect intellectual property. These are patent law, copyright law, trademark law, and trade secret law. Each of these bodies of law may be used to protect different aspects of intellectual property, although there is a great deal of overlap among them.

15.1 Patents

A patent is an official document, issued by the U.S. government or another government, which describes an invention and confers on the inventors a monopoly over the use of the invention. The monopoly allows the patent owner to go to court to stop others from making, selling, or using the invention without the patent owner's permission.

Generally, an invention is any device or process that is based on an original idea conceived by one or more inventors and is useful in getting something done or solving a problem. An invention may also be a non-functional unique design or a plant. But when the word "invention" is used out in the real world, it almost always means a device or process. Many inventions, while extremely clever, do not qualify for patents, primarily because they are not considered to be sufficiently innovative in light of previous developments. The fact that an invention is not patentable does not mean necessarily that it has no value for its owner.

There are three types of patents that can be created: utility, design, and plant patents. Table 15-1 compares the three types of patents and the monopoly each type grants to the author.

15.1.1 What qualifies as a patent

An invention must meet several basic legal tests in order to qualify as a patent. These include:

- patentable subject matter
- usefulness
- novelty
- nonobviousness
- an improvement over an existing invention
- a design
- a plant.

We will concentrate primarily on the utility patent here. The plant patent would be of concern for a design text in agricultural engineering or bioengineering; the design patent is more of concern for those working in

Type of Patent	Legal Test	Length of Monopoly (years)
Utility	Useful/non-obvious/ improvement/novel design of process/machine/matter	20
Design	New, nonobvious design or appearance	14
Plant	New or discovered & asexually reproduced plant or variety, non-tuberous	20

Table 15-1 Patent Monopolies

industrial design. An example of a plant patent would be for a new variety of rose. A design example would be a uniquely shaped bumper on a new car.

15.1.1.1 Patentable subject matter

The most fundamental qualification for a patent is that the invention consists of patentable subject matter. The patent laws define patentable subject matter as inventions that are one of the following:

- a process or method
- a machine or apparatus
- an article of manufacture
- a composition of matter
- a new and useful improvement of an invention in any of these classes.

Computer software is included in the above category, and has been since the early 1990s.

15.1.1.2 Usefulness

Almost always, an invention must be useful in some way to qualify for a patent. Fortunately, this is almost never a problem, since virtually everything can be used for something.

15.1.1.3 Novelty

As a general rule, no invention will receive a patent unless it is different in some important way from previous inventions and developments in the field, both patented or not. To use legal jargon, the invention must be novel over the prior art. As part of deciding whether an invention is novel, the U.S. patent law system focuses on two issues: when the patent application is filed, and when the invention was first conceived.

15.1.1.4 Nonobviousness

In addition to being novel, an invention must have a quality that is referred to as "nonobviousness." This means that the invention would have been surprising or unexpected to someone who is familiar with the field of the invention. And in deciding whether an invention is nonobvious, the United States Patent and Trademark Office (PTO) may consider all previous developments (prior art) that existed when the invention was conceived. Obviousness is a quality that is difficult to define, but supposedly a patent examiner knows when they see it.

As a general rule, an invention is considered nonobvious when it does one of the following:

- solves a problem that people in the field have been trying to solve for some time
- does something significantly quicker that was previously possible
- performs a function that could not be performed before.

15.1.1.5 Improvement of an existing invention

Earlier we noted that to qualify for a patent, an invention must fit into at least one of the statutory classes of matter entitle to a patent - a process, a machine, a manufacture, a composition of matter, or an improvement of any of these. As a practical matter, this statutory class is not very important since even an improvement on an invention in one of the other statutory classes will also qualify as an actual invention in that class. In other words, an invention will be considered as patentable subject matter as long as it fits within at least one of the other four statutory classes - whether or not it is viewed as an improvement or an original invention.

15.1.1.6 A design

Design patents are granted to new, original and ornamental designs that are a part of articles of manufacture. Articles of manufacture are in turn defined as anything made by the hands of humans. In the past, design patents have been granted to items such as truck fenders, chairs, fabric, athletic shoes, toys, tools and artificial hip joints.

The key to understanding this type of patent is the fact that a patentable design is required to be primarily ornamental and an integral part of an item made by humans.

A design patent provides a 14 year monopoly to industrial designs that have no functional use. That is, contrary to the usefulness rule discussed above, designs covered by design patents must be purely ornamental. The further anomaly of design patents is that while the design itself must be primarily ornamental, as opposed to primarily functional, it must at the same time be embodied in something human-made. Design patents are easy to apply for, as they do not require much written description. They require drawings for the design, a short description of each figure or drawing, and one claim that says little more than the inventor claims the ornamental design depicted on the attached drawings. In addition the design patent is less expensive to apply for than a utility patent, lasts for 14 rather than 20 years, and requires no maintenance fees.

15.1.2 The patent process

The design process and the related patent information documentation process consists of the following steps:

- note all problems caused by equipment, supplies, or nonexisting devices when performing a task
- focus on the problem every time you perform the task or use the item
- concentrate on solutions
- keep a detailed, dated diary of problems and solutions; include drawings and sketches
- record the benefits and usefulness of your idea
- evaluate the marketability of your idea. It if does not have a wide application, it may be more advantageous to abandon the idea and focus on another
- do not discuss your idea with anyone except one person you trust who will maintain confidentially.
- prepare an application with a patent attorney
- have a search done, first a computer search, then a hand search.

Purchase a composition book with bound pages for keeping your notes. Start each entry with the date, and include all details of problem identification and solutions. Use drawings or sketches of your idea. Never remove any pages. If you do not like an entry or have made a mistake, simply make an X through the entry or write "error". Sign all entries and have a witness sign and date them as frequently as possible. Your witness should be someone you trust who understands your idea and will maintain confidentiality.

Be sure to understand your rights as an inventor, as your rights depend on your employment agreement if you are developing patentable material within a company, or your status as a student developing material for hire or for an educational experience (see 15.1.4 below.)

The patent document that may come of your effort as filed with the Patent and Trademark Office (PTO) will contain:

- a title for the invention and the names and addresses of the inventors

- details of the patent search made by the PTO
- an abstract that concisely describes the key aspects of the invention
- drawings or flowcharts of the invention
- very precise definitions of the invention covered by the patent (called the patent claims)
- a brief summary of the invention.

Taken together, the various parts of the patent document provide a complete disclosure of every important aspect of the covered invention. When a U.S. patent is issued, all the information in the patent is readily accessible to the public in the PTO and in patent libraries across the U.S. and through on-line patent database services.

As an example of the above, Patent Number 3,359,806, titled "Multicrystal tomographic scanner for mapping thin cross section of radioactivity in an organ of the human body" has the following as an abstract: "ABSTRACT: A multicrystal tomographic scanner is utilized for mapping thin slices or cross sections of radioactivity in an organ of the human body which has been injected or injected with a suitable radioisotope. A plurality of radiation detectors are arranged in a cylindrical monoplanar array with each detector focused in such a manner that the fields of view of all of the detectors intersect at a common point, and the detectors are driven mechanically such that this common point of the detectors is caused to move in a rectilinear raster of about 8 inches square. The distribution of radioactivity measured by the detectors due to the amount of radioisotope within the area being scanned is stored in a computer memory and reproduced on an oscilloscope display, as the section is being examined." Section 23.1 will discuss issues relating to this patent further.

U.S. patents are obtained by submitting to the PTO a patent application and an application fee. Once the application is received, the PTO assigns it to an examiner who is supposed to be knowledgeable in the technology underlying the invention. The patent examiner is responsible for deciding whether the invention qualifies for a patent, and assuming it does, what the scope of the patent should be. Usually, back and forth communications - called patent prosecution - occur between the applicant and the examiner regarding these issues. Clearly the most serious and hard-to-fix issue is whether the invention qualifies for a patent.

Eventually, if all of the examiner's objections are overcome by the applicant, the invention is approved for a patent. A patent issue fee is paid and the applicant receives an official copy of the patent deed. Three additional fees must be paid over the life of the patent to keep it in effect. Note that, though one or more individuals may be listed as inventors, the assignee is the patent holder of record. For the above mentioned patent, four inventors were listed, but the United States Atomic Energy Commission is the assignee, as the invention was done in part with funds from that agency.

15.1.3 Patent claims

Patent claims are the part of the patent application that precisely delimits the scope of the invention - where it begins and where it ends. Perhaps it will help understand what patent claims do if you analogize them to real estate deeds. A deed typically includes a description of the parcel's parameters precise enough to map the exact boundaries of the plot of land in question, which in turn, can be used as the basis of a legal action to toss out any trespassers.

With patents, the idea is to similarly draw in the patent claims a clear line around the property of the inventor so that any infringer can be identified and dealt with. Patent claims have an additional purpose. Because of the precise way in which they are worded, claims also are used to decide whether, in light of previous developments, the invention is patentable in the first place.

Unfortunately, to accomplish these purposes, all patent claims are set forth in an odd, stylized format. But the format has a big benefit. It makes it possible to examine any patent application or patent granted by the PTO and get a pretty good idea about what the invention covered by the patent consists of. While the stylized patent claim language and format have the advantage of lending a degree of precision to a field that badly needs it, there is an obvious and substantial downside to the use of the arcane "patentspeak." Mastering it amounts to climbing a fairly steep learning curve.

For the above-mentioned patent, there exists ten claims, which, when coupled with the technical drawings and proof of concept, serve to describe the invention in very fine detail, and serves to delimit the range of additional patents that might arise from a study of this particular patent. One claim is, for example, "5. The scanner set forth in claim 4, wherein the number of radiation detectors in said monopolar array is at least eight," would seem to limit one's ability to claim a similar patent with nine or ten detectors, for example.

It is when you set out to understand a patent claim that the rest of the patent becomes crucially important. The patent's narrative description of the invention - set out in the patent specification - with all or many of the invention's possible uses, and the accompanying drawings or flowcharts, usually provide enough information in combination to understand any particular claim. And of course, the more patent claims you examine, the more adept you will become in deciphering them.

15.1.4 Protecting your rights as an inventor

If two inventors apply for a patent around the same time, the patent will be awarded to the inventor who came up with the invention first. This may or may not be the inventor who was first to file a patent application. For this reason, it is vital that one carefully document the inventive activities. If two or more pending patent applications by different inventors claim the same invention, the PTO will ask the inventors to establish the date each of them first conceived the invention and the ways in which they then showed diligence in "reducing the invention to practice."

Inventors can reduce the invention to practice in two ways: 1) by making a working model - a prototype - which works as the idea of the invention dictates it should or 2) by constructively reducing it to practice - that is, by describing the invention in sufficient detail for someone else to build it - in a document that is then filed as a patent application with the PTO.

The inventor who conceived the invention first will be awarded the patent if he or she also showed diligence in either building the invention or filing a patent application. If the inventor who was second to conceive the invention was the first one to reduce it to practice - for instance by filing a patent application - that inventor may end up with the patent.

It is often the quality of the inventor's documentation (dated, written in a notebook, showing the conception of the invention and the steps that were taken to reduce the invention to practice) that determines which invention ends up with the patent.

You especially should be aware that you can unintentionally forfeit your right to obtain patent protection. This can happen if you disclose your invention to others, such as a company interested in the invention, and then do not file an application within one year from that disclosure date. Any public disclosure, such as in a speech, poster session, or publication (web or paper) begins a one-year countdown after which patents are precluded in the US. The same one-year period applies if you offer your invention, or a product made by your invention, for sale. You must file your patent application in the United States within one year from any offer of sale.

Even more confusing is the fact that most other countries do not allow this one-year grace period. Any public disclosure before you file your first application will prevent you from obtaining patent protection in nearly every country other than the United States.

15.1.5 Patent infringement

Patent infringement occurs when someone makes, uses, or sells a patented invention without the patent owner's permission. Defining infringement is one thing, but knowing when it occurs in the real world is something else. Even with common technologies, it can be difficult for experienced patent attorneys to tell whether patents have been infringed.

There are multiple steps in deciding whether infringement of a patent has occurred:

- identify the patent's independent apparatus and method claims
- break these apparati and method claims into their elements
- compare these elements with the alleged infringing device or process and decide whether the claim has all of the elements that constitute the alleged infringing device or process. If so, the patent has probably been infringed. If not, proceed to the next step
- if the elements the alleged infringing device or process are somewhat different than the elements of the patent claim, ask if they are the same in structure, function, and result. If yes, you probably have infringement. Note that
- for infringement to occur, only one claim in the patent
- needs to be infringed.

A patent's independent claims are those upon which usually one or more claims immediately following depend. A patent's broadest claims are those with the fewest words and that therefore provide the broadest patent coverage. The patent's broadest claims are its independent claims. As a general rule, if you find infringement of one of the broadest claims, all the other patent's claims that depend on that claim are infringed. Conversely, if you don't find infringement by comparison with a broad claim, then you won't find infringement of claims which depend on it. Although an infringement is declared on a claim-by-claim basis, generally it will be declared that the patent itself is infringed.

In apparatus (machine) claims, the elements are usually conceptualized as the a), b), c), etc. parts of the apparatus that are listed, interrelated, and described in detail following the word "comprising" at the end of the preamble of the claim. Elements in method (process) claims are the steps of the method and sub-parts of those steps.

If each and every element of the patent's broadest claims are in the infringing device, the patent is probably infringed. The reason you start by analyzing the broadest claim is that by definition, that claim has the fewest elements and it is therefore easier to find infringements.

Even if infringement can't be found on the basis of the literal language in the claims, the courts may still find infringement if the alleged infringing device's elements are equivalent to the patent claims in structure, function, and result. Known as the Doctrine of Equivalents, this rule is difficult to apply in practice.

15.1.6 A word or three of warning

There are at least three other considerations regarding patents that we have not addressed. One is the ownership of the patent, another is an invention disclosure, a third involves the cost of filing.

If you are a student developing material for a thesis or for a course, you need to be cognizant of the rules for patents as stated by your school or university. Dependent on the school, you may have complete rights to your invention, even if developed by you as part of a course under the direct supervision of a faculty member, or you may have no rights whatsoever. Often students in graduate courses, who are typically paid a stipend, are considered as having done their work for hire, whereas an undergraduate is paying the university to provide an experience. Do not wait to learn your rights through a lawyer, learn them now by accessing your school's Intellectual Property Statements.

Faculty often face the same challenges, as some universities even claim to own "shower patents" where a faculty has an idea at home and pursues it. Industry seldom claims ownership of ideas not related to an employee's work, but often enforce nondisclosure and noncompete documents.

If you are in an academic setting and are considering getting a patent either through your school or separately, it is advisable to inform your school of your work through an invention disclosure form. Such a form typically contains the following information:

1. Invention title
2. Inventors name(s), contribution(s), contact information
3. Contract or grant numbers
4. Are any IP agreements in place on this work?
5. Were any other parties involved?
6. Earliest date of idea conception
7. Invention description
8. Prior disclosures, nature, dates
9. Invention function (commercial)
10. List of possible licensees
11. Potential impediments to commercialization of invention
12. Signatures of inventor(s) and witnesses.

Filling out such a form will disclose to your university what stake, if any, they have in your invention. Filling out such a form will help protect you if there is a later claim by the university that you did NOT inform them of your work, if the school claims ownership. If there is a question as to whether your work is worth pursuing with a university claim, this document will enable your school to inform you that they do not wish to pursue the matter.

Filing for a patent can be expensive, you may consider an expense of around $10,000 to be a low average for a minimally complicated claim. It may be worth your while to let your school file and share in the proceeds, if applicable.

15.2 Copyrights

A copyright is a legal device that provides the creator of a work of authorship the right to control how the work is used. If someone wrongfully uses material covered by a copyright, the copyright owner can sue and obtain compensation for any losses suffered, as well as an injunction requiring the copyright infringer to stop the infringing activity.

A copyright is a type of tangible property. It belongs to its owner and the courts can be asked to intervene if anyone uses it without permission. Like other forms of property, a copyright may be sold by its owner, or otherwise exploited by the owner for economic benefit.

The Copyright Act of 1976 grants creators many intangible, exclusive rights over their work, including reproduction rights - the right to make copies of a protected work; distribution rights - the right to sell or otherwise distribute copies to the public; the right to create adaptations - the right to prepare new works based on the protected work; performance and display rights - the right to perform a protected work or display a work in public. Copyright law is evolving, the most recent revisions occurred in 1998.

Copyright protects all varieties of original works of authorship, including:

- literary works
- motion pictures, videos, and other audiovisual works
- photographs, sculpture, and graphic works
- sound recordings
- pantomimes and choreographic works
- architectural works.

15.2.1 What can be copyrighted?

Not every work of authorship receives copyright protection. A program or other work is protected if it satisfies all three of the following requirements:

- fixation
- originality
- minimal creativity.

The work must be fixed in a tangible medium of expression. Any stable medium from which the work can be read back or heard, either directly or with the aid of a machine or device, is acceptable.

Copyright protection begins the instant you fix your work. There is no waiting period and it is not necessary to register the copyright. Copyright protects both completed and unfinished works, as well as works that are widely distributed to the public or never distributed at all.

A work is protected by copyright only if, and to the extent, it is original. But this does not mean that copyright protection is limited to works that are novel - that is new to the world. For copyright purposes, a work is "original" if at least a part of the work owes its origin to the author. A work's quality, ingenuity, aesthetic merit, or uniqueness is not considered.

A minimal amount of creativity over and above the independent creation requirement is necessary for copyright protection. Works completely lacking creativity are denied copyright protection even if they have been independently created. However, the amount of creativity required is very slight.

In the past, some courts held that copyright protected works that may have lacked originality and or creativity if a substantial amount of work was involved in their creation. Recent court cases have outlawed this "sweat of the brow" theory. It is now clear that the amount of work put in to create a work of authorship has absolutely no bearing on the degree of copyright protection it will receive. Copyright only protects fixed, original, minimally creative expressions, not hard work.

Perhaps the greatest difficulty with copyrights is determining just what aspects of any given work are protected. All works of authorship contain elements that are protected by copyright and elements that are not protected. Unfortunately, there is no system available to precisely identify which aspects of a given work are protected. The only time we ever obtain a definitive answer as to how much any particular work is protected is when it becomes the subject of a copyright infringement lawsuit. However, there are two tenets which may help in determining what is protected and what is not. The first tenet states that a copyright only protects "expressions," not ideas, systems, or processes. Tenet two states the scope of copyright protection is proportional to the range of expression available. Let us look at both in detail.

Copyright only protects the tangible expression of an idea, system or process - not the idea, system or process itself. Copyright law does not protect ideas, procedures, processes, systems, mathematical principles, formulas, titles, algorithms, methods of operation, concepts, facts and discoveries. Remember, copyright is designed to aid the advancement of knowledge. If the copyright law gave a person a legal monopoly over ideas, the progress of knowledge would be impeded rather than helped.

The scope of copyright protection is proportional to the range of expression available. The copyright law only protects original works of authorship. Part of the essence of original authorship is the making of choices. Any work of authorship is the end result of a whole series of choices made by its creator. For example, the author of a novel expressing the idea of love must choose the novel's plot, characters, locale and the actual words used to express the story. The author of such a novel has a nearly limitless array of choices available. However, the choices available to the creators of many works of authorship are severely limited. In these cases, the idea or ideas underlying the work and the way they are expressed by the author are deemed to " merge". The result is that the author's expression is either treated as if it were in the public domain or protected only against virtually verbatim or "slavish" copying.

15.2.2 The copyright process

15.2.2.1 Copyright notice

Before 1989, all published works had to contain a copyright notice, (the "©" symbol followed by the publication date and copyright owner's name) to be protected by copyright. This is no longer necessary. Use of copyright notices is now optional in the United States. Even so, it is always a good idea to include a copyright notice on all work distributed to the public so that potential infringers will be informed of the underlying claim to copyright ownership. In addition, copyright protection is not available in some 20 foreign countries unless a work contains a copyright notice.

There are strict technical requirements as to what a copyright notice must contain. A valid copyright must contain three elements:

- *The copyright symbol* - use the familiar "©" symbol, i.e., the lower case letter "c" completely surrounded by a circle. The word "Copyright" or the abbreviation "Copr." are also acceptable in the United States, but not in many foreign countries. So if your work might be distributed outside the U.S., always use the "©" symbol.
- *The year in which the work was published* - you only need to include the year the work was first published.
- *The name of the copyright owner* - the owner is 1) the author or authors of the work, 2) the legal owner of a work made for hire, or 3) the person or entity to whom all the author's exclusive copyright rights have been transferred.

Although the three elements of a copyright notice need not appear in a particular order, it is common to list the copyright symbol, followed by the date and owners.

According to Copyright Office regulations, the copyright notice must be placed so as not be concealed from an ordinary user's view upon reasonable examination. A proper copyright notice should be included on all manuals and promotional materials. Notices on written works are usually placed on the title page or the page immediately following the title page.

15.2.2.2 Copyright registration

Copyright registration is a legal formality by which a copyright owner makes a public record in the U.S. Copyright Office in Washington D.C. of some basic information about a protected work, such as the title of the work, who wrote it and when, and who owns the copyright. It is not necessary to register to create or establish a copyright.

Copyright registration is a relatively easy process. You must fill out the appropriate pre-printed application form, pay an application fee, and mail the application and fee to the Copyright Office in Washington, D.C. along with two copies of the work being registered.

15.2.3 Copyright duration

One of the advantages of copyright protection is that it lasts a very long time. The copyright in a protectable work created after 1977 by an individual creator lasts for the life of the creator plus an additional 50 years. If there is more than one creator, the life plus 50 term is measured from the date the last creator dies. The copyright in works created by employees for their employers last for 75 years from the date of publication, or 100 years from the date of creation, whichever occurs first.

15.2.4 Protecting your copyright rights

The exclusive rights granted by the Copyright Act initially belong to a work's author. There are four ways to become an author:

- an individual may independently author a work
- an employer may pay an employee to create the work, in which case, the employer is the author under the work made for hire rule
- a person or business entity may specially commission an independent contractor to create the work under a written work made for hire contract, in which case, the commissioning party becomes the author
- two or more individuals or entities may collaborate to become joint authors.

The initial copyright owner of a work is free to transfer some or all copyright rights to other people or businesses, who will then be entitled to exercise the rights transferred.

15.2.5 Infringement

Copyright infringement occurs when a person other than the copyright owner exploits one or more of the copyright owner's exclusive rights without the owner's permission. A copyright owner who wins an infringement suit may stop any further infringement, obtain damages from the infringer and recover other monetary losses. This means, in effect, that a copyright owner can make a copyright infringer restore the author to the same economic position they would have been in had the infringement never occurred.

Copyright infringement is usually proven by showing that the alleged infringer had access to the copyright owner's work and that the protected expression in the two works is substantially similar. In recent years, the courts have held that the person who claims his work was infringed upon must subject his work to a rigorous filtering process to find out which elements of the work are and are not protected by copyright. In other words, the plaintiff must filter out from his work ideas, elements dictated by efficiency or external factors, or taken from the public domain. After this filtration process is completed, there may or may not be any protectable expression left.

15.3 Trademarks

A trademark is a work, name, symbol, or a combination used by a manufacturer to identify its goods and distinguish them from others. Trademark rights continue indefinitely as long as the mark is not abandoned and it is properly used.

A federal trademark registration is maintained by filing a declaration of use during the sixth year after its registration and by renewal every twenty years, as long as the mark is still in use. The federal law provides that non-use of a mark for two consecutive years is ordinarily considered abandonment, and the first subsequent user of the mark can claim exclusive trademark rights. Trademarks, therefore, must be protected or they will be lost. They must be distinguished in print form from other words and must appear in a distinctive manner.

Trademarks should be followed by a notice of their status. If it has been registered in the U.S. Patent Office, the registration notice "®" or "Reg. U.S. Pat Off," should be used. Neither should be used however, if the trademark has not been registered, but the superscripted letter "TM" should follow the mark, or an asterisk can be used to refer to a footnote starting "a trademark of xxx." The label compliance manager should remember that trademarks are proper adjectives and must be accompanied by the generic name for the product they identify. Trademarks are not to be used as possessives, not in the plural form.

A trademark is any visual mark that accompanies a particular tangible product, or line of goods, and serves to identify and distinguish it from products sold by others and it indicates its source. A trademark may consist of letters, words, names, phrases, slogans, numbers, colors, symbols, designs, or shapes.

As a general rule, to be protected from unauthorized use by others, a trademark must be distinctive in some way.

The word "trademark" is also a generic term used to describe the entire broad body of state and federal law that covers how businesses distinguish their products and services from the competition. Each state has its own set of laws establishing when and how trademarks can be protected. There is also a federal trademark law, called the Lanham Act, which applies in all fifty states. Generally, state trademark laws are relied upon for marks used only within one particular state, while the Lanham Act is used to protect marks for products that are sold in more than one state or across territorial or national borders.

15.3.1 Selecting a trademark

Not all trademarks are treated equally by the law. The best trademarks are "distinctive" - that is, they stand out in a customer's mind because they are inherently memorable. The more distinctive the trademark is, the stronger it will be and the more legal protection it will receive. Less distinctive marks are "weak" and may be entitled to little or no legal protection.

Generally, selecting a mark begins with brainstorming for general ideas. After several possible marks have been selected, the next step is often to use formal or informal market research techniques to see how the potential marks will be accepted by customers. Next, a "trademark search" is conducted. This means that an attempt is made to discover whether the same or similar marks are already in use.

15.3.1.1 What is a distinctive trademark?

A trademark should be created that is distinctive rather than descriptive. A trademark is "distinctive" if it is capable of distinguishing the product to which it is attached from competing products. Certain types of marks are deemed to be inherently distinctive and are automatically entitled to maximum protection. Others are viewed as not inherently distinctive and can be protected only if they acquire "secondary meaning" through use.

Arbitrary, fanciful or coined marks are deemed to be inherently distinctive and are therefore very strong marks. These are words and/or symbols that have absolutely no meaning in the particular trade or industry prior to their adoption by a particular manufacturer for use with its goods or services. After use and promotion, these marks are instantly identified with a particular company and product, and the exclusive right to use the mark is easily asserted against potential infringers.

Fanciful or arbitrary marks consist of common words used in an unexpected or arbitrary way so that their normal meaning has nothing to do with the nature of the product or service they identify. Some examples would be APPLE COMPUTER and PEACHTREE SOFTWARE.

Coined words are words made up solely to serve as trademarks, such as ZEOS or INTEL.

Suggestive marks are also inherently distinctive. A suggestive mark indirectly describes the product it identifies but stays away from literal descriptiveness. That is, the consumer must engage in a mental process to associate the mark with the product it identifies. For example, WORDPERFECT and VISICALC are suggestive marks.

Descriptive marks are not considered to be inherently distinctive. They are generally viewed by the courts as weak and thus not deserving of much, if any, judicial protection unless they acquire a "secondary meaning" - that is, become associated with a product in the public's mind through long and continuous use. There are three types of descriptive marks: 1) marks that directly describe the nature or characteristics of the product they identify (for example, QUICK MAIL), 2) marks that describe the geographic location from which the product emanates (for example, OREGON SOFTWARE), and 3) marks consisting primarily of a person's last name (for example, NORTON UTILITIES). A mark that is in continuous and exclusive use by its owner for a five-year period is presumed to have acquired secondary meaning and qualifies for registration as a distinctive mark.

A generic mark is a word(s) or symbol that is commonly used to describe an entire category or class of products or services, rather than to distinguish one product or service from another. Generic marks are in the public domain and cannot be registered or enforced under the trademark laws. Some examples of generic marks include "computer," "mouse," and "RAM." A term formerly protected as a trademark may lose such protection if it becomes generic. This often occurs when a mark is assimilated into common use to such an extent that it becomes the general term describing an entire product category. Examples would be ESCALATOR and XEROX.

15.3.2 The trademark process

A trademark is registered by filing an application with the PTO in Washington, D.C. Registration is not mandatory. Under both federal and state law, a company may obtain trademark rights in the states in which the mark is actually used. However, federal registration provides many important benefits including:

- the mark's owner is presumed to have the exclusive right to use the mark nationwide
- everyone in the country is presumed to know that the mark is already taken
- the trademark owner obtains the right to put an "®" after the mark
- anyone who begins using a confusingly similar mark after the mark has been registered will be deemed a willful infringer.
- the trademark owner obtains the right to make the mark "incontestable" by keeping it in continuous use for five years.

To qualify for federal trademark registration, a mark must meet several requirements. The mark must:

- actually be used in commerce
- be sufficiently distinctive to reasonably operate as a product identifier
- not be confusingly similar to an existing, federally registered trademark.

A mark you think will be good for your product could already be in use by someone else. If your mark is confusingly similar to one already in use, its owner may be able to sue you for trademark infringement and get you to change it and even pay damages. Obviously, you do not want to spend time and money marketing and advertising a new mark only to discover that it infringes on another preexisting mark and must be changed. To avoid this, state and federal trademark searches should be conducted to attempt to discover if there are any existing similar marks. You can conduct a trademark search yourself, either manually or with the aid of computer databases. You may also pay a professional search firm to do so.

15.3.3 Intent to use registration

If you seriously intend to use a trademark on a product in the near future, you can reserve the right to use the mark by filing an intent to use registration. If the mark is approved, you have six months to actually use the mark on a product sold to the public. If necessary, this period may be increased by six-month intervals up to 24 months if you have a good explanation for the delay. No one else may use the mark during this interim period. You should promptly file an intent to use registration as soon as you have definitely selected a trademark for a forthcoming product.

15.3.4 Protecting your trademark rights

The owner of a valid trademark has the exclusive right to use the mark on its products. Depending on the strength of the mark and whether and where it has been registered, the trademark owner may be able to bring a court action to prevent others from using the same or similar marks on competing or related products.

Trademark infringement occurs when an alleged infringer uses a mark that is likely to cause consumers to confuse the infringer's products with the trademark owner's products. A mark need not be identical to one already in use to infringe upon the owner's rights. If the proposed mark is similar enough to the earlier mark to risk confusing the average consumer, its use will constitute infringement.

Determining whether an average consumer might be confused is the key to deciding whether infringement exists. The determination depends primarily on whether the products or services involved are related, and, if so, whether the marks are sufficiently similar to create a likelihood of consumer confusion.

If a trademark owner is able to convince a court that infringement has occurred, she may be able to get the court to order the infringer to stop using the infringing mark and to pay monetary damages. Depending on whether the mark was registered, such damages may consist of the amount of the trademark owner's losses caused by the infringement or the infringer's profits. In cases of willful infringement, the courts may double or triple the damages award.

A trademark owner must be assertive in enforcing its exclusive rights. Each time a mark is infringed upon, it loses strength and distinctiveness and may eventually die by becoming generic.

15.4 Trade Secrets

Trade secrecy is basically a do-it-yourself form of intellectual property protection. It is based on the simple idea that by keeping valuable information secret, one can prevent competitors from learning about and using it. Trade secrecy is by far the oldest form of intellectual property, dating back at least to ancient Rome. It is useful now as it was then.

A trade secret is any formula, pattern, physical device, idea, process, compilation of information or other information that 1) is not generally known by a company's competitors, 2) provides a business with a competitive advantage, and 3) is treated in a way that can reasonably be expected to prevent the public or competitors from learning about it, absent improper acquisition or theft.

Trade secrets may be used to:

- protect ideas that offer a business a competitive advantage
- keep competitors from knowing that a program is under development and from learning its functional attributes

- protect source code, software development tools, design definitions and specifications, manuals, and other documentation
- protect valuable business information such as marketing plans, cost and price information and customer lists.

Unlike copyrights and patents, whose existence is provided and governed by federal law that applies in all fifty states, trade secrecy is not codified in any federal statute. Instead, it is made up of individual state laws. Nevertheless, the protection afforded to trade secrets is much the same in every state. This is partly because some 26 states have based their trade secrecy laws on the Uniform Trade Secrecy Act (1995), a model trade secrecy law designed by legal scholars.

15.4.1 What qualifies for trade secrecy

Information that is public knowledge or generally known cannot be trade secret. Things that everybody knows cannot provide anyone with a competitive advantage. However, information comprising a trade secret need not be novel or unique. All that is required is that the information not be generally known by people who could profit from its disclosure and use.

15.4.2 Trade secrecy authorship

Only the person that owns a trade secret has the right to seek relief in court if someone else improperly acquires or discloses the trade secret. Only the trade secret owner may grant others a license to use the secret.

As a general rule, any trade secrets developed by an employee in the course of employment belongs to the employer. However, trade secrets developed by an employee on their own time and with their own equipment can sometimes belong to the employee. To avoid possible disputes, it is a very good idea for employers to have all the employees who may develop new technology sign an employee agreement that assigns in advance all trade secrets developed by the employee during their employment to the company.

15.4.3 How trade secrets are lost

A trade secret is lost if either the product in which it is embodied is made widely available to the public through sales and displays on an unrestricted basis, or the secret can be discovered by reverse engineering or inspection.

15.4.4 Duration of trade secrets

Trade secrets have no definite term. A trade secret continues to exist as long as the requirements for trade secret protection remain in effect. In other words, as long as secrecy is maintained, the secret does not become generally known in the industry and the secret continues to provide a competitive advantage, it will be protected.

15.4.5 Protecting your trade secret rights

A trade secret owner has the legal right to prevent the following two groups of people from using and benefiting from its trade secrets or disclosing them to other without the owner's permission:

- people who are bound by a duty of confidentiality not to disclose or use the information
- people who steal or otherwise acquire the trade secret through improper means.

A trade secret owner's rights are limited to the two restricted groups of people discussed above. In this respect, a trade secret owner's rights are much more limited than those of a copyright owner or patent holder.

A trade secret owner may enforce their rights by bringing a trade secret infringement action in court. Such suits may be used to:

- prevent another person or business from using the trade secret without proper authorization
- collect damages for the economic injury suffered as a result of the trade secret's improper acquisition and use.

All persons responsible for the improper acquisition and all those who benefited from the acquisition are typically named as defendants in trade secret infringement actions. To prevail in a trade secret infringement suit, the plaintiff must show that the information alleged to be secret is actually a trade secret. In addition, the plaintiff must show that the information was either improperly acquired by the defendant or improperly disclosed, or likely to be so, by the defendant.

There are two important limits on trade secret protection. It does not prevent others from discovering a trade secret through reverse engineering, nor does it apply to persons who independently create or discover the same information.

15.4.6 A trade secrecy program

The first step in any trade secret protection program is to identify exactly what information and material is a company trade secret. It makes no difference in what form a trade secret is embodied. Trade secrets may be stored on computer hard disks or floppies, written down, or exist only in employees' memories.

Once a trade secret has been established, the protection program should include the following steps:

- maintain physical security
- enforce computer security
- mark confidential documents "Confidential"
- use non-disclosure agreements.

15.4.7 Use of trade secrecy with copyrights and patents

Trade secrecy is a vitally important protection for any medical device, but because of its limitations listed above, it should be used in conjunction with copyright and, in some cases, patent protection.

15.4.7.1 Trade secrets and patents

The federal patent laws provide the owner of a patentable invention with far greater protection than that available under trade secrecy laws. Trade secret protection is not lost when a patent is applied for. The Patent Office keeps patent applications secret unless or until a patent is granted. However, once a patent is granted and an issue feed paid, the patent becomes public record. Then all the information disclosed in the patent application is no longer a trade secret. This is so even if the patent is later challenged in court and invalidated.

If, for example, a software program is patented, the software patent applies only to certain isolated elements of the program. The remainder need not be disclosed in the patent and can remain a trade secret.

21.4.7.2 Trade secrets and copyrights

Trade secrecy and copyright are not incompatible. To the contrary, they are typically used in tandem to provide the maximum legal protection available.

Homework Exercises

1. What are the basic differences between a patent, a copyright, and a trademark? (To include: brief definition, rights included/excluded, lifespan of each.)
2. Give a specific example of material in which the creator would seek a patent, a copyright, a trademark.
3. One method of patent searching is to sift through the many patents in the USPTO (United States Patent and Technology Office) database. Go to http://www.uspto.gov. Do a patent search of a medical device of your choice. Write a brief summary of your search information. Of the six types of subject matter included under a patent, under which category can your material be classified? (Summary to include: exact definition of the item patented, who patented the device, application number, and date filed.) Hint: There are many ways to do a search on the USPTO homepage. One way is to click on Patents, then Issued Years and Patent Numbers, Search, Patent Database, Boolean, then enter MEDICAL into the query. However, you are not bound by these steps to search the database!
4. What are some alternatives to this method (sifting through the USPTO homepage) of patent searching?

5. Do a US patent search using your last name as a search term. Write up a patent found (no result, use Smith.) What does it do?
6. Do a copyright search similar to question 4.
7. One of the authors of this text holds patent number 3,591,806. How many other patents refer to this patent as prior art?
8. Draft an IP agreement with your advisor. Draft an IP disclosure for your work.
9. Outline your patent application for your design project.
10. Find and print out a copy of the first plant patent.
11. Find and print out a copy of the first utility patent. Contrast the reporting style used at this time (1836) with the current required style.

References

American Intellectual Property Law Association, *How to Protect and Benefit From Your Ideas*. Arlington, VA: American Intellectual Property Law Association Inc., 1988.

Banner & Allegretti, *An Overview of Changes to U.S. Patent and Trademark Office Rules and Procedures Effective June 8, 1995*. Chicago: Banner & Allegretti, Ltd., 1995.

Fishman Stephen, *Software Development - A Legal Guide*. Berkeley, California: Nolo Press, 1994.

Fries, Richard C., *Reliable Design of Medical Devices*. New York: Marcel Dekker, Inc., 1997.

Noonan, William D., "Patenting Medical Technology," in *The Journal of Legal Medicine*. Volume 11, Number 3, September, 1990.

Rebar, Linda A., "The Nurse as Inventor - Obtain a Patent and Benefit from Your Ideas," in *AORN Journal*, Volume 53, Number 2, February, 1991.

Sherman, Max, "Developing a Labeling Compliance Program," in *The Medical Device Industry*. New York: Marcel Dekker Inc., 1990.

U.S. Department of Commerce, *General Information Concerning Patents*. Washington, D.C.: U.S. Government Printing Office, 1993.

Web site information from the Library of Congress, http://www.loc.gov/

Web site information for Patents and Trademarks, http://www.uspto.gov/

Chapter 16

Premarket Testing and Validation

"The greatest lesson in life is to know that even fools are right sometimes."
Sir Winston Churchill

The heart of the product development process for hardware and software based systems is the verification and validation phase. During this time, testing indicates how well the product has been designed. The parts count reliability prediction had indicated whether the design would meet the reliability goal. It indicated what parts of the circuit had the potential for high failure rate. Design and tolerance analysis had indicated whether the correct component was being used and if it had been specified properly. None of these exercises had indicated how well the components would work together, once the device became operational. To obtain this information, the device must be tested both in its intended application environment as well as in the worst-case condition.

The product testing process for drugs follows a very different path, this subject will be covered in Section 16.5 and onward.

16.1 Standard Tests

Standard tests are conducted at room temperature, with no acceleration of any parameters. Standard tests are varied, dependent upon their purpose, and include:

- Cycle testing
- Typical use testing
- 10 x 10 testing.

16.1.1 Cycle testing

Cycle testing is usually conducted on individual components, such as switches, phone jacks or cable. Testing consists of placing the component in alternating states, such as ON and OFF for a switch or IN and OUT for a phone plug, while monitoring the operation in each state. One cycle consists of one pass through each state.

Cycle testing could also consist of passing through the state of operation and non-operation of a component or device. Thus a power supply could be power-cycled, with a cycle consisting of going from zero power to maximum power and back to zero. For devices, a cycle could consist of eight hours ON and 16 hours OFF.

16.1.2 Typical use testing

Typical use testing consists of operation of a device as it will be operated in its typical environment. This testing is usually incorporated when conducting a reliability demonstration or for calculating a long term mean time between failures (MTBF) value.

The test unit is tested electrically and mechanically prior to testing and certain parameters are checked at periodic times, such as 2, 4, 8, 24, 48, 72, 96 and 128 hours after beginning the test and weekly thereafter. These recordings aid in determining drift or degradation in certain parameters.

16.1.3 10 x 10 testing

Ten samples of a component or device are subjected to a test where recordings of a particular parameter are taken at 10 different time periods. A chart is created with the ten units listed in the left column and the ten recordings listed across the top (Figure 16-1). Mean and standard deviation values are calculated for each of the ten recordings and ten units.

By reading the horizontal rows of data, the repeatability of the results can be determined. By analyzing the vertical columns, the variability among the units can be measured.

Software verification and validation requires that evidence be collected to demonstrate that the process and the product have met specified requirements. Verification is normally associated with and performed during product development to assure that the software development process, methodology and design has been met by the current version of the software and product. Validation is a terminal activity to software development and demonstrates that the software design and implemented code satisfies the predetermined requirements and specifications for the product. There are other fundamental differences between software verification and validation, but the primary difference is that verification assures that the software was developed according to a documented process and validation assures that the product and software requirements were satisfied.

The application of the principles of quality control, quality assurance, safety and software verification and validation in the medical product manufacturing industry has changed dramatically. Consumer expectations and international competition have increased the pressures to produce goods of the highest quality at a reasonable cost. This expectation for the highest quality product at the most reasonable price is balanced against the consumer and government requirement that medical products must be safe, effective and efficacious at any cost.

Testing the final product for compliance to predetermined specifications is no longer adequate to assure the quality of the product or its software. Manufacturers must assure the quality of the product through the design and development phases of the product life cycle. Software verification and validation should be designed to maximize the assurance of quality and minimize testing.

Unit	1	2	3	4	5	6	7	8	9	10	Mean	S.D.
1	350	380	400	360	340	370	330	340	360	340	357	20
2	200	130	190	200	130	150	250	230	240	160	188	41
3	270	250	270	240	300	230	330	330	300	350	287	39
4	270	140	160	170	160	140	430	130	130	130	186	90
5	230	180	170	150	260	240	210	230	240	210	212	33
6	280	180	70	390	300	210	400	440	370	230	287	110
7	180	210	270	190	210	170	170	270	190	200	206	34
8	190	220	180	190	170	190	200	120	170	130	176	29
9	200	180	160	180	200	120	90	170	140	170	161	33
10	230	190	260	180	290	170	280	220	260	170	225	43
Mean	240	206	213	225	236	199	269	248	240	209		
S.D.	50	66	85	78	67	67	100	95	80	74		

Figure 16-1 10 x 10 test matrix. (From Fries, 1991.)

In the complex regulatory environment of medical products, the only way to satisfy the requirements of the myriad regulatory agencies, international communities and corporate commitments is to establish a systematic approach to medical product software development. This systematic approach must adhere to the basic principles of quality assurance and provide efficient and effective management of commitments. A good software quality assurance program will minimize redundancy, assure access to information and integrate information from all disciplines and levels of the organization. It will also provide the advantage of flexibility, particularly when standards frequently change, where management can impose new directives and products and technologies evolve quickly. A rigorous yet flexible software quality assurance program provides the stability and assurance that can allow a corporation to respond proactively to its market and competition without risking product quality or patient safety.

Software verification and validation must be performed whenever the quality or effectiveness of the product cannot be adequately tested or evaluated in the final product. Verification and validation is also appropriate for 1) utility systems, support software or test equipment and software whose failure could directly affect the safety of the product, patient, consumer or user; 2) any software or equipment and its software that is unique or custom designed; and 3) any software or equipment and its software whose reliability or reproducibility is unknown or suspect.

Software verification and validation requires that evidence be collected to demonstrate that the process and the product have met specified requirements. Verification is normally associated with and performed during product development to assure that the software development process, methodology and design has been met by the current version of the software and product. Validation is a terminal activity to software development and demonstrates that the software design and implemented code satisfies the predetermined requirements and specifications for the product. There are other fundamental differences between software verification and validation but the primary difference is that verification assures that the software was developed according to a documented process and validation assures that the product and software requirements were satisfied.

16.2 Allocation of Software Testing

In order to achieve uniform, consistent and sufficient software test coverage it is of benefit to allocate the various aspects of software testing to corresponding software life cycles activities. During the design process and activities, the software designers perform their design activities and store the resultant design. While the design evolves, the designers should generate test information sheets that will specify the testing to be conducted in order to validate the implemented design. The test information sheets should be used and reviewed as a part of the design walk-through. Since these tests are at the discretion of the designer, they should be prioritized by safety, reliability, effectiveness or performance and then any other appropriate criteria. These tests should target the integrated software components, the interfaces between the integrated tasks or functions and path testing between the various tasks and functions.

When the design has been completed, it is given to the programmers who will create the source code. As the programmers generate the code, they should also generate test information sheets that specify the testing to be conducted in order to validate the implemented design and requirements. the test information sheets should be used and reviewed as a part of the code walk-through. Since these tests are at the discretion of the programmer, they should be prioritized by safety, reliability, effectiveness or performance and then any other appropriate criteria. These tests should target the individually completed components for functionality, robustness and stress testing. The code that is constructed by the programmer will also undergo debug testing. This level of testing is at the function, routine or component level and satisfies path testing, interface testing and logic or branch testing.

After the code has been implemented and integrated the formal testing commences. Both the software development engineers as well as the software verification and validation engineers perform this type of testing. The software developers will execute their testing based on the test information sheets that were generated as the design and code evolved. the software verification and validation engineers will have produced a second set of test information sheets based on the design and code that was documented in the software requirements and software design document. At the conclusion of this formal testing both types of test information sheets are reviewed for adequacy, completeness and coverage and signed off and archived.

16.3 Verification and Validation Test Method Commonality

The safety and performance characteristics of products and their software must be judged by methods that are reliable. Test method verification and validation is a fundamental building block of any software quality assurance program and it begins during the development of a new product or with the integration of new capabilities into an existing product. Not only do correct or passing test results get recorded, but unacceptable or failure results must not be ignored or discounted without adequate rationale or justification. Test results that do not meet their specification must be investigated and the investigation should be appropriate, competent, timely and complete. Most important of all, the investigation results and rationale must be determined.

Software verification by definition requires a stable and defined life cycle. Any organization desiring to create a cohesive and efficient verification and validation effort must first define a software life cycle covering the "cradle to grave" development of the software produced. Once this is accomplished, its application to a project is made. Be prepared for setbacks but do not change the defined process unless absolutely necessary. One implementation of an industry accepted life cycle is as good as another and allowing deviations while executing the new process causes inconsistency which over time places doubt in the minds of the users and ultimately erodes your confidence in the process. Validation requires and assumes that verification is working. In fact, it mandates that there is a defined process that is consistently being followed. It is possible to perform validation without verification, but if validation testing finds a design error late in the software development life cycle, then it is significantly costlier to correct than if it was found during the earlier verification phases.

An efficient verification and validation organization is capable of producing salient results during the validation effort and permeating a common test approach. The first step in establishing this effort requires performing a survey of each product line and the test equipment that the software verification and validation group will support. The outcome of this survey is the generation of two lists that identify the microprocessors and controllers and the software languages that were found. For example, the first list might show 80x86, 8051, and 8085 and the second list would be assembly language for each microprocessor and controller on the first list as well as any high-level languages, such as "C" and "QBASIC."

The second step is to implement a Common Test Set (CTS) containing a suite of static and dynamic test tools that run on all products and equipment undergoing software verification and validation. This is the first step at promoting a commonality of verification and validation intent across the corporation's products and supporting test equipment. The CTS should be employed as soon as software becomes available and should be viewed as both a bench test and a run-time software test tool. The static branch of the CTS tools requires only the source code and functions as the bench test effort. An example of a static tool would be the Lint for "C" software. The dynamic branch of the CTS tools provides the run-time test capability that includes both the computer host environment as well as the target hardware. In the computer host environment, debuggers and simulators will dominate. The tools for the target environment include in-circuit emulators, timing and event diagramming devices and execution profilers.

The third branch of the CTS encompasses the data generator tools that could also be labeled as remote communications tools. Given the pervasive remote communications capability in most medical products, either through RS-232-C or GPIB, support must be provided for this area. A common tool for this is National Instruments LABView that provides the capability to communicate via different protocols. This branch provides a wealth of opportunity to automate software testing of the product being developed because canned batch mode data files can be generated and executed in a fraction of the time that any other method of testing consumes. Taken one step farther, a tool can be developed that acts as an editor in quickly creating a wide variety of test scenarios.

16.4 Validation and Test Overview

Medical companies are faced with validating both products and test and manufacturing equipment. The test and manufacturing equipment spans the range from manufacturer developed hardware and software support equipment at one end to software written or modified by the manufacturer that executes on a host PC or workstation at the other end. While there is a significant difference between products and test and manufacturing equipment, there are basic software standards that are applicable to both and a common approach to software validation should be applied. The only caveat is that the level of validation effort should be adjusted and based on the potential of harm to the customer or user and the view that some equipment will fall under process validation.

Within the phases of software development the generic activities concerned with testing are code and test, integrate and test, and software system testing. The code and test activities include development of the code and debugging the implemented code by the software developers. The integrate and test activities include the integration of software components and the testing of the integrated parts. The software system testing activity typically encompasses the verification and validation testing that is performed by the software verification and validation engineers on the fully integrated software and hardware.

16.4.1 Techniques, methodologies and test approach

The software validation approach and the test categories to be applied to the product and test and manufacturing equipment should be selected based on the categorization of the life cycle that the product or test and manufacturing equipment belongs to. For example, if the product or test and manufacturing equipment is new and deemed to be a high level of concern, then a full software development life cycle process should be adhered to. If the product or test and manufacturing equipment to be produced is based on an existing baseline which has accumulated sufficient runtime to realize a high level of confidence that a majority of the faults have been detected, then an accelerated enhancement development life cycle should be followed.

The test approach to any product or test and manufacturing equipment should be a combination of requirements testing and safety testing. Requirements' testing encompasses a rigorous development effort that includes the production of a requirements design specification. Once the requirements and design are solidified and approved, the software verification and validation engineers can systematically detail the requirements to be tested and trace them to the design in the design specification. The embodiment of this effort is the Requirements Traceability Matrix. Completing the Requirements Traceability Matrix requires that the software verification and validation engineers complete the final column of the Requirements Traceability Matrix that details the testing performed to validate the requirement. This thorough and systematic approach to requirements testing provides high confidence that the test coverage was sufficient.

Safety testing takes a different approach to validation in that the focus is shifted to preventing harm to the user. This approach is aimed at producing a product or equipment that is safe for its intended use. When applied to medical products, a key element to this approach is the production of a hazard analysis. This analysis starts at the system level and decomposes the product into its mechanical, electrical, and software components. This analysis attempts to mitigate single point failures or justify a single error trap by calculating a low probability of occurrence. Safety testing of a medical product requires the utilization of the hazards analysis in the software validation effort. When applied to equipment validation, safety testing takes on a different meaning. Safety in this perspective requires surveying the environment and role that the equipment plays in supporting the production of a safe product. If the equipment is utilized to make a pass or fail determination of a product on a production line then the safety issue is elevated. Furthermore, if the test and manufacturing equipment is the sole check of a function of a product before it leaves the production line and is boxed for shipment, then the safety issue is elevated to the level of the product it supports. By contrast, if the equipment consists of a label generator, then safety testing ensures control of the software and validating that the process in place minimizes the chances of an error occurring due to human intervention.

The preferred software test approach to all products or test and manufacturing equipment is white box testing as opposed to black box testing, but this may not be warranted for all functions such as user interface testing. Furthermore, code inspection as the sole technique for validation is to be avoided unless the change is a hard coded data change such as strings or constants as opposed to a logic change which alters the instruction order.

Software testing of a product or test and manufacturing equipment is normally performed at the software component level and software system level. Software component level testing concentrates on individual components or grouping of components as opposed to software system level testing where the focus is on the performance of the software as a complete entity. Software component level testing is performed during the code and test activities and the integrate and test activities and is best performed by the software developers. Software system level testing is performed during the software system testing activity and should be performed by the software verification and validation engineers.

16.4.2 Software testing requirements

Software component level testing is concerned with subsections of the software product and the integration of these subsections. This level of testing is the responsibility of the software engineers who develop the code. Products that fall into the full development life cycle should address this subject in a software development plan. The software verification and validation engineers should perform software system level testing.

The software systems level testing begins with the software verification and validation engineers completing the requirements traceability matrix except for the test column. The software verification and validation engineers then validate the process that the developers used to create the software system. If necessary, all compiles and links must set the highest warning level flags to produce detailed listings. The verification and validation testing will be performed from a known and controlled test bed. The software verification and validation engineers now perform software fault insertion testing. for embedded software, the verification and validation engineers utilize the in-circuit emulator with the latest software and hardware to perform the functional, robustness, stress, and safety testing. The verification and validation engineers should then remove the in-circuit emulator and perform functional and robustness testing of the user interface and stress testing of the remote communications interface.

The software verification and validation engineers should then execute the appropriate CTS test suite in order to locate software design errors, suspicious coding practices, unused variables, improperly scoped variables and to reverse engineer software in generating test cases. For embedded software, the verification and validation engineers should validate the EPROM burn-in procedure. This should be conducted by using inconsistent memory fill techniques such as all ones, all zeros, halt OPCODE or a jump to an interrupt service routine that handles an illegal address error.

After all testing has been concluded, including the verification of any fixes due to errors produced by the software system tests, the software verification and validation engineers complete and review the requirements traceability matrix in order to verify that all requirements have been tested and satisfied. The software verification and validation engineers then complete the requirements traceability matrix and any necessary reports in order to provide closure. The software verification and validation engineers then complete the software verification and validation report and submit it to a controlled environment. A software verification and validation report includes a version specific identifier, such as the Cyclic Redundancy Check (CRC) identifier. In addition, the software verification and validation report lists all baselined items and specifications that were verified with this version of software.

16.4.3 Verification and validation reporting

The test documentation that is generated for a particular product or equipment depends on the life cycle and its level of concern classification. The verification and validation report summarizes the results of the verification and validation activity. The summary should contain:

- Description of the tasks performed
- Time or number of cycles each activity was run
- Summary of task results
- Summary of errors found and their resolution
- Assessment of the software reliability.

When summarizing the errors found, the report should include:

- Description and location
- Impact

- Criticality
- Rationale for resolution
- Results of retest.

Any deviations from the test plan must be highlighted and justified in the test summary.

16.5 The Essentials of Software Testing

Edward Kit lists six essentials of software testing:

- the quality of the test process determines the success of the test effort
- prevent defect migration by using early life-cycle testing techniques
- the time for software testing tools is now
- a real person must take responsibility for improving the test process
- testing is a professional discipline requiring trained, skilled people
- cultivate a positive team attitude of creative destruction.

16.5.1 The quality of the test process determines the success of the test effort

The quality of a software system is primarily determined by the quality of the software process that produced it. Likewise, the quality and effectiveness of software testing are primarily determined by the quality of the test processes used.

Testing has its own cycle. The testing process begins with the product requirements phase and from there parallels the entire development process. In other words, for each phase of the development process, there is an important testing activity.

Test groups that operate within organizations having an immature development process will feel more pain than those that don't. But regardless of the state of maturity, the test group can and should focus on improving its own internal process. An immature test process within an immature development organization will result in an unproductive, chaotic, frustrating environment that produces low quality results and unsatisfactory products. People effectively renovating a testing process within that same immature organization will serve as a catalyst for improving the development process as a whole.

16.5.2 Prevent defect migration by using early life-cycle testing techniques

More than half the errors are usually introduced in the requirements phase. The cost of errors is minimized if they are detected in the same phase as they are introduced, and an effective test program prevents the migration of errors from any development phase to any subsequent phases.

While many of us are aware of this, in practice we often do not have mechanisms in place to detect these errors until much later - often not until function and system test, at which point we have entered "the Chaos Zone." Chances are that we are currently missing the best opportunity for improving the effectiveness of our testing if we are not taking advantage of the proven testing techniques that can be applied early in the development process.

16.5.3 The time for software testing tools is now

After many years of observation, evaluation, and mostly waiting, we can now say the time for testing tools has arrived. There are a wide variety of tool vendors to choose from, many of which have mature, healthy products.

It is important to have a strategy for tool acquisition and a proper procedure for handling tool selection. While such procedures are based on common sense, they do need to be systematically implemented. Tool acquisition is an area where there may be a strong case for seeking independent expert advice.

16.5.3 A real person must take responsibility for improving the testing process

If the testing group is feeling pain, start campaigning for improvements to a few of the key issues, such as better specifications, and better reviews and inspections. Management should appoint an architect or small core team to prioritize potential improvements and lead the testing improvement effort, and must make it clear that they will give their ongoing support. It is not rocket science - but it takes effort and time. Tools can help tremendously, but they must be used within an overall test process that includes effective test planning and design.

16.5.4 Testing is a professional discipline requiring trained and skilled people

The software testing process has evolved considerably and has reached the point where it is a discipline requiring trained professionals. To succeed today, an organization must be adequately staffed with skilled software testing professionals who get proper support from management. Testing should be independent, unbiased, and organized for the fair sharing of recognition and rewards for contributions made to product quality.

16.5.6 Cultivate a positive team attitude of creative destruction

Testing requires disciplined creativity. Good testing, that is devising and executing successful tests, tests that discover the defects in a product, requires real ingenuity and may be viewed as destructive. Indeed, considerable creativity is needed to destroy something in a controlled and systematic way. Good testers are methodically taking the product apart, finding its weaknesses, and pushing it up to and beyond its limits.

Establishing the proper "test to break" mental attitude has a profound effect on testing success. If the objective is to show that the product does what it shouldn't do, and doesn't do what it should, we're on the way to testing success. Although far from the norm today, the results that we get when practitioners and their managers together cultivate this attitude of disciplined, creative destruction are nothing less than astonishing.

Successful testing requires a methodological approach. It requires us to focus on the basic critical factors: planning, project and process control, risk, management, inspections, measurement, tools, organization, and professionalism. Remember that testers make a vital positive contribution throughout the development process to ensure the quality of the product.

16.6 Drug Development

Over two billion prescriptions per year are filled in the United States for drugs regulated by the Food and Drug Administration. Perhaps an equal number of drugs are purchased over the counter for compounds that once were categorized as prescription based, such as NasalCrom. With the estimated cost of a single new drug making it to market estimated at almost $400,000,000 drug development and sales is a major industry.

Drugs are developed in one of three ways (or combinations thereof). One method involves trial and error testing of a series of developed compounds estimated to have a possible effect on the process to be modified. These compounds are placed in, as appropriate, enzymes, cell cultures, or other cultures to see if there is any effect. A second method involves computer modeling of the chemical structure of receptor sites, blocking enzymes, or chemical structure of enzymes implicated in the process to be modified. Estimated interactions are used to guide the search for candidate compounds to test. A third method involves the acquisition and testing of unusual fungi, viruses, molds, etc. and the testing of these materials for effect on the relevant cell lines or cultures. Samples are collected from all sources, from jungle climates to the oceans.

Once a drug has made it past test tube testing, tests must be done on at least two relevant animal models. These tests are aimed at quantifying the overall drug effect, the processing of the drug by the body, and absorption rates and ranges. At least two relevant animal models are mandated; this is due to past adverse drug experiences with the use of only a single animal model for testing purposes (thalidomide, for example). The main animals used in research are rats, mice and other rodents (85-90% of all experiments), dogs and cats (less than 1%), and nonhuman primates (less than .3%). (Foundation for Biomedical Research data, 1997). Some animal models are good for specific disease studies, for example: armadillos can get leprosy and thus are a good model for this disease, zebrafish are good models for genetic studies, especially since they are transparent.

The structure and function of the facility doing the research on drug development, it is worth noting now, must follow government regulations for "good laboratory practice." This regulation (21CFR Part 58) sets minimal standards for the organization of the testing facility, the animal care and testing procedures, the test and reporting procedures, the requirement for quality assurance, the retention of records, etc. This regulation is equivalent to the ISO9000 series of standards, but explicit for non-clinical laboratory facilities. This structure helps assure that laboratories are properly run and the results of the activity are correctly documented. Failure to properly do so can result in fines and decertification.

16.7 Clinical Trials

If a drug has proven to be effective on animal models of a disease, the testing of the drug may proceed to clinical trials if the FDA is satisfied that the animal model testing has shown potential value for the disease under study. This testing process involves clearance of the protocol through a human patients subject committee and three phases of investigation.

The human patients subject committee is a panel of medical and lay personnel who study the proposed drug test and protocol. The panel will generally include an ethicist and/or clerical personal, as well as others with an interest in the benefit of the study as well as the risks. The panel will take special interest in being sure that the study involves informed consent. The need for randomization of treatment, as well as for placebos will also be scrutinized.

Phase 1 of a clinical trial generally involves a small number of people (20-100), these people are typically healthy volunteers or patients. Phase 1 studies are designed to assess the drug for acute adverse effects and examine the size of doses that patients can take safely without a high incidence of side effects. These studies are also used to determine the best mode of entry of the drug (oral, skin, etc.). Initial clinical studies also are designed to determine what happens to a drug in the human body - whether it's metabolized or stays intact, how much of it (or a metabolite) gets into the blood and various organs, how long it stays in the body, and how the body gets rid of the drug and its effects. These studies should complement the earlier work done on animals, where the use of tracers (radioactive and other) is more easily justified. About 70% of all new drugs pass this first test, these initial studies typically take a few months to perform.

Phase 2 studies involve testing in several hundred patients, mainly to determine short-term safety and effectiveness. About half of all drugs that make it through phase 1 fail at this point. These studies typically take months to years to perform.

Phase 3 tests involve several hundred to several thousand patients, the primary questions being addressed are those of drug safety, dosage, and effectiveness. With such a large sampling, good statistics may be obtained with respect to minor drug reactions, which will be documented in the literature that will accompany the prescription when and if marketed. About 60-70% of drugs tested in phase 2 make it through phase 3, however tracking back to an initial 5000 drugs or compounds studied, only one makes it this far.

Once phase 3 is satisfied, the FDA is petitioned for a new drug approval, which takes an additional two years on average. Phase 4 of the drug process now investigates the continued efficacy and long-term effects of the drug in use.

Homework Exercises

1. You are in charge of setting up the test sequence for a new heart-bypass pump system. The system has a C++ software control scheme for flow control. Maximum expected length of use of the machine will be for surgeries lasting no more than six hours. List some of the test methods you would use for this device.
2. What advantages can you find for the use of LABView as a testing tool? Detail how you would use this package in a testing system.
3. Estimate the types of tests necessary for validation of an implanted defibrillator system. What would be a minimum number of tests be determined by?
4. Purely mechanical systems need not undergo some of the tests that software/hardware systems do. Contrast the types of tests you would perform on an artificial knee vs. the types of tests you would perform on an insulin pump.
5. Visit the Foundation for Biomedical Research home page (www.fbresearch.org), find and list the data for other species (other than cat, dog, etc.) and the uses for these species in research.

6. Find and visit the People for Ethical Treatment of Animals home pages (www.peta.org). Comment on the nature of this site in contrast to the above foundation site.
7. Visit http://www.fda.gov/cdrh/devadvice/part058.html. Look at contents and become familiar with the requirements for good laboratory practice. Write a brief summary of the contents of this web site.
8. Investigate and report on the composition of the Human Subjects Committee at your site.
9. Do a web search and report on at least one drug each in phases 1, 2, and 3.
10. Investigate and report on the history of the drug thalidomide.
11. Investigate and report on the drug diethylstilbestrol (DES).
12. Investigate and report on one "Orphan Drug".

References

Evans, Michael W. and John J. Marciniak., *Software Quality Assurance & Management*. New York: John Wiley & Sons, Inc., 1987.

Fagan, Michael E., "Design and Code Inspections to Reduce Errors in Program Development," *IBM Systems Journal*. Volume 15, Number 3, p. 182-211.

Fairley, Richard E., *Software Engineering Concepts*. New York: McGraw-Hill Book Company, 1985.

Frankel, E. G., *Systems Reliability and Risk Analysis*. The Hague: Martinus Nijhoff Publishers, 1984.

Fries, Richard C., *Reliability Assurance for Medical Devices, Equipment and Software*. Buffalo Grove, IL: Interpharm Press, Inc., 1991.

Fries, Richard C., Paul Pienkowski and Joseph Jorgens III, "Safe, Effective, and Reliable Software Design and Development for Medical Devices," *Medical Instrumentation*. Volume 30, Number 2, March/April, 1996.

IEEE., *IEEE Standards Collection - Software Engineering*. New York: The Institute of Electrical and Electronic Engineers, Inc., 1993.

Ireson, W. Grant and Clyde F. Coombs Jr., *Handbook of Reliability Engineering and Management.* New York: McGraw-Hill Book Company, 1988.

Jensen, F. and N. E. Peterson, *Burn-In.* New York: John Wiley and Sons, 1982.

Kit, Edward, *Software Testing in the Real World - Improving the Process.* Reading, MA: Addison-Wesley Publishing Company, 1995.

Laplante, Phillip, *Real-Time Systems Design and Analysis - An Engineer's Handbook.* New York: The Institute of Electrical and Electronic Engineers, Inc., 1993.

Leveson, Nancy G., "Software Safety: Why, What, and How," *Computing Surveys.* Volume 18, Number 2, June, 1986.

Lloyd, D. K., and M. Lipow, *Reliability Management, Methods and Management.* 2nd Edition. Milwaukee, WI: American Society for Quality Control, 1984.

Logothetis, N. and H. P. Wynn, *Quality Through Design.* London, England: Oxford University Press, 1990.

Mason, R. L., W. G. Hunter, and J. S. Hunter, *Statistical Design and Analysis of Experiments.* New York: John Wiley & Sons, 1989.

MIL-STD-202, *Test Methods for Electronic and Electrical Component Parts.* Washington, DC: Department of Defense, 1980.

MIL-STD-750, *Test Methods for Semiconductor Devices.* Washington, DC: Department of Defense, 1983

MIL-STD-781, *Reliability Design Qualification and Production Acceptance Tests: Exponential Distribution.* Washington, DC: Department of Defense, 1977.

MIL-STD-883, *Test Methods and Procedures forMicroelectronics.* Washington, D.C.: Department of Defense, 1983.

Montgomery, D. C., *Design and Analysis of Experiments*. 2nd Edition. New York: John Wiley & Sons, 1984.

Myers, Glenford J., *The Art of Software Testing*. New York: John Wiley and Sons, 1979.

Neufelder, Ann Marie, *Ensuring Software Reliability*. New York: Marcel Dekker, Inc., 1993.

O'Connor, Patrick D. T., *Practical Reliability Engineering*. 3rd Edition. Chichester, England: John Wiley & Sons, 1991.

Pressman, R., *Software Engineering*. New York: McGraw-Hill Book Company, 1987.

Reliability Analysis Center, *Nonelectronic Parts Reliability Data: 1995*. Rome, NY: Reliability Analysis Center, 1994.

Ross, P. J., *Taguchi Techniques for Quality Engineering*. New York: McGraw-Hill, 1988.

Taguchi, Genichi, *Introduction to Quality Engineering*. Unipub/Asian Productivity Association, 1986.

Taguchi, Genichi, *Systems of Experimental Design*. Unipub/Asian Productivity Association, 1978.

Yourdon, Edward., *Modern Structured Analysis*. Englewood Cliffs, New Jersey: Yourdon Press, 1989.

Chapter 17

System Testing

"You make it, I'll break it"
Sign in Reliability Engineer Richard C. Fries' Lab

System testing is the final stage in the verification and validation of a product. System testing is the first time the full product is together and functioning and is a time to not only check that the unit as a whole functions according to specification, but to check the robustness of the unit when stressed by environmental and customer misuse conditions.

17.1 Purpose

The main purpose of the system test is to ensure the product, as a whole, functions according to its specification. Each requirement in the specification must be verified (see Parsing Requirements in Chapter 16). The compatibility of the hardware and software is verified, both at normal settings of the parameters as well as at the upper and lower limits of each parameter. Any claims made in either operating manuals or advertising must be verified.

In addition to the above testing, the robustness of the unit must be verified. The product is subjected to various stresses, such as:

- temperature
- humidity
- altitude
- shock
- vibration
- electromagnetic interference
- cell phone interference
- power surges
- brownouts
- electrostatic discharge
- spillage
- shipping.

The product is also subjected to potential customer misuse. The project team will hold a brainstorming session to discuss how a customer could misuse the product. Examples of actual misuse include:

- placing a container of liquid on a portion of the product, having the container tip over, and the contents spill into the machine
- a customer sitting on a portion of a product used as a table
- cross-connecting electrical connectors that are not keyed
- connecting a battery in the wrong polarity
- dropping the device on the ground, into a sink full of water, or into a toilet.

A story of the development of the CD illustrates the point. When the first CDs were prototyped, the manufacturer sent some home with employees to use, with the demand that they be returned in one month for analysis. When they were returned, the manufacturer was amazed to find food particles in the grooves of the CD. People had snack food on their hands when they were handling the CDs and this got into the grooves, reducing the playability of the CD. Customer misuse can be one of the more interesting activities conducted during the development cycle.

This is also a good time to test potential hazards which the device may present to the user. For example, there was a metal container which was to be placed in a hospital ceiling through which passed the various electrical, phone, and gas tubes. On the outside of the container were the electrical outlets, gas connections, and phone outlets. When a repair was needed, maintenance personnel were to push up on the box, slide the box forward out of its frame, and lower it. The box was hanging from four chains attached to the frame. The question arose, what happens if the box is pushed up, slid forward, and then dropped, as the maintenance personnel lose their grip on the box? To test this theory, a frame was made and the box inserted. It was then pushed off the frame with a wooden pole and allowed to drop. The first time, all four chains broke. After two more iterations, no chains broke and the maintenance personnel were eternally grateful.

17.2 Failure Definition

For each test and for each device, a failure must be defined. This definition depends on the intended application and the anticipated environment. What is considered a failure for one component or device may not be a failure for another. The test protocol should be as detailed as possible in defining the failure.

17.3 Types of Testing

Types of testing depends on the type of product being developed, and may include event testing, stress testing, environmental testing, time related testing and failure related testing.

17.3.1 Event testing

Event testing consists of repeated testing of equipment through its cycle of operation, either typical application or extreme limits of parameter ranges until failure occurs. This type of testing is analogous to time-to-failure testing. One important parameter developed from this type of test is the number of cycles to failure.

17.3.3 Stress testing

Stress testing involves the application of various stresses, especially input voltage vibration, or temperature. It is important in determining the robustness of a device, but care must be taken in its application. Too much stress may cause the test results to be inconclusive, as excess stress may precipitate a failure that the product would not normally experience during normal usage. Care should also be taken to apply stress in steps, rather than getting to the maximum value immediately. If the device fails, the step method allows the determination of where in the progression of stress applications the failure occurred.

17.3.4 Environmental testing

Environmental testing represents a survey of the reaction of a device to the environmental and shipping environments, it should experience in its daily usage. By investigating a broad spectrum of the environmental space, greater confidence is developed in the equipment than if it was merely subjected to ambient conditions. As with overstress testing, unusually extreme or unrealistic environmental levels should be avoided because of the difficulty in their interpretation.

17.3.4.1 Operating temperature/humidity testing

This test verifies the system operates according to specification at the extremes of its operating temperature and humidity specification.

17.3.4.2 Storage temperature/humidity testing

This test verifies the system operates according to specification after exposure to the extremes of its storage temperature and humidity specification.

17.3.4.3 Altitude testing

This test verifies the system operates according to specification at the extremes of its barometric pressure specifications.

17.3.4.4 Threshold testing

This test verifies a fully loaded system survives crossing a 3/16" threshold. The system is usually subjected to 1,000 cycles of passing over the threshold.

17.3.4.5 Vibration testing

This test verifies the system will survive subjection to random vibration at a typical force of 3 Gs.

17.3.4.6 ISTA shipping test

ISTA is a standards recommending organization dedicated to the development of safe packaging. ISTA stands for International Sate Transit Association. This test verifies the system will survive the stresses of shipping the packaged product via a common carrier. Stresses to be considered in this test are temperature, humidity, vibration, impact, and shock.

17.3.5 Electromagnetic interference

The device must be evaluated according to the various tests listed below for the purpose of both engineering evaluation and for compliance to EN 60601-1-2. Documentation should consist of a brief test report including the following: a description of the test, or related IEC standard, test failure criteria, configuration(s), a discussion of the data obtained, the data itself, and a short conclusion.

The tests described below are essentially the "EN 1000 series (formerly IEC 801 series)" and additional EMC tests that have been found beneficial for product performance evaluation. Testing usually consists of the following:

- Radiated Electric Field Immunity
- Fast Transients Immunity
- Electrical Surge Transients Immunity
- Line Conducted
- Magnetic Field

- Voltage Dips, Short Interruptions and Voltage Variation Immunity
- Voltage and Frequency Fluctuations
- On/Off Power Cycling
- Transparent Surge
- Transparent Sag
- Electro-Surgical Immunity
- Walkie-Talkie and Cellular Phone Immunity
- Radiated and Line Conducted Emissions
- Limits for Harmonic Current Emissions
- Limits for Generated Voltage Flicker
- Electrostatic Discharge (ESD) Immunity.

17.3.6 Life test/reliability demonstration

Life testing or reliability determination is used for two purposes:

- determine early failures which will decrease the efficiency of the device
- determine the long term reliability of the device.

The test is conducted on several units produced according to manufacturing specifications. The functionality of the devices are verified and they are then placed on test in the typical application they will be subjected to at the customer's site. If, for example, a device is operated continuously for 8 hours and turned off for 16 hours, this same cycle may be utilized or the test accelerated by changing the cycle time, but keeping the same ratio of ON and OFF times. Data is collected on a periodic basis.

Tests may be run to indicate various reliability parameters, dependent upon the number of units available to be tested and the amount of time allotted for testing. A typical test would be to test to the equivalent of one year's usage in the field. By this time, feedback should be being received from the field and this data is more realistic than lab data.

17.3.7 Customer misuse

The product, during ordinary usage, is subjected to potential customer misuse. The project team will hold a brainstorming session to discuss how it would be possible for customers to misuse the product. Some typical misuse tests include the following:

17.3.7.1 Fluid spillage

This test verifies the functionality of the device following the pouring of 200 ml of water onto any arbitrary point on the surface of the device or its associated parts.

17.3.7.2 Weight test

This test verifies that if the device contains a surface that could be used as a tabletop, it has been designed to withstand a typical individual sitting on it.

17.3.7.3 Keyed connectors

This test verifies that electrical connectors cannot be misconnected. They should be keyed so that only one possible connection can be made.

17.3.8 Time related

Time related testing is conducted until a certain number of hours of operation or a certain number of cycles has been completed, e.g., a switch test conducted for 100,000 ON/OFF cycles or a monitor operated for 100,000 hours. This type of test will be important in choosing the correct formula to calculate MTBF from the test data. Time testing can also be conducted to determine what part or component fails, when it fails, the mode of failure at that particular time, the mechanism of failure and how much more or less life the equipment has that is required for operational use. This allows priorities of criticality for reliability improvement to be established.

17.3.9 Failure related

A test may be conducted until all test units or a certain percentage of units have failed, e.g., ventilators operated until the first unit fails or power supplies power cycled until all have failed. This type of test will be important in choosing the correct formula to calculate MTBF from the test data.

Homework Exercises

1. You have the responsibility for writing the test protocol for a portable pulse oximeter that will be used in a high school science class. Detail a list of tests that you would use.
2. You must determine why your blood sugar determination kit, which worked so well when tested in Nashville TN., gives erroneous results when used in Salt Lake City. What did you not account for?
3. What common fluid spills would you plan for in testing an ekg machine in use in an operating room? How would this list differ for the same machine in the patient's room?
4. The lobby and part of the immediate exterior of the Vanderbilt University Hospital has a floor made of mortared bricks. On the inside they are shellacked, on the outside they are allowed to weather. What tests can be performed with this flooring?
5. While occupied, an electric wheelchair moved on its own accord in a hospital environment, injuring the occupant. How would you investigate this accident? What tests were probably not run properly on the wheelchair prior to sale?
6. You are placed in charge of specifying shipping containers for a computer based medical device. Investigate how the ISTA can assist you in specification of tests and shipping containers. (Visit the web site for this organization, www.ista.org)

References

Fries, Richard C., *Reliability Assurance for Medical Devices, Equipment and Software*. Buffalo Grove, IL: Interpharm Press, 1991.

Fries, Richard C., *Reliable Design of Medical Devices.* New York: Marcel Dekker, Inc., 1997.

Kit, Edward, *Software Testing in the Real World - Improving the Process.* Reading, MA: Addison-Wesley Publishing Company, 1995.

Laplante, Phillip, *Real-Time Systems Design and Analysis - An Engineer's Handbook.* New York: The Institute of Electrical and Electronic Engineers, Inc., 1993.

Myers, Glenford J., *The Art of Software Testing*. New York: John Wiley & Sons, 1979.

Neufelder, Ann Marie, *Ensuring Software Reliability*. New York: Marcel Dekker, Inc., 1993.

Chapter 18

Regulations Tracking

"The Lord's Prayer is 66 words, the Gettysburg Address is 286 words, and there are 1,322 words in the Declaration of Independence. Yet, government regulations on the sale of cabbage total 26,911 words."
David McIntosh

As a result of revolutionary changes that have occurred around the world, we are part of an inevitable phenomenon: globalization of the economy. Internationalization of competition, deregulation of world trade, the boom of the information economy, and the management revolution move more and more companies to change the way they do business, the way they think, and the way they manage. They are adapting to the new reality to ensure their present survival and future prosperity. Many are reconfiguring their organizations and adopting new political, technical, and cultural values. Business leaders are revolutionizing their management thinking and implementing strategic information management, total quality management, empowerment, reengineering, policy deployment, cross-functional management, activity-based management, and environmental management. Many of these changes are based on the various standards and regulations which exist in various parts of the world. The FDA's role in regulation was discussed in Chapter 14. The remainder of this chapter will deal primarily with regulations and standards outside the United States.

18.1 Regulations

Medical devices are an extraordinarily heterogeneous category of products. The term *medical device* includes such technologically simple articles as ice bags and tongue depressors. On the other end of the spectrum, very sophisticated articles such as pacemakers and surgical lasers are also medical devices. Perhaps it is this diversity of products coupled with the sheer number of different devices that makes the development of an effective and efficient regulatory scheme a unique challenge for the Congress and the Food and Drug Administration (FDA) in the United States and the European Commission (EC) in Europe.

18.1.1 Regulations in the United States

Historically, medical devices have been neglected from a legislative and regulatory perspective. In the early 1900s, Congressional attention focused on food and drugs. The Pure Food and Drug Act of 1906 was passed to prohibit the distribution of adulterated or misbranded food and drugs to interstate commerce. This legislation, however, did not include any provisions to enable the Food and Drug Administration to regulate medical devices. Thus, legitimate and fraudulent medical devices were freely marketed without any effective check on the safety of these articles or the accuracy of their claims.

The most significant rationale for authorizing the FDA to regulate medical devices was the mounting level of consumer fraud. In the years preceding the Federal Food, Drug, and Cosmetic Act of 1938, medical devices were marketed that touted false therapeutic claims. Many of these devices were patently harmful. Others, by virtue of their bogus therapeutic claims, delayed consumers from seeking proper medical attention. Thus, a growing concern evolved - the public welfare was in jeopardy unless a mechanism was established to regulate the safety and reliability of medical devices.

It was not until 1938, when the Pure Food and Drug Act of 1906 underwent extensive revision, that the Congress expressly empowered the federal government to regulate medical devices. The Federal Food, Drug and Cosmetic Act of 1938 expanded the FDA's regulatory control over food and drugs and extended the agency's authority to include medical devices and cosmetics.

The FDA's regulatory authority over medical devices remained unchanged until the mid-1970s. In the late 1960s and early 1970s, there was some interest expressed by administrative officials and members of Congress in improving the regulatory framework for medical devices. Although some of this interest culminated in device regulation bills, formal legislation was not enacted until May, 1976. The Medical Device Amendments to the Federal Food, Drug, and Cosmetic Act, of 1976, established an intricate statutory framework to enable the FDA to regulate nearly every aspect of medical devices, from testing through marketing.

18.1.2 Regulations in Europe

The European Community's program on the completion of the Internal Market has, as the primary objective for medical devices, to ensure Community-wide free circulation of products. The only means to establish such free circulation, in view of quite divergent national systems, regulations governing medical devices, and existing trade barriers, was to adopt legislation for the Community, by which the health and safety of patients, users, and third persons would be ensured through a harmonized set of device related protection requirements. Devices meeting the requirements and sold to members of the Community are identified by means of a CE mark.

Because of the diversity of current national medical device standards, attempts to introduce mutual recognition of device approvals to reconcile the different regimes proved to be fruitless. The European Commission eventually decided that totally new EC legislation, covering all medical devices was needed.

The Active Implantable Medical Devices Directive adopted by the Community legislator in 1990 and the Medical Devices Directive in 1993 cover more than 80% of medical devices for use with human beings. The In-Vitro Diagnostic Medical Devices Directive, which came into force in 1997, addresses the remaining devices. After a period of transition, i.e., a period during which the laws implementing a Directive co-exist with pre-existing national laws, these directives exhaustively govern the conditions for placing medical devices on the market. Through the agreements on the European Economic Area (EEA), the relevant requirements and procedures are the same for all European Community member states and European Free Trade Association (EFTA) countries that belong to the EEA, an economic area comprising more than 380 million people.

18.2 Standards

The degree to which formal standards and procedures are applied to product development varies from company to company. In many cases, standards are dictated by customers or regulatory mandate. In other situations, standards are self-imposed. If formal standards do exist, an assurance activity must be established to guarantee that they are being followed. An assessment of compliance to standards may be conducted as part of a formal technical review or by audit.

Standards simplify communication, promote consistency and uniformity, and eliminate the need to invent yet another solution to the same problem. They are a way of preserving proven practices above and beyond the inevitable staff changes within organizations. Standards, whether official or merely agreed upon, are especially important when talking to customers and suppliers, but it is easy to underestimate their importance when dealing with different departments and disciplines within our own organization.

18.2.1 Standards in the United States

Standards are important in that they impact our industry in many ways. Most of the standards activity relevant to the medical device, diagnostic product, and health care information systems industry, falls into one or more of the four following types:

- regulatory
- national voluntary consensus
- foreign national
- international.

Regulatory standards are those that generally have some basis in law. National voluntary standards are the work products of groups. Foreign national standards are like our own national regulatory and voluntary standards except that they are for other countries. International standards are the attempts by countries to try to reduce the differences in national standards through organizations such as the International Organization for Standardization (ISO) and the International Electrotechnical Commission (IEC).

People who work on medical device standards have been conditioned to think only in terms of voluntary and regulatory standards. While that may be a useful distinction in law, in practice, the distinctions blur because most standards fit into a gray area. From a practical point of view it does not matter very much if a standard is labeled mandatory or voluntary. There are examples of regulatory agency standards being promoted as guidelines and voluntary standards being used as mandatory requirements.

The American National Standards Institute's (ANSI) 1987 *Summary Annual Report of Medical Device Standards Board Activities* identifies over 700 voluntary medical device standards completed or under development. These standards cover everything from needles, syringes, and thermometers to diagnostic test kits, electrical safety, and laboratory computers. Some of these standards are clearly defined and cover only a specific device. Others, however, are so broad - on sterilization, for example - that they cover whole classes of medical devices.

18.2.1.1 Software standards

There are a myriad of software standards to assist the developer in designing and documenting his program. The Institute of Electrical and Electronic Engineers' (IEEE) standards cover documentation through all phases of design. Military standards describe how software is to be designed and developed for military use. There are also standards on software quality and reliability to assist developers in preparing a quality program. The international community has produced standards, primarily dealing with software safety. In each case, the standard is a voluntary document that has been developed to provide guidelines for designing, developing, testing, and documenting a software program.

In the United States, the FDA is responsible for assuring the device utilizing software or the software as a device is safe and effective for its intended use. The FDA has produced several drafts of reviewer guidelines, auditor guidelines, software policy, and Quality System regulations addressing both device and process software. In addition, guidelines for FDA reviewers have been prepared as well as training programs for inspectors and reviewers. The Quality System Regulation addresses software as part of the design phase.

The United States is ahead of other countries in establishing guidelines for medical software development. There is, however, movement within several international organizations to develop regulations and guidelines for software and software controlled devices. For example, ISO 9000-3, *Quality management and quality assurance standards - Part 3: Guidelines for the application of ISO 9001 to the development, supply and maintenance of software,* specifically addresses software development in addition to what is contained in ISO 9001. The Canadian Standards Association (CSA) addresses software issues in four standards covering new and previously developed software in critical and non-critical applications. IEC has a software document currently in development.

18.2.2 International standards

Internationally, standards may be defined as:

> *A technical specification or other document available to the public, drawn up with the cooperation and consensus or general approval of all interests affected by it, based on the consolidated results of science, technology and experience, aimed at the promotion of optimum community benefits and approved by a body on the national, regional, or international level.*

While this definition goes some way to saying what a standard is, it says nothing about the subject matter or purpose, apart from stating that the objectives of the standard must in some way be tied to community benefits.
Standards, however, have a definite subject matter. They include:

- to standardize particular processes,
- to provide a consistent and complete definition of a commodity or process,

- to record good practice regarding the development process associated with the production of commodities,
- to encode good practice for the specification, design, manufacture, testing, maintenance, and operation of commodities.

One of the primary requirements of a standard is that it be produced in such a way that conformance to the standard can be unambiguously determined. A standard is devalued if conformance can not be easily determined or if the standard is so loosely worded that it becomes a matter of debate and conjecture as to whether the requirements of the standard have been met.

Standards also exist in various types:

- De facto and de jure standards. These are usually associated with the prevailing commercial interests in the market place. These de facto standards are often eventually subject to the standardization process.
- Reference models. These provide a framework within
- which standards can be formulated.
- Product versus process standards. Some standards relate to specific products while others relate to the process used to produce products.
- Codes of practice, guidelines, and specifications. These terms relate to the manner in which a standard may be enforced. Codes of practice and guidelines reflect ways of working that are deemed to be *good* or *desirable*, but for which conformance is difficult to determine. Specifications are far more precise and conformance can be determined by analysis or test.
- Prospective and retrospective standards. It is clearly undesirable to develop a standard before the subject matter is well understood scientifically, technically, and through practice. However, it may be desirable to develop a standard alongside the evolving technology.

18.3 Coping with Increased Quality Assurance and Regulatory Issues

A manufacturer has several options available for coping with a changing QA and regulatory environment. These range from participating in shaping the new standards and regulations, to responding to them upon completion. Ignoring them is not considered a viable option.

It is important for manufacturers to be involved in the development process for a new standard or regulation. By being part of the process, they can minimize the impact of the new requirements on their development of a product. They can also present knowledgeable inputs to the discussion, based on experience, that will make the standard or regulation more effective.

Standards and regulatory agencies are very keen to inputs from those subject to the standard or regulation. Agencies are interested in developing good working relationships with organizations that are affected by their rules and regulations. It is in the interest of both parties to develop standards and regulations that are meaningful, effective, and do not present an extraordinary burden.

18.4 Medical Device Directives

The European Community's program on the Completion of the Internal Market has, as the primary objective for medical devices, to assure Community-wide free circulation of products. The only means to establish such free circulation, in view of quite divergent national regulations governing medical devices and existing trade barriers, was to adopt legislation for the Community, by which the health and safety of patients, users and third persons would be ensured through a harmonized set of device related protection requirements. Devices meeting the requirements and sold to members of the Community are identified by means of a CE mark.

The Active Implantable Medical Devices Directive adopted by the Community legislator in 1990 and the Medical Devices Directive in 1993 cover more than 80% of medical devices for use with human beings. After a period of transition, i.e., a period during which the laws implementing a Directive co-exist with pre-existing national laws, these directives exhaustively govern the conditions for placing medical devices on the market. Through the agreements on the European Economic Area (EEA), the relevant requirements and procedures are the same for all European Community (EC) member states and European Free Trade Association (EFTA) countries that belong to the EEA, an economic area comprising more than 380 million people.

18.4.1 Definition of a medical device

The various Medical Device Directives define a medical device as:

"any instrument, appliance, apparatus, material or other article, whether used alone or in combination, including the software necessary for its proper application, intended by the manufacturer to be used for human beings for the purpose of:

- *diagnosis, prevention, monitoring, treatment or alleviation of disease*
- *diagnosis, monitoring, alleviation of or compensation for an injury or handicap*
- *investigation, replacement or modification of the anatomy or of a physiological process*
- *control of conception;*

and which does not achieve its principal intended action in or on the human body by pharmacological, immunological or metabolic means, but which may be assisted in its function by such means."

One important feature of the definition is that it emphasizes the "intended use" of the device and its "principal intended action." This use of the term *intended* gives manufacturers of certain products some opportunity to include or exclude their product from the scope of the particular Directive.

Another important feature of the definition is the inclusion of the term *software*. The software definition will probably be given further interpretation, but is currently interpreted to mean 1) software intended to control the function of a device is a medical device, 2) software for patient records or other administrative purposes is not a device, 3) software which is built into a device, e.g., software in an electrocardiographic monitor used to drive a display, is clearly an integral part of the medical device or 4) a software update sold by the manufacturer, or a variation sold by a software house, is a medical device in its own right.

18.4.2 The medical device directives process

The process of meeting the requirements of the Medical Device Directives is a multi-step approach, involving the following activities:

- analyze the device to determine which directive is applicable
- identify the applicable Essentials Requirements List
- identify any corresponding Harmonized Standards
- confirm that the device meets the Essential Requirements/Harmonized Standards and document the evidence
- classify the device
- decide on the appropriate conformity assessment procedure
- identify and choosing a notified body
- obtain conformity certifications for the device
- establish a Declaration of Conformity
- apply for the CE mark.

This process does not necessarily occur in a serial manner, but iterations may occur throughout the cycle. Each activity in the process will be examined in detail.

18.4.3 Choosing the appropriate directive

Because of the diversity of current national medical device regulations, the Commission decided that totally new Community legislation covering all medical devices was needed. Software or a medical device containing software may be subject to the requirements of the Active Implantable Medical Device Directive or the Medical Device Directive.

Three directives are envisaged to cover the entire field of medical devices:

Active Implantable Medical Device Directive (AIMDD)

This directive applies to a medical device which depends on a source of electrical energy or any source of power other than that directly generated by the human body or gravity, which is intended to be totally or partially introduced, surgically or medically, into the human body or by medical intervention into a natural orifice, and which is intended to remain after the procedure. This directive was adopted in June, 1990, implemented in January, 1993 and the transition period ended January, 1995.

Medical Device Directive (MDD)

This directive applies to all medical devices and accessories, unless they are covered by the Active Implantable Medical Device Directive or the In Vitro Diagnostic Medical Device Directive. This directive was adopted in June, 1993, was implemented in January, 1995 and the transition period ends June, 1998.

In Vitro Diagnostic Medical Device Directive (IVDMDD)

This directive applies to any medical device that is a reagent, reagent product, calibrator, control kit, instrument, equipment or system intended to be used in vitro for the examination of samples derived from the human body for the purpose of providing information concerning a physiological state of health or disease or congenital abnormality, or to determine the safety and compatibility with potential recipients. This directive is currently in preparation.

18.4.4 Identifying the applicable essential requirements

The major legal responsibility the Directives place on the manufacturer of a medical device requires the device meet the Essential Requirements set out in Annex I of the Directive which applies to them, taking into account the intended purpose of the device. The Essential Requirements are written in the form of 1) general requirements which always apply and 2) particular requirements, only some of which apply to any particular device.

The general requirements for the Essential Requirements List take the following form:

- the device must be safe. Any risk must be acceptable in relation to the benefits offered by the device
- the device must be designed in such a manner that risk is minimized
- the device must perform in accordance with the manufacturer's specification
- the safety and performance must be maintained throughout the indicated lifetime of the device.
- the safety and performance of the device must not be affected by normal conditions of transport and storage.
- any side effects must be acceptable in relation to the benefits offered.

The particular requirements for the Essential Requirements List address the following topics:

- chemical, physical, and biological properties
- infection and microbial contamination
- construction and environmental properties
- devices with a measuring function
- protection against radiation
- requirements for devices connected to or equipped with an energy source
- protection against electrical risks
- protection against mechanical and thermal risks
- protection against the risks posed to the patient by energy supplies or substances
- information supplied by the manufacturer.

The easiest method of assuring the Essential Requirements are met is to establish a checklist of the Essential Requirements from Appendix I of the appropriate Directive, which then forms the basis of the technical dossier.

The Essential Requirements checklist includes:

- a statement of the Essential Requirements
- an indication of the applicability of the Essential Requirements to a particular device
- a list of the standards used to address the Essential Requirements
- the activity that addresses the Essential Requirements,
- the clause(s) in the standard detailing the applicable test for the particular Essential Requirement
- an indication of whether the device passed/or failed the test
- a statement of the location of the test documentation or certificates.

18.4.5 Identification of corresponding harmonized standards

A "harmonized" standard is a standard produced under a mandate from the European Commission by one of the European standardization bodies, such as CEN (the European Committee for Standardization) and CENELEC (the European Committee for Electrotechnical Standardization), and which has its reference published in the *Official Journal of the European Communities*.

The Essential Requirements are worded such that they identify a risk and state that the device should be designed and manufactured so that the risk is avoided or minimized. The technical detail for assuring these requirements is to be found in Harmonized Standards. Manufacturers must therefore identify the Harmonized Standards corresponding to the Essential Requirements which apply to their device.

With regard to choosing such standards, the manufacturer must be aware of the hierarchy of standards which have been developed:

- Horizontal Standards: generic standards covering fundamental requirements common to all, or a very wide range of medical devices
- Semi-Horizontal Standards: group standards which deal with requirements applicable to a group of devices

- Vertical Standards: product-specific standards which give requirements to one device or a very small group of devices.

Manufacturers must give particular attention to the horizontal standards since, because of their general nature, they apply to almost all devices. As these standards come into use for almost all products, they will become extremely powerful.

Semi-horizontal standards may be particularly important as they have virtually the same weight as horizontal standards for groups of devices, such as orthopedic implants, IVDs, or X-ray equipment.

Vertical standards might well be too narrow to cope with new technological developments when a question of a specific feature of a device arises. Table 18-1 lists some common harmonized standards for medical devices and medical device electromagnetic compatibility standards.

18.4.6 Identification and choice of a notified body

Identifying and choosing a Notified Body is one of the most critical issues facing a manufacturer. A long-term and close relationship should be developed and time and care spent in making a careful choice of a Notified Body should be viewed as an investment in the future of the company.

Notified bodies must satisfy the criteria given in Annex XI of the Medical Device Directive, namely:

- independence from the design, manufacture or supply of the devices in question
- integrity
- competence
- staff who are trained, experienced, and able to report
- impartiality of the staff

Standard	Areas Covered
EN 60 601 Series	Medical Electrical Equipment
EN 29000 Series	Quality Systems
EN 46000 Series	Quality Systems
EN 55011 (CISPR 11)	EMC/Emission
EN 60801 Series	EMC/Immunity
EN 540	Clinical Investigation of Medical Devices
EN 980	Symbols on Medical Equipment
IEC 601-1-2	Medical Device Emission and Immunity
IEC 801-2	Electrostatic Discharge
IEC 801-2	Immunity to Radiated Radio Frequency Electromagnetic Fields
IEC 801-4	Fast Transients/Burst
IEC 801-5	Voltage Surge Immunity

Table 18-1 Important Harmonized and EMC Standards (From Fries, 1997.)

- possession of liability insurance
- professional secrecy.

In addition, the bodies must satisfy the criteria fixed by the relevant Harmonized Standards. The relevant Harmonized Standards include those of the EN 45000 series dealing with the accreditation and operation of certification bodies.

The tasks to be carried out by Notified Bodies include:

- audit manufacturers; quality systems for compliance with Annexes II, V and VI
- examine any modifications to an approved quality system
- carry out periodic surveillance of approved quality systems
- examine design dossiers and issue EC Design Examination Certificates
- examine modifications to an approved design
- carry out type examinations and issue EC Type Examination Certificates
- examine modifications to an approved type
- carry out EC verification
- take measures to prevent rejected batches from reaching the market
- agree with the manufacturer time limits for the conformity assessment procedures
- take into account the results of tests or verifications already carried out
- communicate to other Notified Bodies (on request) all relevant information about approvals of quality systems issued, refused, and withdrawn
- communicate to other Notified Bodies (on request) all relevant information about EC Type Approval Certificates issued, refused, and withdrawn.

Notified bodies must be located within the European Community in order that effective control may be applied by the Competent Authorities that appointed them, but certain operations may be carried out on behalf of Notified Bodies by subcontractors who may be based outside the European Community. Competent Authorities will generally notify bodies on their own territory, but they may notify bodies based in another Member State provided that they have already been notified by their parent Competent Authority.

There are several factors to be taken into account by a manufacturer in choosing a Notified Body, including:

- experience with medical devices
- range of medical devices for which the Notified Body has skills
- possession of specific skills, e.g., EMC or software
- links with subcontractors and subcontractor skills
- conformity assessment procedures for which the body is notified
- plans for handling issues, such as clinical evaluation
- attitude to existing certifications
- queue times/processing times
- costs
- location and working languages.

Experience with medical devices is limited to a small number of test houses and their experience is largely confined to electromedical equipment. Manufacturers should probe carefully the competence of the certification body to assess their device. Actual experience with a product of a similar nature would be reassuring. The certification body should be pressed to demonstrate sufficient understanding of the requirements, particularly where special processes are involved (e.g., sterilization) and/or previous experience.

18.4.7 Establishing a declaration of conformity

Of all documents prepared for the Medical Device Directives, the most important may be the declaration of conformity. Every device, other that a custom-made or clinical investigation device, must be covered by a declaration of conformity.

The general requirement is that the manufacturer must draw up a written declaration that the products concerned meet the provisions of the Directive that apply to them. The declaration must cover a given number of the products manufactured. A strictly literal interpretation of this wording would suggest that the preparation of a declaration of conformity is not a once-and-for-all event with an indefinite coverage, but rather a formal statement that products which have been manufactured and verified in accordance with the particular conformity assessment procedure chosen by the manufacturer do meet the requirements of the Directive. Such an interpretation would impose severe burdens on manufacturers, and the Commission is understood to be moving to a position where a declaration of conformity can be prepared in respect of future production of a model of device for which the conformity assessment procedures have been carried out. The CE marking of individual devices after manufacture can then be regarded as a short-form expression of the declaration of conformity in respect of that individual device. This position is likely to form part of future Commission guidance.

Even so, the declaration remains a very formal statement from the manufacturer and accordingly, must be drawn up with care. The declaration must include the serial numbers or batch numbers of the products it covers and manufacturers should give careful thought to the appropriate coverage of a declaration. In the extreme, it may be that a separate declaration should be prepared individually for each product or batch.

A practical approach is probably to draw up one basic declaration that is stated to apply to the products whose serial (batch) numbers are listed in an Appendix. The Appendix can then be added to at sensible intervals. A suggested format is shown in Figure 18-1.

18.4.8 Application of the CE mark

The CE marking (Figure 18-2) is the symbol used to indicate that a particular product complies with the relevant Essential Requirements of the appropriate Directive, and as such, that the product has achieved a satisfactory level of safety and thus may circulate freely throughout the Community.

It is important to note that it is the manufacturer or his authorized representative who applies the CE marking to the product, and not the Notified Body. The responsibility for ensuring that each and every product conforms to the requirements of the Directive is that of the manufacturer and the affixing of the CE marking constitutes the manufacturer's statement that an individual device conforms.

The CE marking should appear on the device itself, if practicable, on the instructions for use, and on the shipping packaging. It should be accompanied by the identification number of the Notified Body which has been involved in the verification of the production of the device. It is prohibited to

DECLARATION OF CONFORMITY

We: Company Name
Company Address

Declare that the product(s) listed below:

Product to be declared

Hereby conform(s) to the European Council Directive 93/42/EEC, Medical Device Directive, Annex II, Article 3. This declaration is based on the Certification of the Full Quality Assurance System by NAME OF NOTIFIED BODY, Notified Body # XXXX.

Name (*Print or type*) : ______________________
Title : ______________________
Signature: ______________________
Date: ______________________

Figure 18-1 Declaration of Conformance. (From, Fries, 1997.)

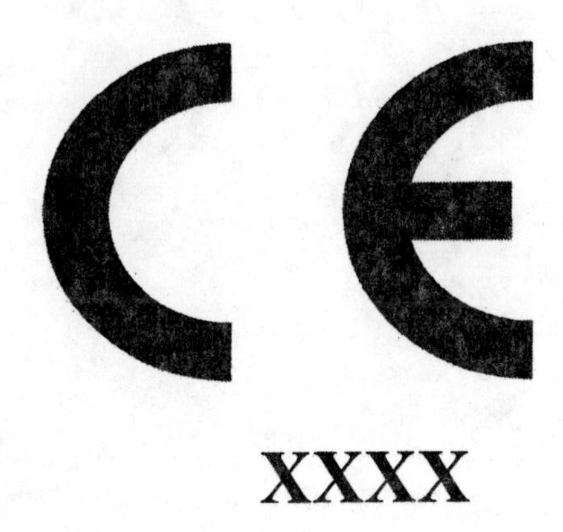

Figure 18-2 CE mark. (From, Fries, 1997.)

add other marks which could confuse or obscure the meaning of the CE marking. The XXXX noted in Figure 18-2 is the identification number of the Notified Body.

18.5 ISO 9000

The ISO 9000 set of standards is used to develop the elements necessary to maintain an efficient quality system at any company. They can be used by manufacturing and service industries alike because they are not specific to any given product. The standards focus on controlling the process an organization uses to develop and produce their products rather than dictating specific requirements for the finished product.

The series really encompass a set of five standards:

ISO 9000-1	Provides guidelines for selection and use of the remaining standards.
ISO 9001	The most comprehensive of the standards. Covers Design, Development, Production, Installation and Servicing.
ISO 9002	Covers Production Installation and Servicing.

ISO 9003	Least comprehensive. Only covers Final Inspection.
ISO 9004-1	A Guide to Quality Management Elements

There are 20 elements or clauses that make up the core of the ISO 9001 standard. The differences in 9001 – 9003 are illustrated in Table 18-1.

18.6 Canadian Regulations

All Medical Devices sold in Canada must be in compliance with the *Food and Drugs Act, Medical Device Regulations*, published in July, 1998, Registration SOR/98-282 7 May, 1998. The *Medical Devices Regulations* prepared by the Medical Device Bureau, Health Protection Branch, set out the requirements governing the sale, importation, and advertisement of medical devices. The goal of the Regulations is to ensure that medical devices distributed in Canada are both safe and effective. In developing these regulations, emphasis was placed on developing requirements, which are harmonious with those of Canadian international trading partners and eliminating, to the greatest extent possible, requirements unique to Canada. Harmonization allows meaningful negotiations toward Mutual Recognition Agreements (MRA) to occur, thereby eliminating barriers to trade. MRAs, once operational, will allow devices to be assessed in one jurisdiction and placed on the market in all other jurisdictions party to the agreement without further assessment.

The *Medical Devices Regulations* are administrated by theTherapeutic Products Programme (TPP), which recognizes and strongly endorses the importance of harmonization as a key factor of these Medical Devices Regulations. Harmonization of requirements to the greatest extent possible with the European Union and United States, would facilitate mutual recognition agreements (MRAs) with both these jurisdictions, which in turn would lead to elimination of duplication of third party audits and significant cost savings to industry and regulators. Canada has signed an MRA with the EU, and the *Medical Device Regulations* are similar with the EU *Medical Device Directive* (MDD). The groundwork is also being laid to facilitate similar agreement with the FDA. In the broader international scheme Canada is participating in the Global Harmonization Task Force (GHTF).

All of these activities, schemes, and agreements would eventually lead the designer to design the product which would comply with the single standard

ISO 9001	ISO 9002	ISO 9003
	All of ISO 9001 except:	*All of ISO 9002 except:*
4.1 Management Responsibilities		
4.2 Quality System	Design Control	Purchasing
4.3 Contract Review		Process Control
4.4 Design Control		Servicing
4.5 Document Control		
4.6 Purchasing		
4.7 Control of Customer Supplied Product		
4.8 Product Identification and Traceability		
4.9 Process Control		
4.10 Inspection and Testing		
4.11 Inspection Measuring and Test Equipment (Calibration)		
4.13 Nonconforming Product		
4.14 Corrective and Preventive Action		
4.15 Handling, Storage, Packaging, Preservation and Delivery		
4.16 Control of Quality Records		
4.17 Internal Audits		
4.18 Training		
4.19 Servicing		
4.20 Statistical Techniques		
Total # of Clauses = 20	19	16

Table 18-1 ISO 9001 Elements

and the single regulation, which would be acceptable worldwide. The *Medical Device Regulations* are harmonized as closely as possible with those of the EU and the US. However, it must be noted that the systems of administration and enforcement are different. The intent of this chapter is to highlight, explain, and provide the rationale for these unique requirements in Canada.

18.6.1 Fundamental safety and effectiveness principles

The design of medical devices imported or sold in Canada must meet the following principles, appropriate to the device, on which regulatory requirements would be based:

- Devices must not, when used under the conditions and for the purposes intended, compromise the clinical condition or the safety of patients, or the safety and health of users or, where applicable, other persons, provided that any risk which may be associated with their use constitute acceptable risks when weighed against the benefits to the patient and are compatible with a high level of protection of health and safety.
- A manufacturer must take measures reasonable and prudent to ensure that the design and manufacture of a device conforms to safety principles, taking into account the generally acknowledged state of the art. The measures should, with respect to the use of the device: identify and eliminate or reduce risks as far as possible (inherently safe design and construction), where appropriate take adequate protection measures, including alarms, if necessary, in relation to risks that cannot be eliminated, inform users of the residual risks due to any shortcomings of the protection measures adopted, and minimize the danger from any potential failure during the lifetime of the device.
- The device must perform as intended by the manufacturer, and must be effective for the medical conditions, purposes or uses for which it is recommended or intended.
- The characteristics and performance of the device must not be adversely affected to such a degree that the clinical conditions and safety of patients and, where applicable, of other persons, are compromised during the lifetime of the device as indicated by the manufacturer, when the device is subjected to the stresses which can occur during normal conditions of use.

- The performance of a device shall not be compromised by transport or conditions of storage, taking into account the instructions and information provided by the manufacturer.
- Device materials should be compatible with each other and with materials (biological and non-biological). They may contact during normal use and should not pose unnecessary risks to patients, users and other persons.
- The design, manufacture and packaging of a device should minimize risk to patients, users, and other persons from, for example:
- Flammability or explosion,
- Chemical or microbial contamination and residues,
- Radiation emissions,
- Electrical, mechanical, and thermal hazards,
- Fluids leaking from the device, or the ingress of fluids into the device.
- Sterile devices must have been manufactured and sterilized by an appropriate validated method and under appropriately controlled environment conditions.
- Devices intended to be used as part of a system must be compatible with other components of the total system.
- Devices with a measuring function must be designed to perform with a degree of accuracy and stability suitable for the intended purpose.
- Devices, which are or contain software, must be designed to perform as intended, and the performance must be tested and validated.
- Every device must be accompanied by the information needed to use it safely and effectively, taking into account the training and knowledge of the potential users.

The above fundamental safety and effectiveness principles are considered to be equivalent to the Essential Requirements in the *Medical Device Directives* (Council Directive 93/42/EEC of June 1993), taking into account the differences between the use of the term *effectiveness* in the Canadian Regulations and the use of the term *performance* in the European Directive. The Therapeutic Product Program (TPP) interprets effectiveness to mean that the device will produce the effect represented or intended by the manufacturer relative to the medical conditions, purposes or uses for which the device is recommended or intended.

The TPP has also adopted the spirit and intent of the United States FDA 510(k) safety and effectiveness principles. The TPP consider the European principles too lengthy and has condensed them. Furthermore, whereas the European document uses performance, the TPP must key on the term effectiveness to be consistent with its mandate. The FDA 510(k) does not iterate their principles in the same detail nor identify their principles in one common location.

18.6.2 Device classification

The Medical Devices Regulations distinguish medical devices under a risk-based classification system. Devices are grouped into four classes, with Class I representing the lowest risk devices and Class IV representing the highest risk devices. Where a medical device can fit into multiple classes, it is placed in the highest applicable class. Detailed rules to classify medical devices are set out in Schedule I of the Medical Devices Regulations. Factors that are used to classify medical devices include:

- the invasiveness or non-invasiveness of the device and its contact with the user;
- if invasive, the part of the user's body that is penetrated;
- the purpose of the device;
- whether the device is active, i.e., whether its operation depends on a source of energy other than energy generated by the human body or gravity; and
- whether the device is an *in vitro* diagnostic device.

Dental or surgical instruments and devices placed in the oral or nasal cavities, as far as the pharynx or in the ear canal up to the eardrum are examples of Class I devices. Devices used to disinfect or sterilize other devices and non-invasive calibrators are examples of Class II devices. Surgically invasive devices that are intended to be absorbed by the body or that are intended to remain in the body for thirty (30) days or more are examples of Class III devices. Surgically invasive devices used to diagnose, monitor, correct or control a defect of the central cardiovascular system, of the central nervous system or of fetus *in utero* are examples of Class IV devices.

18.6.4 Standards and the design process

In the process in designing of medical equipment the knowledge, use and application of applicable standards are essential. The safety, efficacy and performance of the medical device must be introduced during the design process, using all know and applicable standards. The Medical Devices Regulations do not include any standards except *National Standard of Canada CAN/CSA – ISO 13485-98, Quality systems – Medical Devices- Particular requirements for the application of ISO 9001,* and *National Standard of Canada CAN/CSA – ISO 13488- 98, Quality systems –Medical Devices- Particular requirements for the application of ISO 9002,* as amended from time to time.

Policy Documents are used to reference internationally recognized standards, which the Therapeutic Product Program (TPP) considers as being minimum acceptable standards for meeting the Safety and Effectiveness requirements set out in the *Medical Devices Regulations.* Policy Documents are developed for any risk class of device. The TPP uses standards in Policy Documents as a basis for enforcement action based on the following:

- All devices must meet the Safety and Effectiveness requirements set out in the Medical Devices Regulations.
- Standards are a means of stating minimum acceptable requirements respecting the safety and effectiveness requirements applicable to a device or group of devices.
- Where a standard is referenced in a Policy Document by the TPP, the TPP would deem that the manufacturer has demonstrated that their device complies with the applicable safety and effectiveness requirements covered by the standard, where compliance with the standard is demonstrated. A statement to this effect is placed in the *Medical Devices Regulations.*

Where a standard is referenced in a Policy Document and the manufacturer uses an alternate standard, the manufacturer must provide justification that the standard that is used provides equivalent assurance of safety and effectiveness. Standards set out in the Policy Document prescribe an acceptable means of meeting the Safety and Effectiveness requirements set out in the *Medical Devices Regulations.* The option remains open to a manufacturer to propose any alternate means, but the burden of proof required to establish acceptability of the alternate means rest with the manufacturer.

The TPP is not in a position to equip itself with the test equipment and personnel necessary to conduct all the different manufacturer's test methods. Therefore, whenever the TPP would conduct compliance testing, the TPP would use the test method or methods as set out in the Policy Document. Where a manufacturer has chosen to use a standard referenced in a Policy Document, and compliance testing to the device by the TPP to that standard demonstrates that the device does not meet the standard, the TPP would take any necessary enforcement action to resolve the issue. The TPP's action would be based on the fact that compliance with the standard demonstrates that the applicable provisions of the Safety and Effectiveness requirements have been met.

A second case would be where a manufacturer has chosen not to use a standard referenced in a Policy Document, and has demonstrated to the TPP that the standard which they do use provides an equivalent assurance of safety and effectiveness as the standard referenced in a Policy Document. With this case, where compliance testing of the device by the TPP to the standard referenced in the Policy Document demonstrated that the device does not meet the standard, the TPP would discuss with the manufacturer the results of the testing and try to resolve any concerns which are raised as a result of the compliance testing. The TPP is referencing internationally recognized standards such as IEC and ISO where possible and use of uniquely Canadian standards is minimized. The Policy Documents are similar to the FDA Policy on Recognition of Standards.

18.7 Pacific Rim

The far-reaching economic and political turmoil that has rocked Asia for the past few years continues to have profound repercussions both in the countries of the region and throughout the rest of the world. Touched off by a devaluation of the Thai currency and expanding in a ripple effect that grew to tidal-wave proportions, the crisis roiled world financial markets, plunged national economies into recession, and threatened the existence of a new middle class created as a result of rapid economic growth. For foreign companies, including medical device firms, that had looked to Asia both as a site for expanding manufacturing operations and as a market of enormous potential, the crisis was a rude awakening.

In addition, there is the question of what is being done in Asia with regard to standards and regulation. Is the area moving toward harmonization? All developed nations are rapidly moving toward the same level of sophistication when it comes to the evaluation of medical devices, be they Class I, II, or III. The European Union (EU) has created a regulatory mechanism that ensures the highest level of safety for patients, while quickly moving beneficial products to the market. The EU has already established a very credible review system for medical devices through efforts such as basing the process on quality system standards, using the world-class, globally recognized ISO 9000 series of standards. In fact, as countries update their regulatory procedures, most are following the lead of Europe.

The EU is aggressively pursuing mutual recognition agreements (MRAs) with many non-EU partners, including Switzerland, Canada, Australia, and some Asian countries. Even without an MRA with the EU, some Asian countries, notably China, are unilaterally adopting an EU-style regulatory approach.

Homework Exercises

1. Compare the EU and the FDA definition of a medical device. What is similar? What differs?
2. Perform a web search with ISO9000 as the search term. You likely will turn up several companies that offer ISO9000 and related services. What are the companies really offering (guidance/advice/consulting)? Justify your answer.
3. You have developed a portable device that monitors the eeg of patients prone to grand mal seizures. If one is predicted, your device automatically injects a drug to stop the impending seizure. How would this device be classified in the US? In the European Union?
4. Same as question 3, but the device only warns the patient.
5. Visit the web site: http://www.ghtf.org/. Briefly report on the purposes of the four study groups listed. Why do you think such a group is needed?
6. You manufacture a device currently accepted by the FDA. Why would you wish to get CE certification?

References

The Active Implantable Medical Devices Directive. 90/385/EEC, 20 June, 1990.

Appler, William D. and Gaile L. McMann, "Medical Device Regulation: The Big Picture," in *The Medical Device Industry: Science, Technology, and Regulation in a Competitive Environment.* New York: Marcel Dekker, Inc., 1990.

American National Standards Institute, *Summary Annual Report of Medical Device Standards Board Activities.* New York: American National Standards Institute, 1987.

Canadian Electrical Code, Part I.

Canadian Electrical Code, Part II, Life Sciences Standards

Deming, W. Edward, *Out of the Crisis.* Cambridge, MA: MIT Center for Advanced Engineering Studies, 1986.

Department of Defense, *MIL-Q-9858.* Washington, D.C., April 4, 1959.

Extract Canada Gazette. Part II, May 27, 1998 Department of Health.

Fries, Richard C., editor, *Handbook of Medical Device Design.* New York: Marcel Dekker, 2001.

Fries, Richard C., *Medical Device Quality Assurance and Regulatory Compliance.* New York: Marcel Dekker, 1998.

Fries, Richard C., *Reliable Design of Medical Devices.* New York: Marcel Dekker, Inc., 1997.

Fries, R.C. and M. Graber, "Designing Medical Devices for Conformance with Harmonized Standards," *Biomedical Instrumentation & Technology.* Volume 29, Number 4, July/August, 1995.

Halverson, Fred S., "Global Harmonization and Mutual Recognition Efforts: Keeping Up The Pace," in *Medical Device and Diagnostic Industry,* April, 1999.

Higson, Gordon R., *The Medical Devices Directives - A Manufacturers' Handbook.* Brussels: Medical Technology Consultants Europe Ltd., 1993.

Information Institute of Technical Supervision, *China – Information Institute of Technical Supervision.* Chinanet Infotech & Service, Inc., 1998.

ISO 9001, *Quality systems - Model for quality assurance in design, development, production, installation and servicing.* Geneva, Switzerland: International Organization for Standardization, 1994.

ISO 9001:2000, *Quality Management Systems, First Committee Drafts.* Milwaukee, WI: American Society for Quality. 1998.

Japanese Regulations, Standards, Quality Marks, and Certification Systems. Tokyo, Japan: 1994.

Maksimova, Ludmila, *Registration and Certification of Medical Devices and Pharmaceuticals in Russia.* Washington, D.C.: U.S. Foreign Commercial Service and U.S. Department of State, January, 1997.

The Medical Devices Directive. 93/42/EEC, 14 June, 1993. *Draft Proposal for a Council Directive on In Vitro Diagnostic Medical Devices, Working Document.* III/D/4181/93, April, 1993.

The Medical Devices Directive. 93/42/EEC, 14 June, 1993. *Draft Proposal for a Council Directive on In Vitro Diagnostic Medical Devices, Working Document.* III/D/4181/93, April, 1993.

Naisbitt, John, *Global Paradox.* New York: Avon Books, 1995.

Olsson, John E., "Trends in International Regulations and Their Growing Impact." In *The Medical Device Industry.* Norman F. Estrin, editor. New York: Marcel Dekker, Inc., 1990.

Shepard, Stephen, "Defining the Q-word," in *Business Week*, Special Issue, 1991.

Steudel, H.J & Associates, Inc,. *What every Employee needs to know about ISO 9000.* Madison, WI: 1995.

SWBC, Organization for the European Conformity of Products, *CE-Mark: The New European Legislation for Products.* Milwaukee, WI: ASQC Quality Press, 1996.

Todorov, Branimir, *ISO 9000 Required: Your Worldwide Passport to Customer Confidence.* Portland, OR: Productivity Press, 1996.

Willingmyre, George T., "Industry's Role in Standards Development," in *The Medical Device Industry - Science, Technology, and Regulation in a Competitive Environment.* New York: Marcel Dekker, Inc., 1990.

Chapter 19

Manufacturing and Quality Control

"When one find's oneself in a hole of one's own making,
it is a good time to examine the quality of the workmanship."
John Renmerde

The FDA promulgated the Good Manufacturing Practices (GMP) for medical devices regulations in 1978, drawing authority from the Medical Devices Amendments to the Federal Food, Drug, and Cosmetic Act of 1976. The GMP regulations represented a total quality assurance program intended to control the manufacture and distribution of devices. It allows the FDA to periodically inspect medical device manufacturers for compliance to the regulations.

Manufacturers must operate in an environment in which the manufacturing process is controlled. Manufacturing excellence can only be achieved by designing products and processes to address potential problems before they occur. Manufacturers must also operate in an environment that meets GMP regulations. This requires proof of control over manufacturing processes.

19.1 A History of GMPs

Two years after the Medical Device Amendments of 1976 were enacted, FDA issued its final draft of the medical device good manufacturing practices (GMP) regulation, a series of requirements that prescribed the facilities, methods, and controls to be used in the manufacturing, packaging, and storage of medical devices. Except for an update of organizational references and revisions to the critical device list included in the 1978 final draft's preamble, these regulations have remained virtually unchanged since they were published in the *Federal Register* on July 21, 1978. That does not mean that their interpretation has not changed.

Several key events since that date have influenced the way FDA has interpreted and applied these regulations. The first occurred in 1987 with FDA's publication of the "Guidelines on General Principles of Process Validation," which not only provided guidance but advised industry that device manufacturers must validate other processes when necessary to assure that these processes would consistently produce acceptable results.

In 1989, FDA published a notice of availability for design control recommendations titled "Preproduction Quality Assurance Planning: Recommendations for Medical Device Manufacturers." These recommendations fulfilled a promised made by the Center for Devices and Radiological Health (CDRH) director to a congressional hearing committee to do something to prevent device failures that were occurring due to design defects, resulting in some injuries and deaths. It was also a warning to industry that FDA was moving to add design controls to the GMP regulation.

The next year, FDA moved closer to adding design controls, publishing the "Suggested Changes to the Medical Device Good Manufacturing Practices Regulation Information Document," which described the changes the agency was proposing to make to the GMP regulation. Comments asserted that FDA did not have the authority to add design controls to the GMPs, a point that became moot later that year when the Safe Medical Devices Act of 1990 (SMDA) became law. SMDA amended section 520(f) of the Federal Food, Drug, and Cosmetic Act to add "preproduction design validation" controls to the device GMP regulation.

SMDA also added the FD&C Act a new section 803, which encouraged FDA to wok with foreign countries toward mutual recognition agreements for the

GMP and other regulations. Soon afterward, FDA began to actively pursue the harmonization of GMP requirements on a global basis.

Over the following two years, FDA took steps to assure that manufacturers with device applications under review at the agency were also in compliance with GMPs. The first step was taken in 1991, when CDRH established its "reference list" program for manufacturers with pending premarket approval (PMA) applications, ensuring that no PMA would be approved while the device maker had significant GMP violations on record. In 1992, the program was extended to all 510(k)s. Under this umbrella program, 510(k)s would not be processed if there was evidence on hand that the site where the 510(k) device would be manufactured was not in compliance with GMPs.

On November 23, 1993, FDA acted on comments it had received three years earlier regarding its "Suggested Changes" document, publishing a proposed revision of the 1978 GMPs in the *Federal Register*. The proposal incorporated almost all of the 1987 version of ISO 9001, the quality systems standard compiled by the International Organization for Standardization. While supporting adoption of ISO 9001, most of the comments received from industry objected to the addition of proposals such as applying the GMP regulation to component manufacturers.

In July 1995, FDA published a working draft of the proposed final revised GMP regulation. As stated in that draft, the two reasons for the revision were to bring about the addition of design and servicing controls, and to ensure that the requirements were made compatible with those of ISO 9001 and EN46001 (ISO 13485), the quality standard that manufacturers must meet if they select the European Union directives' total quality system approach to marketing.

Among the proposals in this version that drew the most fire from industry were the application of GMPs to component manufacturers and used of the term *end of life*, which was intended to differentiate between servicing and reconditioning. FDA agreed to delete most but not all of the objectionable requirements during an August, 1995 FDA-industry meeting and the GMP Advisory Committee meeting in September, 1995. The end-of life concept was deleted from the GMPs, but was retained in the medical device reporting regulation.

As the 1995 working draft now stands, it is very similar to the proposed ISO 13485 standard. To further harmonize the two documents, FDA's July 1995 working draft includes additions that incorporate the requirements of the 1994 version of ISO 9001 that were not in the 1987 version. FDA published a final GMP regulation in October 1996 (also called "quality system regulation

In addition, FDA has indicated that GMP inspections might be made by third parties. If that happens, these inspections would probably begin on a small scale with third parties doing follow-up to non-violative inspections. But eventually, third parties could play an important role in mitigating delays from FDA's reference list, which, while not now referred to by that name, is still in effect and not likely to be dropped by the agency. Although review of a 510(k) is not affected by the manufacturer being on the list, a 510(k) will not be approved until the manufacturing site is found to be in GMP compliance. The availability of the third party auditors to inspect those sites might speed the review process under those circumstances.

Also in the future, is a training course for GMP specialists being prepared by the Association for the Advancement of Medical Instrumentation (AAMI). If this course were incorporated into the FDA investigator certification training, it could help assure that the GMP regulation is interpreted and applied uniformly by FDA, consultants, and the device industry.

19.2 The GMP Regulation

The latest draft of the GMP regulation was published for comment in the Federal Register on November 23, 1993. They were established to replace quality assurance program requirements with quality system requirements that include design, purchasing, and servicing controls, clarify record keeping requirements for device failure and complaint investigations, clarify requirements for qualifying, verifying, and validating processes and specification changes, and clarify requirements for evaluating quality data and correcting quality problems. In addition, the FDA has also revised the Current Good Manufacturing Practice (CGMP) requirements for medical devices to assure they are compatible with specifications for quality systems contained in international quality standard ISO 9001.

The following changes were made from previous regulations.

19.2.1 Design controls

Over the past several years, the FDA has identified lack of design controls as one of the major causes of device recalls. The intrinsic quality of devices, including their safety and effectiveness, is established during the design phase. The FDA believes that unless appropriate design controls are observed during preproduction stages of development, a finished device may not be safe nor effective for its intended use. Based on experience with administering the CGMP regulations, which currently do not include preproduction design controls, the FDA is concerned that the current regulations provide less than an appropriate level of assurance that devices will be safe and effective. Therefore, the FDA is proposing to add general requirements for design controls to the device CGMP regulations for all Class III and II devices, and several Class I devices.

19.2.2 Purchasing controls

The quality of purchased product and services is crucial to maintaining the intrinsic safety and effectiveness of a device. Many device failures due to problems with components that result in recall are due to unacceptable components provided by suppliers. The FDA has found during CGMP inspections that the use of unacceptable components is often due to the failure of the manufacturer of finished devices to adequately establish and define requirements for the device's purchased components, including quality requirements. Therefore, the FDA believes that the purchasing of components, finished devices, packaging, labeling, and manufacturing materials must be conducted with the same level of planning, control, and verification as internal activities. The FDA believes the appropriate level of control should be achieved through a proper mixture of supplier and in-house controls.

19.2.3 Servicing controls

The FDA has found, as a result of reviewing service records that the data resulting from the maintenance and repair of medical devices provide valuable insight into the adequacy of the performance of devices. Thus, the FDA believes that service data must be included among the data manufacturers use to evaluate and monitor the adequacy of the device design, the quality system, and the manufacturing process. Accordingly, the FDA is proposing to add general requirements for the maintenance of servicing records and for the review of these records by the manufacturer. Manufacturers must assure that the performance data obtained as a part of servicing product are fed back into the manufacturer's quality system for evaluation as part of the overall device experience data.

19.2.4 Changes in critical device requirements

The FDA is proposing to eliminate the critical component and critical operation terminology contained in the present CGMP regulation. The increased emphasis on purchasing controls and on establishing the acceptability of component suppliers assures that the intent of the present critical component requirement is carried forward into the revised CGMP. The addition of a requirement to validate and document special processes further ensures that the requirements of the present critical operation requirements are retained. FDA is proposing to retain the distinction between critical and noncritical devices for one regulatory purpose. Traceability will continue to be required only for critical devices.

19.2.5 Harmonization

The FDA is proposing to reorganize the structure of the device CGMP regulations and modify some of their language in order to harmonize them with international quality standards. FDA is proposing to relocate and combine certain requirements to better harmonize the requirements with specifications for quality systems in the ISO 9001 quality standard and to use as much common language as possible to enhance conformance with ISO 9001 terminology. By requiring all manufacturers to design and manufacture devices under the controls of a total quality system, the FDA believes the proposed changes in the CGMP regulations will improve the quality of medical devices manufactured in the United States for domestic distribution or exportation as well as devices imported from other countries. The proposed changes should ensure that only safe and effective devices are distributed in conformance with the act. Harmonization means a general enhancement of CGMP requirements among the world's leading producers of medical devices.

19.3 Design for Manufacturability

Design for Manufacturability (DFM) assures that a design can be repeatably manufactured while satisfying the requirements for quality, reliability, performance, availability, and price. One of the fundamental principles of DFM is reducing the number of parts in a product. Existing parts should be simple and add value to the product. All parts should be specified, designed, and manufactured to allow 100% usable parts to be produced. It takes a concerted effort by Design, Manufacturing, and vendors to achieve this goal.

Design for Manufacturability is desirable because it is less costly. The reduction in cost is due to:

- a simpler design with fewer parts
- simple production processes
- higher quality and reliability
- easier to service.

19.3.1 The DFM process

The theme of DFM is to eliminate nonfunctional parts, such as screws or fasteners, while also reducing the number of functional parts. The remaining parts should each perform as many functions as possible. The following questions help in determining if a part is necessary:

- Must the part move relative to its mating part?
- Must the part be of a different material than its mating part or isolated from all other parts?
- Must the part be separate for disassembly or service purposes?

All fasteners are automatically considered candidates for elimination.

A process that can be expected to have a defect rate of no more that a few parts per million consists of:

- Identification of critical characteristics
- Determining product elements contributing to critical characteristics

- For each identified product element, determining the step or process choice that affects or controls the required performance
- Determining a nominal value and maximum allowable tolerance for each product component and process step.
- Determining the capability for parts and process elements that control required performance
- Ensuring that the capability index (Cp) is greater than or equal to 2, where

$$Cp = (\text{specification width})/\text{process capability}$$

19.4 Design for Assembly

Design for Assembly is a structured methodology for analyzing product concepts or existing products for simplification of the design and its assembly process. Reduction in parts and assembly operations, and individual part geometry changes to ease assembly are the primary goals. The analysis process exposes many other life cycle cost and customer satisfaction issues which can then be addressed. Design and assembly process quality are significantly improved by this process.

Most textbook approaches to Design for Assembly (DFA) discuss elimination of parts. While this is a very important aspect of DFA, there are also many other factors that affect product assembly. A few rules include:

<u>Overall Design Concept</u>

- the design should be simple with a minimum number of parts
- assure the unit is light weight
- the system should have a unified design approach, rather than look like an accumulation of parts
- components should be arranged and mounted for the most economical assembly and wiring
- components that have a limited shelf life should be avoided
- the use of special tools should be minimized

- the use of wiring and harnesses to connect components should be avoided.

Component Mounting

- the preferred assembly direction is top down
- repositioning of the unit to different orientations during assembly should be avoided
- all functional internal components should mount to one main chassis component
- mating parts should be self aligning
- simple, foolproof operations should be used.

Test Points

- pneumatic test point shall be accessible without removal of any other module
- electrical test points shall include, but not be limited to:
- reference voltages
- adjustments
- key control signals
- power supply voltages
- all electronic test points shall be short-circuit protected and easily accessible.

Stress Levels and Tolerances

- the lowest possible stress levels should be used
- the maximum possible operating limits and mechanical tolerances should be maximized
- operations of known capability should be use.

Printed Circuit Boards (PCBs)

- adequate clearance should be provided around circuit board mounting locations to allow for tools
- components should be soldered, not socketed
- PCBs must be mechanically secured and supported

- there must be unobstructed access to test and calibration points
- exposed voltages should be less than 40 volts.

Miscellaneous

- all air intakes should be filtered and an indication that the filter needs to be changed should be given to the user
- the device shall be packed in a recyclable container so as to minimize the system installation time.

19.4.1 Design for assembly process

- Develop a multi-functional team before the new product architecture is defined. This team should foster a creative climate which will encourage ownership of the new product's design and delivery process.
- Establish product goals through a benchmarking process or by creating a model, drawing, or a conception of the product.
- Perform a design for assembly analysis of the product. this identifies possible candidates for elimination or redesign, as well as highlighting high cost assembly operations.
- Segment the product architecture into manageable modules or levels of assembly.
- Apply design for assembly principles to these assembly modules to generate a list of possible cost opportunities.
- Apply creative tools, such as brainstorming, to enhance the emerging design and identify further design improvements.
- As a team, evaluate and select the best ideas, thus narrowing and focusing the team's goals.
- Make commodity and material selections. Start early supplier involvement to assure economical production.
- With the aid of cost models or competitive benchmarking, establish a target cost for every part in the new design.

- Start the detailed design of the emerging product. Model, test, and evaluate the new design for form, fit, and function.
- Re-apply the process at the next logical point.
- Share the results.

19.5 The Manufacturing Process

The process of producing a new product may be said to be a multi-phased process consisting of:

- pre-production activity
- the pilot run build
- the production run
- delivery to the customer.

19.5.1 Pre-production activity

Prior to the first manufacturing build, Manufacturing is responsible for completing a myriad of activities. Manufacturing and Engineering should work together to identify proposed technologies and to assure that the chosen technology is manufacturable.

The selection of suppliers should begin by consulting the current approved suppliers listing to determine if any of the existing suppliers can provide the technology and/or parts. A new supplier evaluation would be necessary if a supplier is being considered as a potential source for a component, subassembly, or device.

A Pilot Run plan must be developed that specifies the quantity of units to be built during the pilot run, the yield expectations and contingency plans, the distribution of those units, the feedback mechanism for problems, the intended production location, staffing requirements, training plan, post production evaluation, and any other key issues specific to the project.

The Manufacturing strategy needs to be developed. The strategy must be documented and communicated to appropriate personnel to ensure it is complete, meets the business objectives, and ultimately is reflected in the design for the product. Developing a strategy for producing the product involves work on five major fronts:

- the production plan
- the quality plan
- the test plan
- the materials plan
- the supplier plan.

The Production Plan details how Manufacturing will produce the product. The first step is defining the requirements of the production process. Some of these requirements will be found in the business proposal and product specification. A Bill of Materials structure is developed for the product which best meets the defined requirements. Based on this Bill of Materials, a process flow diagram can be developed along with specific details of inventory levels and locations, test points, skills, resources, tooling required, and processing times.

The Quality Plan details the control through all phases of manufacture, procurement, packaging, storage, and shipment which collectively assures that the product meets specifications. The plan should cover not only initial production, but also how the plan will be matured over time, using data collected internally and from the field.

The Test Plan specifies the "how" of the Quality Plan. This document must have enough technical detail to assure that the features are incorporated in the product design specification. Care must be taken to ensure that the manufacturer's test strategies are consistent with those of all suppliers.

The Materials Plan consists of defining the operating plan by which the final product, parts, accessories, and service support parts will be managed logistically to meet the launch plans. This involves product structure, lead times, inventory management techniques, inventory phasing/impact estimates, and identification of any special materials considerations that must be addressed. Any production variants which will be in production as well as potentially obsolete product would be detailed.

The Supplier Plan consists of a matrix of potential suppliers versus evaluation criteria. The potential suppliers have been identified using preliminary functional component specifications. The evaluation criteria should include business stability, quality systems, cost, engineering capabilities, and test philosophy.

The Design for Manufacture and Assembly (DFMA) review should be held when a representative model is available. This review should be documented, with action items assigned.

19.5.2 The pilot run build

The objective of this phase is to complete the pilot run and validate the manufacturing process against the objectives set forth in the manufacturing strategy and the product specification.

The pilot run build is the first build of devices using the Manufacturing documentation. It is during this phase that training of the assembly force takes place. All training should be documented so no employee is given a task without the appropriate training prior to the task.

The pilot run build will validate the manufacturing process against the strategy and the Manufacturing documentation. The validation will determine if Manufacturing has met its objectives, including:

- standard cost
- product quality
- documentation
- tooling
- training
- process control.

The validation will also determine if the production testing is sufficient to ensure that the product meets the specified requirements.

The pilot run build also validates the supplier plan and supplier contracts. The validation will determine if the manufacturing plan is sufficient to control the internal processes of the supplier. The method and ground rules for communication between the two companies must be well defined to ensure that both parties keep each other informed of developments which impact the other. It should also confirm that all points have been addressed in the supplier contract and that all the controls and procedures required by the agreement are in place and operating correctly.

Internal failure analysis and corrective action takes place, involving investigating to the root cause all failures during the pilot run. The information should be communicated to the project team in detail and in a timely manner. The project team determines the appropriate corrective action plans.

A pilot run review meeting is held to review all aspects of the build, including the Manufacturing documentation. All remaining issues must be resolved and documentation corrected. Sufficient time should be allowed in the project schedule for corrective action to be completed before the production run.

19.5.3 The production run

The objective of this phase is to produce high quality product on time, while continuing to fine tune the process using controls which have been put in place.

During this phase, the first production order of units and service parts are manufactured. The training effort continues, as new employees are transferred in or minor refinements are made to the process. Line failures at any point in the process should be thoroughly analyzed and the root cause determined. Product cost should be verified at this time.

19.5.4 Customer delivery

The objective of this phase is to deliver the first production units to the customer, refine the manufacturing process based on lessons learned during the first build, and finally to monitor field unit performance to correct any problems.

Following production and shipment of product, continued surveillance of the production process should take place to measure its performance against the manufacturing strategy. The production process should be evaluated for effectiveness as well as unit field performance. Feedback from the field on unit problems should be sent to the project team, where it may be disseminated to the proper area.

Homework Exercises

1. Year 2000 (Y2k) problems were a concern for medical device manufacturers, especially those that dealt with imbedded microprocessors. Investigate this statement using a web search. How might the GMP regulation have avoided this problem?
2. Visit the web site http://www.fda.gov/cdrh/dsma/gmp_man.html and briefly look at the manual listed here. How does this differ from the GMP regulation?
3. Perform a web search for DFMA, report on the best site you can find.
4. Find and report on at least one good example of DFA or DFMA.
5. A related term involves Design for the Environment. Find information on this type of process and report on its value.
6. A related activity involves Design for Life Cycle, report on this concept.
7. Investigate a typical blood pressure unit that may be purchased at your corner drug store. What improvements can you suggest with respect to DFA?
8. As in Exercise 7, but investigate an in-the-ear temperature unit.

References

Boothroyd Dewhurst, Inc., *Design for Manufacture and Assembly/Service/Environment and Concurrent Engineering (Workshop Manual).* Wakefield, RI: Boothroyd Dewhurst, Inc, 1966.

Food and Drug Administration, *21 CFR Part 820 Medical Devices; Current Good Manufacturing Practice (CGMP Regulations; Proposed Revisions.* Rockville, MD: November 23, 1993.

Fries, Richard C., *Reliability Assurance for Medical Devices, Equipment and Software.* Buffalo Grove, IL: Interpharm Press, Inc., 1991.

Fries, Richard C., *Reliable Design of Medical Devices.* New York: Marcel Dekker, Inc., 1997.

Hooten, W. Fred, "A Brief History of FDA Good Manufacturing Practices," in *Medical Device & Diagnostic Industry.* Volume 18, Number 5, May, 1996.

Chapter 20

Product Issues

"An error doesn't become a mistake until you refuse to correct it."
Orlando A. Battista

20.1 Product Safety and Legal Issues

When designing for safety, there are two aspects to consider. The first is risk assessment that addresses the questions: What failure could cause harm to the patient or user? What misuse of the device could cause harm? These failures must be analyzed using such methods as fault tree analysis or failure mode analysis and must be designed out of the device.

The second aspect of safety is liability assessment. This addresses the questions: Have all possible failure modes been explored and designed out? Have all possible misuse situations been addressed? Court cases have special punitive judgements for companies that have knowledge about an unsafe condition and do nothing about it.

20.1.1 Definition of safety

Safety may be defined as:

freedom from accidents or losses.

Some people have argued that there is no such thing as absolute safety, and therefore safety should be defined in terms of acceptable losses. Using this argument, an alternative definition of safety would be:

a judgement of the acceptability of risk, with risk, in turn, as a measure of the probability and severity of harm to human health.

A product is safe if its attendant risks are judged to be acceptable. This definition of safety implies that hazards cannot be eliminated, when they often can. While in most instances, all hazards cannot be eliminated, specific hazards can be totally eliminated from a product or system.

System safety is a subdiscipline of systems engineering that applies scientific, management, and engineering principles to ensure adequate safety throughout the system life cycle, without constraints of operational effectiveness, time, and cost. Although safety has been defined as freedom from those conditions that can cause death, injury, occupational illness, or damage to or loss of equipment or property, it is generally recognized that this is unrealistic. By this definition, any system that presents an element of risk is unsafe. But almost any system that produces personal, social, or industrial benefits contains an indispensable element of risk.

The problem is complicated by the fact that attempts to eliminate risk often result in risk displacement rather than risk elimination. Benefits and risks often have trade-offs, such as trading off the benefits of improved medical diagnosis capabilities against the risks of exposure to diagnostic X-rays. Unfortunately, the question "How safe is safe enough?" has no simple answer.

Safety is also relative in that nothing is completely safe under all conditions. There is always some case in which a relatively safe material or piece of equipment becomes hazardous. The act of drinking water, if done to excess, can cause kidney failure. Thus safety is a function of the situation in which it is measured. One definition might be that safety is a measure of the degree of freedom from risk in any environment. To understand safety better, it is helpful to consider the nature of accidents in general.

An accident is traditionally defined by safety engineers as an unwanted and unexpected release of energy. However, a release of energy is not involved in some hazards associated with new technologies and potentially lethal chemicals. Therefore the term mishap is often used to denote an unplanned event or series of events that result in death, injury, occupational illness, damage to or loss of equipment or property, or environmental harm. The term mishap includes both accidents and harmful exposures.

Mishaps are almost always caused by multiple factors and the relative contribution of each factor is usually not clear. A mishap can be thought of as a set of events combining in random fashion, or alternatively, as a dynamic mechanism that begins with the activation of a hazard and flows through the system as a series of sequential and concurrent events in a logical sequence until the system is out of control and a loss is produced. The high frequency of complex, multifactorial mishaps may arise from the fact that the simpler potentials have been anticipated and handled. However, the very complexity of the events leading up to a mishap implies that there may be many opportunities to interrupt the sequences.

Mishaps often involve problems in subsystem interfaces. It appears to be easier to deal with failures of components than failures in the interfaces between components.

How do engineers deal with safety problems? The earliest approach to safety, called operational or industrial safety, involves examining the system during its operational life and correcting what are deemed to be unacceptable hazards. In this approach, accidents are examined, the causes determined, and corrective action initiated. In some complex systems, however, a single accident can involve such a great loss as to be unacceptable. The goal of system safety is to design an acceptable safety level into the system before actual production or operation.

System safety engineering attempts to optimize safety by applying scientific and engineering principles to identify and control hazards through analysis, design, and management procedures.

20.1.2 Safety and reliability

There is some confusion in the industry about the difference between safety and reliability. Both are good things to which systems should aspire. They remain, however, distinct concepts. They may at times even be conflicting concerns. The literature has muddied the picture by using these terms imprecisely, particularly the term safety.

A safe system is one that does not incur too much risk to persons or equipment. A risk is an event or condition that can occur, but is undesirable. Risk is measured both in terms of severity and probability. Safety only concerns itself with failures that introduce hazards. The probability of failure of a device to meet its requirements defines its reliability. Safety takes a broader view - it is possible to write requirements so that they do not consider all safety concerns. The concept of safety is not defined in terms of meeting requirements, but on a level of risk.

A safe system is one in which damage to persons or property doesn't happen often or, when it does, the damage is minor. If the damage potential is small, then it can happen more frequently and still be considered safe. If the damage potential is great, then the chance for a mishap must be correspondingly small for the system to be safe. Note that the availability of the system does not appear in the definition of safe. A system can fail all the time, but provided that it fails in a safe way, that is, in a way that does not lead to mishaps, the system is still safe. Conversely, a system can be up and running all the time and consistently put people at risk. Such a system is reliable, but not safe.

Consider the example of a pacemaker. For the vast majority of pacemaker patients, the pacemaker provides an assistance only. When the sino-atrial (SA) node, the normal pacemaker of the heart, fails to function properly, some other area of cardiac tissue takes over its role. However, the SA node provides the best rate for physiological control, typically 60 to 80 beats per minute. When other portions of the heart assume the pacing function, the rates are typically much less and can be as low as 30 beats per minute. Patients with this condition have a reduced cardiac output and have difficulty performing tasks that require increased cardiac flow, such as climbing stairs.

A pacemaker solves this problem by artificially pacing the heart at some minimum programmed rate. A pacemaker that paces at 110 beats per minute continuously no matter what, is very reliable. However, if the patient is in cardiac failure, a high pacing rate is medically inappropriate. Thus, this is a reliable but unsafe device.

An unreliable pacemaker would be one that didn't always pace at the programmed rate. However, not pacing is not a safety concern, except for a small minority of patients. In this case, we have an unreliable but safe device.

Hardware components and subsystems usually have known failure histories and there are published values for such reliability measures as mean time to failure (MTTF) and mean time between failures (MTBF). When a system is entirely composed of components whose reliability statistics are known, the reliability of the entire system can be estimated by combining the reliability of the components according to the mathematical laws of probability Such calculations are the source of assertions that certain safety-critical systems, such as aircraft controls, have a very low probability of failure.

For software, there are no sound foundations for quantitative statistical failure estimates, such as MTBF. Software faults are design errors, not random equipment failures. Control software is customized for each product. A new control program is therefore a unique artifact with no performance history of any kind. That is why object oriented design and programming have suggested the reuse of software objects that have been tested and used in the field and thus have a history of success or failure.

Failure data should be collected during development and early field experience. It is usual to discover many faults early in a product's lifetime. The fault discovery rate gradually declines as more subtle problems are unearthed. There exist statistical software reliability models that attempt to predict the number of undiscovered faults remaining, based on the past history of failures, but these models are necessarily less trustworthy than statistics gathered from mass-produced items. In practice, it is not possible to predict when a program will next fail, and it is not realistic to assign failure probabilities or measures to programs just entering service. The main practical lessons of the software reliability models is that a program that has recently exhibited many failures is likely to continue to fail. It is also important to note that a new version of a program may need to be considered a completely new program from the point of view of failure history.

The concerns for safety and reliability can be at odds with each other. To improve reliability, marginally operating systems may be allowed to continue to function. At the same time, devices are not automatically beneficial, and they, like all technology, are associated with risk. Recent examples include ultrasound equipment that often does not comply with electrical safety guidelines, leakage of insulin pumps, defective artificial cardiac valves and reactions of the body to materials used in implants.

20.1.3 The legal aspects of safety

Limiting legal liability is one of the goals of system safety. Ideally, tort law complements safety regulation by deterring the production of harmful products, along with its primary purpose of compensating injured individuals. The impact of product liability judgements and the increase in insurance rates as a consequence have been highly controversial. While data are difficult to acquire, it is clear that new theories of liability have expanded the number of potential lawsuits and that there has been a trend toward larger compensatory and punitive damage awards. Medical devices have been the focus of several mass tort actions, including thousands of cases brought against the producers of tampons for toxic shock injuries and against A. H. Robbins, the manufacturer of the Dalkon Shield. There is no question that product liability has increased the costs of doing business in some sectors of the medical device industry.

The three most common theories of liability for which a manufacturer may be held liable for personal injury caused by its product are

- negligence
- strict liability
- breach of warranty.

These are referred to as common-law causes of action, which are distinct from causes of action based on federal or state statutory law. Although within the last decade federal legislative action that would create a uniform federal product liability law has been proposed and debated, no such law exists today. Thus, such litigation is governed by the laws of each state.

The basic idea of negligence law is that one should have to pay for injuries that he or she causes when acting below the standard of care of a reasonable, prudent person participating in the activity in question. This standard of conduct relates to a belief that centers on potential victims: that people have a right to be protected from unreasonable risks of harm. A fundamental aspect of the negligence standard of care resides in the concept of foreseeability. In one of the most famous torts opinions, in what today would be called a products liability case, it was written that there is a duty "to use ordinary skill and care to avoid...danger" when "one person is by circumstances placed in such a position with regard to another... that every one of ordinary sense who did think would at once recognize" the risk of danger "if he did not use ordinary care and skill." It is interesting that in this nineteenth century opinion, long before the coinage of the term "products liability," this formulation emerged from a case dealing with a ship painter's allegation that the failure of a rope on a scaffold caused him to fall.

Under the theory of negligence, a manufacturer that does not exercise reasonable care or fails to meet a reasonable standard of care in the manufacture, handling, or distribution of a product may be liable for any damages caused. For example, if it can be established that not having a reliability program constitutes a failure to meet an industry-wide practice that is found to be an applicable standard of care, then the manufacturer may be subject to liability for negligence.

Unlike the negligence suit, in which the focus is on the defendant's conduct, in a strict liability suit, the focus is on the product itself. The formulation of strict liability states that one who sells any product in a defective condition unreasonably dangerous to the user or consumer or to his property is subject to liability for physical harm thereby caused to the ultimate user or consumer or to his property if the seller is engaged in the business of selling such a product, and it is expected to and does reach the user or consumer without substantial change to the condition in which it is sold. Therefore, the critical focus in a strict liability case is on whether the product is defective and unreasonably dangerous. A common standard applied in medical device cases to reach that determination is the risk/benefit analysis - that is, whether the benefits of the device outweigh the risks attendant with its use.

Strict Liability in tort had its modern origins in warranty and in the tort doctrine of res ipsa loquitur. The rationales for imposing strict liability are based on the fact that the manufacturer is in the best position to reduce the risk. The loss may be overwhelming to the injured person, but it can be effectively insured against by the manufacturer and distributed among the public as a cost of doing business. The manufacturer, even if not negligent, is responsible for the product being on the market.

There are three types of breaches of warranty that may be alleged:

- breach of the implied warranty of merchantability
- breach of the implied warranty of fitness for a particular purpose
- breach of an express warranty.

An express warranty is one which is stated explicitly, either orally, in a contract of sale, or in the labeling. For instance, let us assume that a clinical engineer requests and receives a written or oral statement that the medical device manufacturer followed a certain reliability protocol or that the medical device and its software will perform in a specific fashion. If the device causes an injury because it was not developed according to the stated reliability protocol or because it did not function as warranted, the manufacturer faces liability under the express warranty theory.

Sometimes, a warranty is not stated explicitly. By introducing a product into commercial distribution, the manufacturer implicitly warrants that the product is reasonably fit for the purposes that similar products are intended to serve. For instance, if all pacemaker manufacturers have reliability programs to ensure proper functioning of their products, and a new pacemaker manufacturer begins commercial distribution, there may be an implied warranty that the new manufacturer has a similar program in place.

These warranty causes of action do not offer any advantages for the injured plaintiff that cannot be obtained by resort to negligence and strict liability claims and, in fact, pose greater hurdles to recovery. Thus, although a breach of warranty claim is often pled in the plaintiff's complaint, it is seldom relied on at trial as the basis for recovery.

As a general proposition, a plaintiff is entitled to plead and prove as many counts or causes of action as they wish. The plaintiff is usually entitled to recover all foreseeable damages in a products liability suit. Such damages may cover the areas of emotional distress, punitive damages, and joint and several liability.

There is a division of authority as to whether recovery for emotional distress alone is allowable, where there is no accompanying physical injury. Courts have held that recovery for emotional distress without physical injury is permissible where the defendant's conduct is intentional or outrageous. A distinction is drawn between recovery for fear of future injury, and recovery for the risk of the injury itself. Some courts will not allow recovery for the risk of future injury, even where the chance that the risk will result in greater injury is greater than 50%. Others allow for recovery if the risk is more probable than not.

Perhaps no subject in tort law has generated more heated controversy in recent years that the recoverability of punitive damages in tort, including products liability. The evidence indicates that only a small fraction of cases result in punitive damages and many of these are business torts, rather than personal injury cases. A few cases have received disproportionate attention, however, and the specter of potentially large punitive recoveries has probably contributed significantly to substantial increase in products liability insurance premiums, as well as to the enactment at the state level of various restrictions on punitive recoveries. The statutory restrictions vary widely, from raising the burden of proof to clear and convincing evidence to requiring actual malice, to placing a cap on the amount of recovery, to requiring bifurcation of trial of the compensatory and punitive aspects of a case, to requiring managerial involvement in the misconduct, to requiring part of the recovery to be paid to the state, and other variations.

Another area in which extensive efforts have been made to modify the common law by statute is with regard to joint liability - whereby one tortfeasor is held liable for all damages suffered by a claimant, even though other tortfeasors may also have contributed to the injury. If the damages are readily divisible, the tortfeasor would normally be liable only for his share. But liability for the full amount of damages is usually imposed when the damages are practically indivisible, as is often the case when there are multiple tortfeasors.

As can be seen, safety, as evidenced through products liability, will have an effect on a manufacturer, both in terms of finances and in reputation. The topic of products liability is discussed in greater detail in Chapter 13.

20.1.4 System safety

Every system, no matter how complex it is, should be fail-safe, that is, it should be designed to fail into a safe and harmless state. Only a few simple functions should be required to enter or preserve the safe states by terminating or preventing potentially hazardous conditions. These functions, usually called interlocks, lockouts, or shutdown systems, should be designed to work properly despite the failure of other functions. Many regulations and guidelines specify that these safety functions should not be performed by the same computer system that provides normal operating functions and should perhaps not be performed by computers at all.

A very important part of the design process is identifying the safe states. A radiation therapy machine is in a safe state when the beam is turned OFF and all motions are stopped. An automatic drug infusing device is in a safe state when the infusion is stopped or, depending on the drug, when the infusion rate is at some constant, low value. Unlike some applications, like aviation, which require backup computers with considerable functionality, in medicine it is usually sufficient to provide a simple safety system that disconnects the computer, achieves the safe state, and turns on an alarm when faults are discovered. It can then be left to a human operator to correct the problem.

20.1.5 Hardware safety

Computer hardware is less robust than electromechanical hardware. Modern solid-state electronics, including discrete logic modules and microprocessors are far more vulnerable to environmental stresses than are relays, for example. Extremes of heat and cold, modest electronic over voltages, even static electric charge carried on an operator's clothing can temporarily disrupt or permanently damage solid-state circuitry. Extremely brief electronic transients or "noise spikes" which can only be detected by special test equipment, may cause mystifying and unreproducible systems behavior. Control programs stored in what is supposed to be permanent, read-only memory may fade away as components age. Electrical interferences from unexpected sources can induce serious hazards.

Because solid-state electronics are more delicate than electromechanical devices, it is usually not possible to simply replace electromechanical controls with functionally equivalent solid-state equipment. the new equipment often fails because it proves to be vulnerable to electrical interference and other environmental disturbances that the older equipment could easily tolerate. It is usually necessary to provide the computer with a more protected electrical environment, constructed according to good packaging, grounding and shielding practices. In addition, special signal conditioning and isolation circuitry is often required. Techniques sufficient for personal computers and other consumer electronics are not always adequate for more demanding process control environments.

Electromechanical components usually fail one at a time. Consequently, many functions may continue to work even after one or more components have failed. Therefore, each component in a device must be analyzed for potential failures and safety concerns. There are several methods which aid in the analysis of components. Fault tree analysis is a methodology where potential failures are traced back to the components causing them. Failure Mode Analysis looks at each component and determines the effect of a failure of that component on the system.

Once the component has been analyzed, there are techniques that can be employed to reduce the potential for the failure of that component. Such techniques include:

- component derating
- safety margin
- load protection.

The methodologies and techniques for analyzing and assuring component safety are discussed in detail in Chapter 11.

20.1.6 Software safety

Software is not, in itself, unsafe. Only the physical systems that it may control can do damage. Safety considerations hardly arise for programs that perform conventional data processing or scientific computation. In these applications, the computer only displays results on paper or on video screens. It is presumed that the users will review these results, bringing their informed judgement to bear before acting upon them. It is only when computers are used to directly control systems that are themselves potentially unsafe, that safety issues arise.

It is not unusual for all software functions to fail simultaneously. In computer-controlled systems, many different functions are usually performed by a single processor. Distributed or multiprocessor control systems having more than one computer usually have more functions than they have processors. Different functions are controlled by different parts of the control program, which are run in rapid sequences on a single processor. This control program replaces, in effect, a large number of relays or other discrete components. Concentrating so much complexity into software provides much of the economy and flexibility of computer-controlled systems, but also makes then more vulnerable to errors.

Most programming languages provide some way to divide a program text into sections variously called subroutines, procedures, functions, modules, tasks, or processes. These sections are sometimes called software components, but this analogy is misleading. Even when the text of two program sections appear to be completely independent, they are in fact much more tightly coupled than is usual for electronic components. They share a vital resource - the processor itself.

Certain kinds of software errors can cause the process to interrupt its normal sequence of operations and enter an abnormal state that prevents it from doing useful work. Such an event is colorfully termed a "crash." Crashes can be caused by many programming errors that are easy to commit: attempting to divide by zero, attempting to compute a number larger or smaller than can be accommodated by the processor hardware, attempting to read or write into a memory location that is not populated by a memory chip, attempting to use an array element whose subscript is larger than the size of the array, and so forth. Crashes can also be induced by hardware failures, such as intermittent faults or electrical interference.

The behavior of a crashed program is completely unpredictable. It may halt in some apparently random state, or it may continue on, generating random output. Another kind of global program failure occurs when a particular program section seizes control of the processor and will not release it. These occurrences, in which the computer appears to be "stuck" or "hung" result from common programming errors, such as infinite loops and deadlocks. All functions in a crashed or hung program stop working, not just the one containing the error. System in which several processors share common memory can be vulnerable because errors in one processor's program may cause it to corrupt instructions or data needed by other processors.

In data processing and scientific computing, program crashes do not contribute to accidents because they do not release energy directly. In these environments, programs run under control of a supervisory program called an operating system, which can usually recover control from a crashed or stuck program. If the operating system itself crashes, the operator can shut down and restart the computer, which often clears the problem. Process control systems, on the other hand, often have no operating system or include customized program sections that perform some of the functions of the operating system. There may be no opportunity for the operator to intervene in any useful way. Consequences of failure can be very serious. A runaway program could drive a radiation therapy machine gantry into a patient. A hung program could fail to terminate a radiation exposure and deliver an overdose.

The expanded use of software in medical devices has offered the promise of increased product functionality and more efficient manufacturing. The type of failures caused by poor design practices, however can result in costs that can easily exceed projected benefits. One way to prevent this is to study past software safety-related failures and develop methods to prevent those failures.

Fortunately, there are enough sources of information available detailing past software safety failures to construct of history of such occurrences. FDA's "Device Recalls: A Study of Quality Problems" documents 85 preproduction quality problems caused by software design. It also relates 93 episodes in which a change in some aspect of the device or its manufacturing process led ultimately to a recall. Another FDA publication titled "Evaluation of Software Related Recalls for the Period FY83-FY89" identifies 116 problems in software quality that resulted in medical device recalls.

20.1.7 Verification and validation of safety

A proof of safety involves a choice or combination of 1) showing that a fault cannot occur, that is, the device cannot get into an unsafe state, or 2) showing that if a fault occurs, it is not dangerous. It has been argued that verification systems that prove the correspondence of devices to concrete specifications are only fragments of verification systems. Verification systems must capture the semantics of the hardware, the software code, and the system behavior.

Another verification methodology for safety involves the use of fault tree analysis. Once the design is completed, fault tree analysis procedures can be used to work backward from critical faults determined by the top levels of the fault tree through the device to verify whether the device can cause the top level event or mishap.

Since the goal of in safety verification is to prove that something will not happen, it is helpful to use proof by contradiction. That is, it is assumed the device has produced an unsafe action and it is shown that this could not happen since it lead to a logical contradiction. Although a proof of correctness should theoretically be able to show that a device is safe, it is often impractical to accomplish this because of the sheer magnitude of the proof effort involved and because of the difficulty of completely specifying correct behavior.

20.1.8 An effective safety program

Any effective safety program requires procedures and expertise in formal hazard identification and analysis techniques. In addition, several expected-hazard mitigation controls should be implemented in any medical device system. These controls include checking the status of hardware on start-up, monitoring hardware equipment during runtime, checking data ranges to reduce the likelihood of operator entry errors, defining system fail-safe states in the case of failures, implementing securing controls, and conducting formal low-level testing and review of safety-critical functions. Applying hazard mitigation controls that adhere to good engineering practices is essential for developing an effective safety program.

A truly effective safety program includes implementation of internal hazard analysis procedures, a firm grasp of regulatory and other standards, and an awareness of the current industry practices regarding safety controls. Such programs consume considerable time and resources, but failing to make the investment increases the risk of product recalls for medical device manufacturers.

Safety analysis begins when the project is conceived and continues throughout the product development life cycle. Due to the variety of medical devices with many degrees of complexity, the following should be included in a safety analysis program:

- Safety review personnel must have a thorough understanding of the operation of the device. Personnel should review pertinent documentation, such as drawings, test reports and manuals prior to the analysis.
- Make a representative device available for the review. It will be subject to disassembly.
- Use a checklist for the analysis especially prepared for the particular device
- Address all areas of concern immediately. Safety release is not granted until the device has no apparent areas of concern
- Safety release the device via a release letter only after all areas of concern are addressed.
- Retain the checklist and release letter as part of the product file.

Specifically prepare a comprehensive checklist for the device under analysis. Areas to be addressed in the checklist include, but are not limited to:

- Voltages
- Operating frequencies
- Leakage currents
- Dielectric withstand
- Environmental specifications
- Grounding impedance
- Power cord and plug
- Electrical insulation
- Abnormal operations
- Physical stability
- Corrosion protection
- Circuit breakers and fuses
- Color coding
- Ergonomic specifications

- Standards Conformance
- Alarms, warnings and indicators
- Mechanical design integrity.

The checklist should be signed by the analyst(s) after completion of the analysis. Figure 20-1 shows an example of one page of such a checklist.

20.2 Accident Reconstruction and Forensics

Biomedical engineers, due to their generally broad-based education, may sometimes be called upon to analyze accidents. Analysis of medical device accidents will first be discussed, followed by a brief discussion on biomechanics and accident (physical injury due to car, etc impact) investigation. Both of these have implications for improved designs of devices and processes that biomedical engineers may be involved in.

20.2.1 Medical device accidents

Medical device accident investigation follows a fairly typical chain of events, of which most are in common for accidents in general. The overall process for a medical device accident investigation takes roughly the following outline:

- An incident occurs, someone is injured, and a cause for action is established.
- You are contacted by the wronged person, by his/her lawyer, or by one of the parties or their representative needing an investigation.
- After an initial familiarization with the problem, you may opt to work on the problem, or opt out (see section 21.5).
- You need to collect data. This means you must inspect the scene (if any), photograph and/or sketch the environment as necessary, gather evidence, and read whatever written documentation exists at this point. This may include operative notes, nurses notes, some preliminary testimony, machine charts, etc.

Characteristic	Comments
Operating voltages	
Operating frequencies	
Leakage currents	
Dielectric withstand	
Environmental specs	
Grounding impedance	
Power cord and plug	
Electrical insulation	
Abnormal operations	
Physical stability	
Corrosion protection	
Circuit breakers/fuses	
Color coding	
Ergonomic specs	
Standards conformance	
Alarms and warnings	
Mechanical design integrity	
Cleaning solutions	

Figure 20-1 Safety analysis checklist. (From Fries, 1997.)

- You need to research the device or process in question. This means that you will use MAUDE if necessary. You will need to access the operators' manual for the device, as necessary. You will need to investigate maintenance manuals, if necessary. You will need to run simulations on the device, if necessary. You likely will need to use the web, other than just MAUDE for keyword searches. You will need to obtain agreement for the use of specialists, such as personnel who perform calibration or maintenance on the devices as necessary. You may need to do some basic research and mockups of the device as necessary.
- As a result of your work, you will need to estimate causes and their likelihood. If you can demonstrate the error, so much the better.
- A branching point is reached here. A report (oral or written, this should be pre-agreed to) should be submitted to the person who contacted and contracted you. You must be prepared to continue the investigation, await further court action, or be released from further work. The latter is generally the case when you find for someone other than those who hired you.
- You must be prepared to answer questioning from opposition lawyers if necessary. This can take the form of both oral and written testimony as to the current status of the investigation.
- Most of the time, a final formal report designating the fault will end your work. On a small number of occasions, expect to go to court, get sworn in, and testify regarding your work.

Two brief cases below will serve to illustrate the range of efforts that may come of a medical device accident.

- Scene: A patient was sent home from a nursing facility with an enteral feeding pump (direct to stomach tube feeding), a supply of feeding compound, and a supply of enteral feeding pump tubes. On the first use of the pump, the patient wound up with too high a flow of food such that food filled the stomach and entered the lungs. She expired due to pneumonia induced by the flow within a few days.

- Resolution: After a very brief overview of the material, a panel was convened comprised of representatives of the nursing facility, a biomedical engineer from academia, a representative from the company that manufactured the pump, and the opposition lawyers. Within five minutes the determination was made that the pump had been sent home with the wrong pump tubing installed, the tubing that was in place allowed for gravity feed of the feeding fluid independent of the pump speed. Thus a direct cause of the accident was found in a timely manner.

- Scene: A pressure limited pump was used to ventilate a very young child who had a very small plastic airway directly in place in the throat. The child was found asphyxiated after the airway had withdrawn from the child. The unit, though the nursing service has presumably properly set the upper and lower pressure controls, was not alarming.
  - Resolution: The unit was retested and still did not alarm. Various settings were tried. It was determined that the extremely small airway element enabled sufficient backpressure to the system that the recommended pressure settings were meaningless.

20.2.2 Biomechanics and traffic accident investigations

A very basic understanding of biomechanics is necessary prior to any undertaking in which a Bioengineer may be involved in design or accident investigation. Some of the concepts that need to be understood are the following:

Data collection: data for analyses involving traffic accidents involve data collected from reported and analyzed accidents. Large data sets are collected by individual states, some of which is recollected and analyzed by the National Highway Transportation Safety Administration (NHTSA). The agency also specifically maintains data on fatal accidents, including information on vehicle type, rollover, ejection, alcohol use, etc. A smaller data set includes data for cases specifically investigated by the agency, data that includes medical information as well as more specific conclusions as to the cause of the accident and many other details. Other related data sets have been obtained from cadaver studies, anthropometrical dummy studies, animal studies, and mathematical modeling analyses. Much of the data obtained and related issues may be found on the NHSTA web site (http://www.nhtsa.dot.gov/) and in the *Proceedings of the Annual STAPP Car Crash Conferences.*

Injury Estimation: In studies of human survival following trauma an early scheme involved the development of an abbreviated injury scale (AIS), this scale ranges from 0 (minor sprain) to 6 (unsurvivable injury.) This scale is developed for each of the six body regions of interest in survivability, the head, face, chest, abdomen, extremities (including pelvis) and external. The highest squared scores from the three most injured areas are added together to generate a new score, the Injury Severity Score. With the exception that any "6" AIS rating automatically yields the maximum ISS score of 75, this score relates linearly to rates of mortality, morbidity, and length of hospital stay.[1]

Impact Analyses: Often, an engineer must estimate the relative speeds of the vehicles and personnel involved. This means that the engineer must, from the data involved in the accident report, crush patterns on the vehicles involved, vehicle data sheets, weather conditions reported, etc, estimate the relative speeds, angles of impact, and probable outcome of an accident. For example, working backward from skid length data, one can find that a vehicles initial velocity prior to the skid is directly related to the square root of twice the product of skid length, skid friction coefficient, and the value of gravity, or "g". The skid friction coefficient is a function of the type of surface (pavement v dirt road, for example), the weather conditions (dry, wet, or icy), and the type of braking system the vehicle has (2 or 4 wheel, anti-lock, etc.) If a subject has been thrown or ejected from a vehicle, simple trajectory analysis can be used to determine the initial velocity, if sufficient information exists. If there is little body damage on two vehicles, a combination of conservation of momentum analysis and elastic collision analysis might apply, along with skid analysis. Alternatively, damage analysis combined with inelastic collision analysis must be used.

The biomedical engineer doing design or doing forensic analysis after the fact in on matters involving vehicular accidents must understand the above, and be able to apply background material learned in a biomechanics class to real life problems. A few examples follow:

- Occupant restraint systems may be design to absorb energy during an impact. Consider the alternatives for air bags, especially for situations with low body weight passengers.
- During a motorcycle-truck accident, the helmet of the motorcyclist came off, resulting in death of the motorcyclist due to blunt head trauma. Where was the error in the design of the helmet system?
- Current seat belts are a trade-off between convenience and safety. Determine the "ideal" design.

Homework Exercises

1. Visit the new car assessment pages at the NHTSA web site (http://www.nhtsa.dot.gov/NCAP/Info.html), copy the frequently asked questions list, and comment on five of the particular items.
2. Visit the Stapp Conference website (www.stapp.org), determine the history of the conferences.
3. Do a MAUDE search for deaths caused by Enteral Feeders Print out and discuss at least one case.
4. Do a MAUDE search for deaths caused in one week of the year. Comment on your results.
5. One of the authors of this book owns a 1996 Chrysler Voyager Van and a 1995 Volvo 950. Visit the NHSTA site to determine which is the safer car.
6. Find data for the chance of survival for a patient with a major liver laceration and a closed tibial fracture as a result of a vehicular injury.
7. A lawyer asks you to testify about an injury that was received during a low-speed (10 mph or less) two-vehicle collision. Specifically he asks that you testify that no data exists that can prove the correct speeds of the vehicles and the likelihood of injury. Is this correct?
8. A three-year-old female sustained neck injuries on a child roller coaster at a theme park. What would you do to prove or disprove this claim? By the way, the father has a videotape of the injury occurring, and the girl seemed to have a "long neck". This particular ride had been in use for ten years.
9. A child sustained a severe cut on his nose due to him falling off of a motorbike. The helmet he was wearing caused the cut. What was the design flaw here, and who was at fault?

10. Find and report on the use of the Apgar score. Compare this to the AIS score in this section.
11. How might tissue engineering change the field of trauma care?
12. The brain poses a special case when studying injury patterns. Research the term contrecoup; report on its significance.

References

[1] See www.trauma.org for more information

Boardman, Thomas A. and Thomas DiPasquale, "Product Liability Implications of Regulatory Compliance or Noncompliance," in *The Medical Device Industry - Science, Technology, and Regulation in a Competitive Environment*. New York: Marcel Dekker, Inc., 1990.

Boumil, Marcia M. and Clifford E. Elias, *The Law of Medical Liability in a Nutshell*. St. Paul, MN: West Publishing Co., 1995

Department of Defense, MIL-STD-882: System Safety Program Requirements. Washington DC: U.S. Government Printing Office, 1984.

Food and Drug Administration, *Device Recalls: A Study of Quality Problems*. Rockville, MD: FDA, 1990.

Food and Drug Administration, *Evaluation of Software Related Recalls for the Period FY83-FY89*. Rockville, MD: Food and Drug Administration, Center for Devices and Radiological Health, 1990.

Fries, Richard C., *Reliable Design of Medical Devices*. New York: Marcel Dekker, Inc., 1997.

Fries, Richard C., *Reliability Assurance for Medical Devices, Equipment and Software*. Buffalo Grove, IL: Interpharm Press, Inc., 1991.

Goel, A. L., "Software Reliability Models: Assumptions, Limitations, and Applicability," in *IEEE Transactions on Software Engineering*. Volume SE-11, Number 12, 1985.

Jahanian, F. and A. K. Mok, "Safety Analysis of Timing Properties in Real Time Systems," *IEEE Transactions on Software Engineering*. Volume SE-12, Number 9, September, 1986.

Jacky, Jonathan, "Safety of Computer-Controlled Devices," in *Developing Safe, Effective and Reliable Medical Software*. Arlington, VA: Association for the Advancement of Medical Instrumentation, 1991.

Jorgens III, Joseph , "The Purpose of Software Quality Assurance: A Means to an End," in *Developing Safe, Effective and Reliable Medical Software*. Arlington, VA: Association for the Advancement of Medical Instrumentation, 1991.

Levenson, Nancy G., *Safeware*. Reading, MA: Addison-Wesley Publishers, 1995.

Levenson, Nancy G., "Software Safety: Why, What and How," *Computing Surveys*. Volume 18, Number 2, June, 1986.

Musa, John D., Anthony Iannonio and Kazuhira Okumoto, *Software Reliability: Measurement, Prediction, Application*. New York: McGraw-Hill, 1987.

Nahum, Alan M., Melvin, John W. "*Accidental Injury, Biomechanics and Prevention*", Springer, New York, 2002.

Olivier, Daniel P., "Software Safety: Historical Problems and Proposed Solutions," *Medical Device and Diagnostic Industry*. Volume 17, Number 7, July, 1995.

Phillips, Jerry J., *Products Liability in a Nutshell*. St. Paul, MN: West Publishing Co., 1993.

Shapo, Marshall S., *Products Liability and the Search for Justice*. Durham, NC: Carolina Academic Press, 1993.

Chapter 21

Professional Issues

"A man's ethical behavior should be based effectually on sympathy, education, and social ties; no religious basis is necessary. Man would indeed be in a poor way if he had to be restrained by fear of punishment and hope of reward after death."
Albert Einstein

This chapter will discuss several professional issues relating to professionalism in Biomedical Engineering. Specifically it will cover some of the alphabet soup of professional societies that many biomedical engineers are members of and/or need to be familiar with as they are also standards setting groups. Next it will cover licensing of engineers and the ramifications for practicing biomedical engineers, especially those working in the area of forensics. Lastly, it will briefly discuss issues relating to continuing education for both licensed and unlicensed engineers.

21.1 BME Related Professional Societies

Society memberships, properly chosen, can be an invaluable aid in professional pursuits. Memberships should allow for one to meet others with related professional interests, assist in professional advancement through relevant newsletters and professional magazines, and should allow for the sharing of knowledge and the acquisition of new knowledge through regularly scheduled reasonably convenient national meetings. Most will also have a web presence and a means for distribution of job opportunities. The results of these meetings should be archived and be a part of the membership benefits of the organization. Some of the groups also provide standards setting functions; the ability to sit on such committees should be a function of experience with the group and its goals. These groups will be re-listed as necessary in the next section.

21.1.1 Biomedical engineering societies

Many campuses have a small number of societies that relate directly to Biomedical Engineering, the choice of societies can widen dramatically upon graduation and a first or later job. Some of the major societies are as follows:

- AAMI – The Association for the Advancement of Medical Instrumentation, this society is aimed at designers, managers, users, and regulators of medical technologies. As such it is heavily hospital user and medical industry oriented, with a large clinical engineering emphasis. For product and process design engineers, it is a comprehensive and useful organization in which to be a member. See www.aami.org for more information.
- ACM – The Association for Computing Machinery has a special interest group – SIGBIO which emphasizes medical informatics and other topics such as multimedia and molecular databases. This group sponsors several workshops and conferences each year. (See www.acm.org, search for sigbio).
- AMIA – The American Medical Informatics Association is a society devoted "to developing and using information technologies to improve health care" and is composed of individual, institutional, and corporate members. This group holds one major and one minor congress each year devoted to the application of informatics to problems in heath care, and collaborates with the international medical

informatics association. (See www.amia.org and www.imia.org for additional information).

- BMES – The Biomedical Engineering Society, the society aims to "promote the increase of biomedical engineering knowledge and its utilization." This group is heavily academic (students to professors) oriented, provides two national meetings and one newsletter and one annals. See www.bmes.org for additional information.
- IBE – Institute of Biological Engineering, this society aims to encourage interest and promote inquiry into biological engineering in its broadest manner, with potential application to the improvement of the human condition. This group is very broad in nature and includes many participants from agricultural engineering. Many of their yearly conferences are held in conduction with other groups that have some overlap in interests, such as the BMES. See www.ibeweb.org for additional information.
- IEEE-EMBS - The Institute of Electrical and Electronics Engineers is a multinational society that represents many working in the electronics and related industries, one of its 36 societies is the Engineering in Medicine and Biology Society (EMBS), the membership in this group exceeds 10,000, with about 25% of this membership outside the U.S. The group publishes transactions on Biomedical Engineering, Rehabilitation Engineering, and on Information Technology, as well as a bi-monthly magazine. It collaborates on three other publications, one on medical imaging, one on neural networks, and one on machine intelligence. This society also sponsors one international conference each year. This full-service group represents the largest number of biomedical engineers of any organization. (See www.ieee.org, search for the EMBS group).
- RESNA – The Rehabilitation Engineering and Assistive Technology Society of North America "is an interdisciplinary association of people with a common interest in technology and disability." As might be expected from the title, this group is composed of a broad range of professionals interested in various aspects of assistive care and technology. (See www.resna.org)

- SPIE – The Society of Photo-Optical Instrumentation Engineers is an international society specializing in photo-optical systems, many of which have biomedical applications (see www.spie.org).

Several of the major classical discipline-oriented groups have focus groups relating to biomedical engineering. The American Society for Mechanical Engineers has a bioengineering division as one of its many subdivisions, this group holds a small conference each year, other papers are part of the yearly ASME presentation series (see www.asme.org/bed/). The American Society of Civil Engineers and the American Institute of Chemical Engineers do not have specific subdivisions relating to Biomedical Engineering, but they do publish papers relevant to various aspects of the field (see www.asce.org and www.aiche.org). The American Society for Engineering Education sponsors a biomedical engineering division; this group sponsors a number of sessions at the yearly conferences (see www.asee.org). The site www.biomat.net is a resource for those working with biomaterials.

21.2 Standards Setting Groups

In order to establish minimal standards for biomedical devices and some processes many groups have established written standards in areas within their areas of expertise. These standards are then typically available for purchase; documentation that standards have been met then becomes a part of the continuing certification that a process or product meets specifications.

In the United States, standards setting is done by a mixture of professional societies, nongovernmental agencies, and governmental agencies. For example, AAMI sets standards in the areas of biomedical equipment, dialysis equipment, and sterilization. The American National Standards Institute (www.ansi.org), an independent organization, coordinates U.S. voluntary standards and is the U.S. representative to the International Organization for Standardization (ISO). ANSI has a small number of standards that are uniquely theirs; they co-list with many of the other standards as being in agreement with those standards. The major governmental organization involved in standards is the Occupational Safety and Health Organization (OSHA), the majority of the standards here relate to health and safety of workers in the workplace. Specific standards apply to the health industry. A partial listing of U.S. Standards setting agencies and groups may be seen in Table 21.1

Agency	Web site
American Heart Association	www.aha.org
American Dental Association	www.ada.org
American Medical Association	www.ama-assn.org
American Society for Quality Control	www.asqc.org
American Society for Testing of Materials	www.astm.org
American Society of Mechanical Engineers	www.asme.org
Association for the Advancement of Medical Instrumentation	www.aami.org
Federal Communications Commission	www.fcc.gov
Institute of Electrical and Electronic Engineers	www.ieee.org
Joint Commission On Accreditation of Healthcare Organizations	www.jcaho.org
National Council on Radiation Protection and Measurements	www.ncrp.com
National Electrical Manufacturers Association	www.nema.org
National Fire Protection Association	www.nfpa.org
National Safety Council	www.nsc.org
Occupational Safety and Health Administration	www.osha.gov
Underwriters Laboratory	www.ul.com

Table 21.1 Representative U.S. Standards Setting Organizations

Many nations have the majority of their standards setting functions imbedded in a governmental sponsored standards body. For a partial listing of such sites and representative standards, a good starting point is the publication *The Guide to Biomedical Standards* (Aspen Publishers, Inc., Gaithersburg MD, ISBN 0-8342-1692-2, 1999).

The most influential international standards organization is the International Organization for Standardization (ISO) (http://www.worldyellowpages.com/iso/) which is a worldwide federation of national standards bodies from some 110 countries, one from each country (ANSI in the US). The mission of the ISO is the development of consensus standards in order to facilitate the international exchange of goods and services, and to developing cooperation in the spheres of intellectual, scientific, technological and economic activity. ISO's work results in international agreements that are published as international Standards. If successful, these standards will supplant the potentially 110 or more individual standards as time progresses.

21.3 Professional Engineering Licensure

An extremely important decision in an engineer's career is that of applying for professional licensure. All states in the United States have statutes that establish the registration requirements for architects, engineers, landscape architects and interior designers, and describes the size and scope of projects for which a registrant is needed. To improve the level of professional conduct and to establish a standard of care, the licensing board also enacts Rules of Professional Conduct. A typical state licensure board holds its purpose one of safeguarding life, health, and property, and the promotion of the public welfare through the establishment of standards and regulating the practice of engineering within the state. It does this through general requirements regarding educational attainment, participation in practice, examination and licensure, continuing education requirements, and the publication and enforcement of codes of conduct for the practice of engineering.

The implications of licensure are increased earnings, better employment possibilities, and a legal status for private practice opportunities, such as consulting and expert witnessing. According to the National Council of Examiners for Engineering and Surveying, licensed engineers enjoy salaries 15% to 25% higher than non-licensed engineers. State regulations specify the conditions under which a licensed engineer must be supervisory, certain projects cannot be undertaken without this supervision, which includes certification with a signature and stamp. If called upon to testify in court regarding areas of your expertise, for example medical device accidents, the professional engineering license is generally enough to convince a judge that you are a credible witness.

21.3.1 Engineering internship

To become an engineering intern (also known as an engineer-in-training) the following conditions must (typically) be satisfied:

1. Graduation (or a senior in good standing) from a minimum 4-year undergraduate engineering curriculum accredited by the Accreditation Board for Engineering and Technology or substantially equivalent; AND
2. Business in the state to be licensed in; AND
3. Passage of residence or principal place of the Fundamentals of Engineering Examination (a full day general comprehensive exam).

Fees for the exam are reasonable. Pass rates vary by state, dependent in part on whether or not the exam is mandatory for graduation from college. A pass rate of 60% or better is not uncommon.

21.3.2 Registration as a professional engineer

The following requirements must typically be satisfied for professional engineering licensure:

1. Graduation from a minimum 4-year undergraduate engineering curriculum accredited by the Accreditation Board for Engineering and Technology or substantially equivalent; AND
2. Four years of progressive engineering experience satisfactory to the Board (often certified via plans developed, etc); AND
3. Certification as an Engineer Intern or 12 years of progressive engineering experience satisfactory to the Board; AND
4. Passage of the Principles and Practice of Engineering Examination in one of the areas tested (Mechanical, Electrical, etc., a major day-long exam)

Fees for this exam are reasonable. Pass rates vary considerably by state and by discipline.

Once a person has passed the above registration process, the license must be maintained by:

1. yearly license renewal fee payment
2. yearly or other privilege tax payment (if mandated)
3. proof of continuing education efforts (if requested)
4. abiding by the rules of conduct as set forward by the state.

21.3.3 Rules of professional conduct

The following are general guidelines regarding the rules of professional conduct for the practice of engineering:

1. The registrant must recognize that the welfare of the public is paramount. If it is felt that the decisions made by one's employer (or client, etc.) are counter to this it is the registrant's responsibility to report the decision to the appropriate authorities and to refuse to carry out the decision.
2. The registrant must perform service only in areas of personal competence. This service will typically be noted by the affixing of his/her signature and seal to documents prepared in this way. The affixing of this seal or signature to other documents can lead to dismissal and/or fines. Similar punishments will ensue due to violation of any regulations and acts of incompetence due to malpractice or disability.
3. Professional reports and expert testimony made by the registrant must be objective and truthful. If the registrant is speaking on behalf of another party that fact must be clearly enunciated.
4. Registrants must avoid conflicts of interest, if any arise it must be disclosed to the employer or client. Compensation must be above board and only for services performed. (No acceptance of bribes, perks, kickbacks, etc.).
5. Registrants must be honest in all matters regarding their professional qualifications. Registrants must not offer any gift of any kind for the awarding of a contract.

State licensing boards has the power to fine and suspend engineers violating the rules above, or assisting others to violate the rules. Suspension typically can also occur if the registrant is convicted of a felony, or has had his/her license suspended in another state (for cause).

21.4 Code of Ethics

Most major societies prominently post and endorse a code of ethics. In general these amount to reiterations and refinements of the above stated five rules of professional conflict.

The IEEE code of ethics has ten points, the IEEE makes explicit the additional ethical rules of non-discrimination, rules against slander, and suggests the role of mentor for associations with co-workers (see http://www.ieee.org/about/whatis/code.html for details). The National Society for Professional Engineers (see http://www.nspe.org/ethics/eh1-code.asp) reiterates the above 5 rules as 6 fundamental canons. They then refine and expand each of these terms in a "rules of practice section", which is then followed by an interesting section on professional obligations. This section suggests such topics as participation in public affairs for the common good, and publication in the lay press, along with sections that further refine the above rules of practice section. This site further has links to case studies and the engineers' creed.

Several online web sites offer links to codes of ethics and case studies. One of the larger relating to engineering is http://www.onlineethics.org/. Should the need arise, this center offers assistance in solving ethical questions.

21.5 Forensics and Consulting

At some point in many engineer's career, they may acquire sufficient knowledge in an area that they can become forensic engineers and/or consulting engineers. Both can be very interesting and highly remunerative careers.

Forensic engineers typically research, in order to assist in the determination of "fault", the cause of an accident. Finding fault, or placing blame allows one to proceed with litigation, if necessary or justified. In the field of Biomedical Engineering, cases can run the gamut from determination of the potential for injury in a low speed auto accident, to the determination as to who is at fault for a death due to an air embolus. The first case would require that the engineer be well versed in biomechanics and accident reconstruction and the databases maintained on automobile accident injuries. The second case would require an in-depth look at all the instrumentation used in the case, the personnel involved, all records kept, etc.

A typical case involving a medical device accident involves an initial telephone contact between a lawyer (or sometimes a relative of the injured party) and the engineer (or firm). An initial familiarization with the accident being investigated is strongly recommended. Often this involves a review of the operative notes from a case, or other documentation involving the injury or death. During this initial review the forensics engineer must determine if the work is in his/her area of competence and if assistance is likely. If the engineer agrees to investigate, details such as timing (when might this go to court, how fast a response do you need, etc.) and payment schedule (rates per hour, contingencies, expense payments, etc) need to be agreed to. Other details, such as the need for access to records and devices need to be taken care of as soon as feasible.

There is no typical investigation. A broken device may be investigated and documented with data taken from the FDA MAUDE database system (medical device error reporting system). The clinical engineering services group in a related hospital may be queried about similar incidents. The device in question may be linked up to a patient simulator in order to determine error conditions in an assumed scenario. Determination of the fault is often a function of the imagination and resourcefulness of the investigating engineer.

In a significant fraction of cases, the engineer will find fault with the conduct of the clients of the lawyer who retained the engineer, at which point the engineer is typically relieved of further duty and employment on the case. If the data obtained is sufficient and for the case of the employer, negotiations will often become the job of the lawyer, with an out-of-court settlement generally a goal. Rarely do cases make it to trial. When and if they do, it behooves the engineer to have the credentials of licensing and adequate proof of experience with the device or process in question.

A typical hourly rate for a forensic engineer is on the order of 1/1000 of the engineers' annual gross salary, or more. Daily rates generally are capped at 1/100 of the annual salary in order to not overcharge for time spent waiting for a court appearance, traveling, etc. Other reasonable fees (mileage, meals, hotel) are charged as applicable. Additional charges (for technician help, etc.) need to be negotiated in advance. With fees in this range, the engineer's fees will be near, but typically slightly lower, than the lawyer's fees.

Consulting practices generally involve the use of an expert in a particular area as an assistant in the solution of a "closed end" problem. Thus an expert in Optics might be hired by an anesthesia machine development company to assist in the correction of a system to measure CO_2 in expired air. An expert in BioInformatics may be asked to advise on the development of a new database system. A biotechnologist may be called in to help advise on a new pharmaceutical generation system.

Consultants can be paid on an hourly basis, with rates negotiated by the consultants. These are often higher than those of the forensic engineer, due to the specialization of the task(s). Often consultants are kept on a retainer basis, and their expertise requested on an as-needed basis.

21.6 Continuing Education

In order to maintain licensure, many states require that licensed engineers obtain a minimum of relevant continuing education hours per year (24 hours per year, for example, in Tennessee). These may be via attendance at technical or professional meetings, via seminars (corporate or correspondence), or via attendance in college or university courses. The courses must be relevant to the practice of engineering as the licensee practices it.

Membership in at least one relevant society and attendance at one three day society meeting per year would meet this minimum requirement, and is strongly recommended. Additional attendance at trade shows and related seminars (for example the Medical Design and Manufacturing Show, held three times a year) is highly recommended as a means of staying current.

Homework Exercises

1. Perform a web search using the terms engineer and "code of ethics". Briefly document the number and variety of sources you find.
2. Perform a web search using the term "forensic engineering". Summarize your data. Discuss one firm or case of interest to you.
3. As a forensic engineer, you are called in on a case to determine how air entered a patient who was undergoing heart catheterization. What sources would you use to determine the cause of death?
4. As a forensics engineer, you have been "let go" by the client that hired you, as your results were not conducive to them winning their case. The opposition lawyers ask to hire you. What is your answer and why?

5. You have submitted a written report detrimental to the company that hired you as a consultant. Their lawyer asks that all further discussions with them be oral rather than written. Why?
6. Search the web for the details on licensure in your home state. Compare these data to those mentioned in the text (TN).

Chapter 22

Miscellaneous Issues

"When you get right down to it, one of the most important tasks of a leader is to eliminate his people's excuse for failure."
Robert Townsend

22.1 Learning from Failure

It is important to recognize that the engineering profession has learned from failures and the study of their causes. An exposure to such classical failures as the Tacoma Narrows Bridge, the Shuttle Challenger, the Hyatt Regency Walkway Collapse, Three Mile Island, the Bhopal Chemical Plant disaster, and more recently, the World Trade Center disasters, amongst others, should be a part of every engineers' education.[1] Most disasters are the result of a combination of unexpected circumstances, poor design, and/or ethical failures, but not all.[2]

A brief mention of a number of Biomedical Engineering related failures should help point out some of the considerations that students in Bioengineering should consider in the process of design activities. Other examples are in various sections of this text to assist in a sensitization to the need for safe design procedures.

A computer programming glitch on a Therac-25 radiation therapy machine allowed a technician to deliver over 125 times the required therapeutic dose of radiation to a patient. The error message "Malfunction 54" did not convey the correct message that the technician should not repeat the dose. Needless to say, the patient died. [3]

Technicians in an ambulance taking a heart attack victim to a hospital lost use of their heart machine every time they attempted to use their radio transmitter. (Unshielded RF interference.) The patient died.[4]

Toxic shock syndrome plagued some users of super absorbency tampons in the late 1970s. It also caused some deaths. There had been no FDA or other guidelines as to the composition, degree of absorbency, or recommendations on length of use (time) until this occurred.

Thalidomide was sold in Europe in the late 1950s, causing over 8,000 births of malformed children. The drug had not been tested adequately prior to market release.

Laetrile, a substance that can be extracted from apricot seeds (or synthesized) has been touted as a cancer cure since the 1960s. Banned in the U.S. by the FDA, it can still be obtained in Mexico.

In 1938 107 deaths of (primarily) children were caused due to ingestion of Elixir of Sulfanilamide, a toxic combination of diethylene glycol and sulfa. This one disaster is one of the prime initiators of the early FDA drug (especially patent drug) enforcement activities.

Quack medical devices have plagued the US population for years. Most advertisers claims for devices or drugs that have claims for medical benefits come under the scrutiny of the FDA, which has the power to fine and recall for false claims.

22.2 Design for Failure

It is important to consider, when designing systems and devices, that sometimes you must consider and plan for failure. One must often be proactive, rather than reactive, when considering failure. Designing for failure can be for the purposes of safety and for convenience. We will examine several examples of each, both in terms of system design and in terms of Biomimetics.

22.2.1 Safety considerations

Safety considerations are paramount in many design problems and an understanding of several examples is important. A few examples follow:

- Fuses – current flow through a fine wire or a low temperature melt point wire causes it to vaporize or melt, protecting the circuit beyond the fuse point.
- Shear pins – many devices have a section that will break, rather than ruin the entire system. Many lawnmowers have a shear pin, which breaks before the main crankshaft can.
- Sprinkler systems – the increase in temperature due to a fire causes melting of a metal plug and the opening of a sprinkler or gas quenching system to put out the fire.
- The coating on a medicine "lasts long enough" in the stomach to deliver a drug to the intestines, where it is needed or causes no harm compared to direct stomach delivery (enteric coatings, a variation on the M&M melts in your mouth, not your hands philosophy).
- Individually bubble packed drugs stay isolated from the atmosphere (generally used with hydroscopic drugs) until the bubble is "burst."
- A humidification/heating system is allowed to operate until a bimetallic element snaps a vent shut at a given temperature (too hot or too cold).
- In the event of a power failure, a lead shield drops in front of a cobalt therapy delivery unit.
- A current limiter is placed between a patient and a medical device; the patient is protected from excessive currents.
- Bottle tops can be fashioned to require a minimal amount of squeezing and/or manipulation before they open, thus protecting the weak or young (typically for dispensing of medicines).

- Plastic or real peanuts used for packing deform during impacts, protecting the packaged item.
- Graphite rods are designed to drop into reactors to quell runaway reactions.
- Feathers protect a bird but pull out in order to enable a bird to escape a predator.
- Eggshells protect an embryo but can be shattered from within by a chick ready to hatch.
- Pine seed can sit dormant for years, opening after a fire when there exists a chance for sunlight and growth.

For systems such as computer security systems, the goal of a safe design would be to do the following items: deter intrusion, detect intrusions, delay intrusions, warn of intrusions, and perhaps redirect intrusions to a "honey pot" system which can collect information on the intruder. Military systems – design so that in case of the failure of an outer system, an inner ring picks up on the challenge.

22.2.2 Design for convenience

Many items are designed to fail in a particular manner only for the convenience of the user, a quick listing of a few of these items include:

- Postage stamps – sheets of postage stamps typically contain individual stamps separated by perforations. A slightly skilled user can easily separate out an individual stamp by causing failure along the perforations. Obviously this same concept has been applied to toilet paper, paper towels, and checkbooks.
- Waffles in family and other packs typically are packed two or four to a sheet, the connections between the waffles being much thinner than any other part in order to allow ease of separations.
- Scoring of a surface to enhance breakage is a common way to ensure easily opened bags of coffee and pop-top cans of various designs.

22.3 Product Life Issues

The goal of the Product Development process is to put a safe, effective and reliable medical device in the hands of a physician or other medical personnel where it may be used to improve health care. The device has been designed and manufactured to be safe, effective and reliable. The manufacturer warranties the device for a certain period of time, usually one year. Is this the end of the manufacturer's concern about the device? It shouldn't be. There is too much valuable information to be obtained.

Analysis of field data is the means of determining how a product is performing in actual use. It is a means of determining the reliability growth over time. It is a measure of how well the product was specified, designed and manufactured. It is a source of information on the effectiveness of the shipping configuration. It is also a source for information for product enhancements or new designs. Field information may be obtained in any of several ways, including:

- Analysis of Field Service Reports
- Failure Analysis of Failed Units
- Warranty Analysis.

22.3.1 Analysis of field service reports

The type of data necessary for a meaningful analysis of product reliability is gathered from Field Service Reports (FSR). The reports contain such vital information as:

- Type of product
- Serial number
- Date of service activity
- Symptom of the problem
- Diagnosis
- List of parts replaced
- Labor hours required
- Service representative.

The type of product allows classification by individual model. The serial number allows a history of each individual unit to be established and traceability to the manufacturing date. The date of service activity helps to indicate the length of time until the problem occurred.

The symptom is the problem, as recognized by the user. The diagnosis is the description of the cause of the problem from analysis by the service representative. The two may be mutually exclusive, as the cause of the problem may be remote from the user's original complaint. The list of parts replaced is an adjunct to the diagnosis and can serve to trend parts usage and possible vendor problems. The diagnosis is then coded, where it may later be sorted.

The required labor hours help in evaluating the complexity of a problem, as represented by the time involved in repair. It, along with the name of the Service Representative, acts as a check on the efficiency of the individual representative, as average labor hours for the same failure code may be compared on a representative to representative basis. The labor hours per problem may be calculated to assist in determining warranty cost as well as determining the efficiency of service methods.

The only additional data, which is not included in the Field Service Report is the date of manufacture of each unit and the length of time since manufacture that the problem occurred. The manufacturing date is kept on file in the Device History Record. The length of time since manufacture is calculated by subtracting the manufacturing date from the date of service.

22.3.1.1 The database

Field Service Reports are sorted by product upon receipt. The report is scanned for completeness. Service representatives may be contacted where clarification of an entry or lack of information would lead to an incomplete database record. The diagnoses are coded, according to a list of failures, as developed by Reliability Assurance, Design Engineering and Manufacturing Engineering (Figure 22-1). Manufacturing date and the length of time since manufacture are obtained. The data is then ready to be entered into the computer.

The data is entered into a computer database, where it may be manipulated to determine the necessary parameters. Each Field Service Report

Failure Code	Failure
Base Machine	
101	Missing parts
102	Shipping Damage
103	Circuit Breaker Wiring Damage
104	Regulator Defect
105	Shelf Latch Broken
Monitor	
201	Display Problems
202	Control Cable Defect
203	Power Board Problem
204	Control Board Problem
205	Unstable Reference Voltage

Figure 22-1 List of failure codes. (From Fries, 1997.)

is input to a single database record, unless the service report contains multiple failure codes. Figure 22-2 shows a sample database record.

The data is first sorted by service date, so trending can be accomplished by a predetermined time period, such as a fiscal quarter. Data within that time frame is then sorted by problem code, indicating the frequency of problems during the particular reporting period. A pareto analysis of the problems can then be developed. Data is finally sorted by serial number, which gives an indication of which devices experienced multiple service call and or experienced continuing problems.

Field	Field Content
1	Service date
2	Device serial number
3	Manufacturing date
4	Time in use (hours)
5	Failure code
6	Failed parts 1
7	Failed parts 2
8	Failed parts 3
9	Failed parts 4
10	Failed parts 5
11	Time to repair (hours)
12	Service representative ID

Figure 28-2 Sample database record. (From Fries, 1997.)

Percentages of total problems are helpful in determining primary failures. Spread sheets are developed listing the problems versus manufacturing dates and the problems versus time since manufacturing. The spreadsheet data can then be plotted and analyzed.

22.3.1.2 Data analysis

The most important reason for collecting the field data is to extract the most significant problem information and put it in such a form that the cause of product problems may be highlighted, trended and focused upon. The cause of the problem must be determined and the most appropriate solution implemented. A "band-aid" solution is unacceptable.

Pareto analysis is used to determine what the major problems are. The individual problems are plotted along the x-axis and the frequency on the y-axis. The result is a histogram of problems, where the severity of the problem is indicated, leading to the establishment of priorities in addressing solutions.

Several graphical plots are helpful in analyzing problems. One is the plot of particular problems versus length of time since manufacturing. This plot is used to determine the area of the life cycle in which the problem occurs. Peaks of problem activity indicate infant mortality, useful life or wearout, depending on the length of time since manufacture.

A second plot of interest is that of a particular problem versus the date of manufacture. This plot is a good indication of the efficiency of the manufacturing process. It shows times where problems occur, e.g., the rush to ship product at the end of a fiscal quarter, lot problems on components, or vendor problems The extent of the problem is an indication of the correct or incorrect solution.

Another useful plot is that of the total number of problems versus the date of manufacture. The learning curve for the product is visible at the peaks of the curve. It can also be shown how the problems for subsequent builds decrease as manufacturing personnel become more familiar and efficient with the process.

Trending of problems, set against the time of reporting is an indicator of the extent of a problem and how effective the correction is. Decreasing numbers indicate the solution is effective. Reappearing high counts indicate the initial solution did not address the cause of the problem.

The database is also useful for analyzing warranty costs. The data can be used to calculate warranty expenses, problems per manufactured unit and warranty costs as a percentage of sales. A similar table can be established for installation of devices.

22.3.2 Failure analysis of field units

Most failure analysis performed in the field is done at the board level. Service Representatives usually solve problems by board swapping, since they are not equipped to troubleshoot at the component level. Boards should be returned to be analyzed to the component level. This not only yields data for trending purposes, but highlights the real cause of the problem. It also gives data on problem parts or problem vendors.

The most important process in performing field failure analysis is focusing on the cause of the problem, based on the symptom. It does no good to develop a fix for a symptom, if the cause is not known. To do so only creates additional problems. Analysis techniques, such as fault tree analysis of FMEA may help to focus on the cause.

Once the component level analysis is completed, pareto charts may be made, highlighting problem areas and prioritizing problem solutions. The major problems can be placed in a spread sheet and monitored over time. Graphical plots can also be constructed to monitor various parameters over time.

22.3.3 Warranty analysis

Warranty analysis is an indication of the reliability of a device in its early life, usually the first year. Warranty analysis (Figure 22-3) is a valuable source of information on such parameters as warranty cost as a percentage of sales, warranty cost per unit, installation cost per unit and percentage of shipped units experiencing problems. By plotting this data, a trend can be established over time.

22.4 Product Testing Issues

Analysis of field data is also a significant means of reviewing the testing completed during the product development cycle to determine if it was sufficient for the intended use of the device. If field reports indicate a litany of problems, the types and severity of the testing performed need to be reviewed. HALT testing may have needed to be performed, as this type of testing may indicate problems early in the testing that would take some time to occur in the field. The severity of the test parameters needs to be reviewed to determine if more severe parameters could have indicated a problem was present. If the failure was caused by customer misuse of the product, the type and severity of the misuse testing needs to be reviewed.

Product Code	Parameters	Cost 1/95	Cost 2/95	Cost Year to Date
xxxxx	Normal Warranty	$	$	$
xxxxx	Recall Warranty	$	$	$
xxxxx	Total Warranty	$	$	$
xxxxx	Setup Cost	$	$	$
xxxxx	Total Cost	$	$	$
xxxxx	Sales	$	$	$
	Warranty/Sales			
	Setup/Sales			
	Total/Sales			
	Number of Units Shipped			
	Number of Units Setup			
	Number Warranty Units			
	Number of Recall Units			
xxxxx	Warranty/Unit	$	$	$
xxxxx	Recall/Unit	$	$	$
xxxxx	Setup/Unit	$	$	$
xxxxx	Total/Unit	$	$	$

Figure 22-3 Warranty analysis. (From Fries, 1997.)

When reviewing the tests that were performed, it is important to analyze test severity, as you want the test parameters to be severe enough to indicate a weakness in the design or component, yet you don't want the parameters so severe that they cause problems that would not occur under ordinary use of the device.

Homework Exercises

1. Find and report on heart valve failure history. What valves and valve types are still in the development phase?
2. Find information on the health effects of the Chernobyl accident; report on the current state of this event.
3. Your Volvo hits a guardrail at high speed. How many systems are involved in the incident as a design to fail device? Detail these (at least three).
4. The was a significant social outcry associated with the lack of patient informed consent in a long term study of Syphilis in the U.S. South in the 1900s. Find and discuss information on this event.
5. Illegal medical experimentation was detected during World War II. Find information on this and report on the outcomes.
6. There are a few excellent web sites dealing with ethical issues in the United States. Find one and document what is at the site.
7. Find and discuss at least one good university web site relating to medical ethics.
8. Find and report on the Bhopal incident. What elementary safety rule was violated in this case?
9. Find and discuss at least one new design for failure example.
10. Find and discuss at least one design for convenience example.

References

[1] See, for example http://www.matscieng.sunysb.edu/disaster/
[2] "The Importance of Failure", Vicky Hendley, ASEE Prism, October 1998, pgs. 18-23.
[3] Casey, Steven, *Set Phasers on Stun*, Aegean Publishing, 1993.
[4] Geddes, Leslie. *Medical Device Accidents*, CRC Press, 1998, pg 27.

AAMI, *Guideline for Establishing and Administering Medical Instrumentation.* Arlington, VA: Association for the Advancement of Medical Instrumentation, 1984.

Fries, Richard C., *Reliable Design of Medical Devices.* New York: Marcel Dekker, Inc., 1997.

Fries, R. C. et. al., "A Reliability Assurance Database for Analysis of Medical Product Performance," in *Proceedings of the Symposium on e Engineering of Computer-Based Medical Systems*. New York: The Institute of Electrical and Electronic Engineers, 1988.

MIL-HDBK-472, *Maintainability Prediction.* Washington, DC: Department of Defense, 1966.

Chapter 23

Design Case Studies

"When possible make the decisions now, even if action is in the future. A reviewed decision usually is better than one reached at the last moment."
William B. Given, Jr.

The goal of this chapter is the review of a mixture of design case studies with the aim of illuminating the design processes elaborated on in the previous twenty two chapters. Each example is assumed to be at the level of a senior Biomedical Engineering student, with the required course or experience in their background. It is not meant to be complete in its coverage; this text is too small to be that comprehensive.

23.1 Multidetector Brain Scanning System Development

23.1.1 Background

Nuclear Medicine is a branch of Radiology whereby radioactive elements are injected into a study subject. The elements are typically such that they are concentrated in the body in known processes, this information is mapped using radiation detectors in order to diagnose normal or abnormal function. For example, technetium 99-m is a gamma emitter with chemical characteristics similar to calcium. Thus, it will concentrate in areas with a high metabolism, such as in tumors. In the early days of Nuclear Medicine, these distributions were mapped with single detector systems, which were translated in a rectilinear grid.

The detection system consisted of a collimator (typically lead) section, shielding, a scintillation crystal, and a photodetector system. Shielding allowed the system to have directional sensitivity, cutting holes in the collimator allowed the system to have a sensitivity which is depth (distance from collimator) dependent. Figure 23-1 shows a typical point source response for a focusing collimator with a 3-inch depth of focus. The lead shielding is on the left (cross-hatched), the detector crystal and electronics would be on the far left.

The depth response of the collimator assists in determining how deep in the body a system can sense radiation. A straight bore collimator shows strict adherence to an inverse square of the distance sensitivity, the collimator above would show an enhanced response to radiation (hence tumors) at a depth of about three inches.

23.1.2 Problem Statement

The design problem to be addressed is this: "Given one or more focusing collimators (and related electronics), develop a brain scanning system that shows increased sensitivity compared to a rectilinear scan using a single detector, and which gives a cross sectional image of the brain more suited for surgical planning than rectilinear scans."

Solution 1: Multicrystal Tomographic Scanner

An initial solution attempt (1) may be seen in Figure 23-2. Eight detectors were placed on pivot points on an annular support structure. Each of the eight detectors was slaved to a common drive point through a series of slotted guide bars. The patient's head was to be placed in the apparatus, the level at which the scanners were placed determined the section to be scanned. The slave point was then scanned in a rectilinear raster and data collected and displayed on a computer screen. The data obtained from all eight detectors was simply stored together at the current raster data point in computer memory.

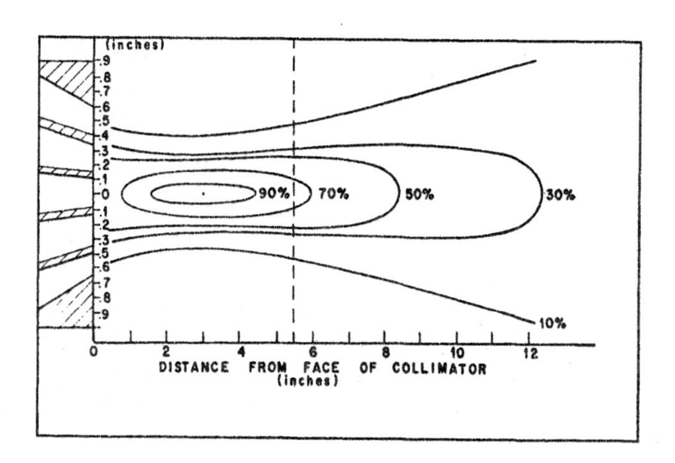

Figure 23-1 Point source response map for a converging focus collimator.

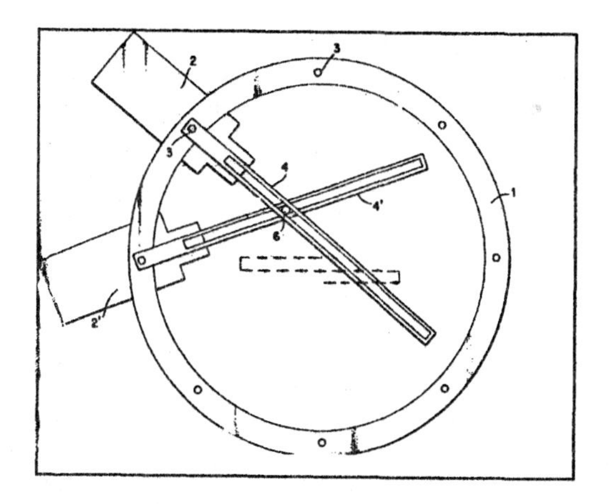

Figure 23-2 Schematic of early tomographic scanner, U.S. Patent Number 3,591,806.

This early system was used for a small number of patient studies, and did prove to be a useful construct. However, additional sensitivity was desired. As configured, the drive point (#6 in diagram) needed to traverse a roughly 9"x7" rectangle in order to scan an adult head, this forced the diameter of the annulus to be roughly 20", which severely decreased the response of the detectors to information from points "far away" during the scanning procedure.

Solution 2: Mutually Orthogonal Multicrystal Tomographic Scanner

Figure 23-3 shows the next iteration of the attempts to obtain a good tomographic image of the human head. Based upon the work above, it was reasoned that the detector system could be replaced by four sets of three mutually orthogonal detector systems (12 in all, compared to the eight above). The overall construct could be done such that each of the four sets of detectors need only scan one fourth of the patient in the raster scan, the data could then be properly placed in the correct x-y location in memory (2). The common scanning point for each of the triads was to be the focal point of the collimators used.

One enhancement of this apparatus is the fact that one is no longer constrained to a horizontal cross sectional scan, the device can scan in any plane desired as long as it does not contact the patients' head. Further, the data obtained by the detectors could be signal processed to enhance the final image by looking at the individual rates and making some inference about the data actually contained in the source. For example - if one detector has a high count rate and the other two do not, the detector with a high count rate is likely getting data from off-focal point sources and the data to be stored should be related to the minimum of the count rates, rather than the sum.

This system too was tested on patients, and did prove to be a useful improvement over the original system. It never made it to production as a useful clinical tool as Computerized Axial Tomography soon appeared as a clinical tool. Other developments, such as the Anger camera, also supplanted this technology due to higher count rates and better spatial sensitivity.

The basic concept in both of these instruments is quite simple: additional data is always useful, this was achieved by "combining in space homogenous objects destined for contiguous operations " (TRIZ principle 5).

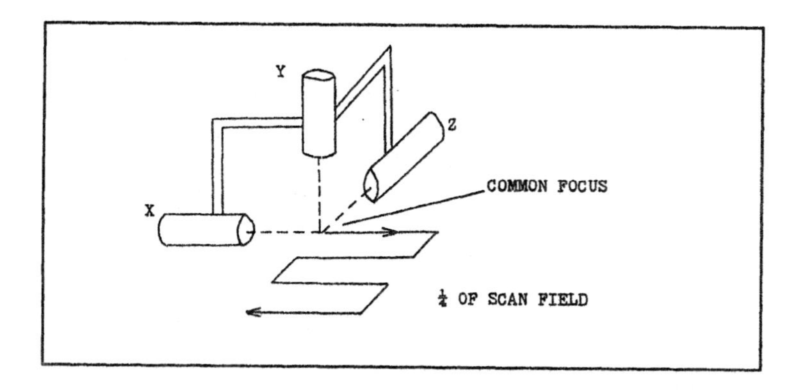

Figure 23-3 Mutually orthogonal schematic arrangement.

Data collection in scanning devices may be enhanced by proper geometry. Such a straightforward conclusion has led to the original work being cited in twelve subsequent patents that were granted.

23.2 Testing of Anesthetists

23.2.1 Background

The major job of an anesthetist is the preservation of a patient's well being during surgical procedures. This implies that the patient will not react during the insults of surgery, that the patient will not hear or otherwise respond or remember anything that occurs during a procedure, and that the patient is medicated, ventilated, and transfused, etc in order to maintain a somewhat status quo physiological state. Anesthetists include CRNAs, who are graduates from Nurse Anesthetist training programs and medical doctors who have just begun to those who have completed a residency specializing in Anesthesiology.

Training for anesthetists begins with didactic classroom and laboratory work in nursing or medical school. The hands-on portion is typically a gradual affair, new residents (post M.D.) typically spend three years under the supervision of practicing anesthesiologists with extensive experience in the field, gradually taking more and more responsibility for the care of the patient.

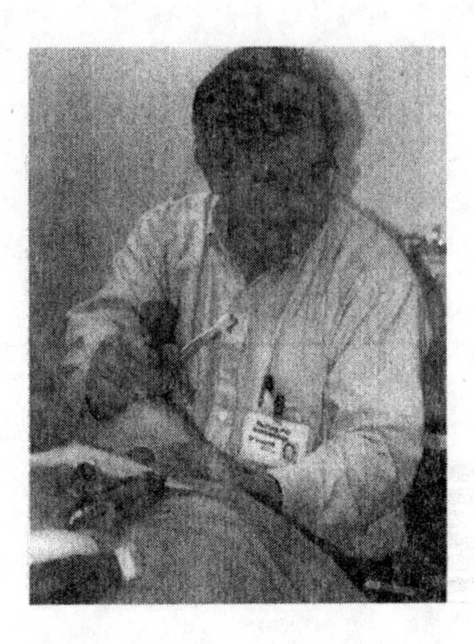

Figure 23-4 Human patient simulator (METI).

Training aids have been developed to assist in the education of these personnel, these aids range from simple plastic models of the throat to full scale human patient simulators (3). Of interest to this chapter is the human patient simulator, specifically the METI unit, which may be seen in Figure 23-4.

The METI simulator consists of a full-scale plastic manikin and associated sensors, actuators, and computer system. The manikin has an airway and "lungs", gas exchanges simulate normal and abnormal human responses. The simulator additionally has a heart beat and breath sounds that are audible at the surface, pulses at the wrists and neck, and a "hand" that responds to a neuromuscular stimulator. The computer system, through various transducers and actuators, simulates responses to drugs (administered through a flow sensor with bar code reader) and gas mixture administration (anesthesia machine, bagging, or room air) and controls gas exchange and other "physiological responses". The patient may be programmed to be one of a multitude of patients (standard man ("STAN"), truck driver, etc.), the system will respond to the drugs and gasses administered in a mathematically modeled manner. The system is powered by both electrical and pneumatic methods, an anesthesia machine is necessary to administer agents and to display simulated vital signs approximating what might be seen in surgery. Data are archived on a regular basis (every 5 seconds) by the simulator. Various protocols or simulations may be run under the control of the simulation computer and/or by anyone adept at using the provided interfaces.[4]

23.2.2 Problem statement

Given an Anesthesiology department, a METI simulator, and the requisite personnel, devise a means to "test the competency" of residents and others involved in the provision of anesthesia care. Scores are to be numeric, and will hopefully indicate the level of training and therefore presumed competency of the person being tested.

23.2.3 Problem solution

The above problem statement actually implies two elements. The first is the development of a test or testing method, the second is development of a method of quantification of the test results.

A review of the literature for testing methods yielded that most were aimed at "stressing" the examinee. Many included scenarios whereby the examinee was put "in charge" of a patient in midcase. Something would then go wrong and the examinee was expected to react properly.

The design decision was made to generate a standardized scenario that would be independent of the need for multiple actors and the potential for variability between examiners. Rather the computerized protocol would be consistent between exams, variability would only be introduced into the process through the simulated patients' response to medications given by the examinee as the case progressed. A moderately stressful procedure (abdominal surgery) was generated as a testing protocol, testing took roughly 30 minutes per candidate.[5]

The second design decision was to let the data speak for itself, rather than to use a mixture of subjective (examiner) and objective data. As recorded blood pressures, heart rate, and pulse oximetry data are normally recorded parameters in the operating room, only this data was used to quantify the tightness of control by the examiners. For a normotensive human, for example with a preoperative blood pressure of 120/70, a +/-20% variation in systolic blood pressure will put the blood pressures from clinically hypertensive to hypotensive. Hypertensive events in surgery have been linked to postoperative cardiac and kidney problems, hypotensive episodes can lead to oxygenation problems. This 20% bound was applied to blood pressure and heart rate, any deviation below or above the preoperative value plus or minus this value was considered "out of range". For pulse oximetry data, a tighter range of +/-5% was used, as variation in this parameter is more critical.

This protocol has been tested on a novice, a second year, and a postgraduate anesthetist. There was a clear demarcation of their abilities to hold patient parameters within the above-defined ranges.

23.3 Apnea Detection System

23.3.1 Background

In the United States, the current emphasis on reduction of labor costs in hospital care has excluded many patients with risk factors for respiratory depression from being cared for in traditional respiratory monitoring suites in Critical Care Units (CCU). Many types of hospital patients are at risk for respiratory failure, those who are receiving postoperative opioids (morphine) are most at risk. Such patients are those who have undergone major joint surgery and need opioids for pain relief. They are often placed post surgically in hospital environments where surveillance by hospital personnel is periodic, rather than continuous.

23.3.2 Problem statement

A means of monitoring patients for potential respiratory depression needs to be found, such that the patient in a step-down unit may be better monitored than just with simple periodic visits by hospital personnel.

Solution (partial):

A partial solution included the following items:

- CO2 monitoring was selected as the indicator of choice for respiratory depression. Too low a CO2 level as detected by a commercial unit, or no waveform (apnea) as detected by the unit was selected as the measurement system of choice. Sampling was initially achieved with a single capillary tube placed near the patient's nostrils. The units used had an alarm level that could be set manually; the alarm signal could be accessed for use in other devices.
- A chance conversation with a person installing an autodialing motion detection alarm system in the author's offices led to the acquisition of an autodialing system that was connected to the capnometer. The system would then dial the charge a nurses' beeper when the system alarmed. The beeper was unique to the patient being monitored.
- The basic system had to be modified with an on/off switch that could be activated when the patient was talking (seen as a high respiration rate) or eating.
- A special cannula had to be obtained to sample air from both nostrils and from near the mouth. This was necessary for patients who mouth breathed due to snoring and/or stuffy noses.

Twenty-two patients were studied with this system; these patients were selected as being at risk due to recent surgery and the prescription of opioids, either through epidural injection or patient controlled analgesia. Alarms were generated on twenty-one patients during the period of the study. Several of the alarms were due to a displaced cannula (7 patients), a few were due to talking or mouth breathing (3) which led to the above change in cannula type and the on/off switch, several were due to legitimate concerns (apnea, occlusions, 8 patients).

Due to a variety of reasons, this study only made it to the feasibility stage, and was formally presented at only one meeting.[6] The complete solution, perhaps utilizing the technologies mentioned here, remains to be determined.

23.4 Cancer Clinic Charting

23.4.1 Background

Many hospital clinics service a mixture of well to ill patients. Such clinics are multiuse, serving as a screening clinic for the majority of the clients and as a triage and referral clinic for others. One such clinic that has been the subject of a design study is the Breast Diagnostic Center at Vanderbilt[7]. The clinic patient pathway was in need of study to determine areas for improvement in services and in patient perceptions of the process.

23.4.2 Problem statement

While charting the pathway of patients through a screening clinic (breast cancer screening) a means had to be found to display not only the process but also the patient perception of the process.

23.4.3 Problem solution

The student involved in the process painstakingly tracked patients through the clinic. The final flowchart for the process was very comprehensive, six pages in Micrografx FlowCharter (see web site.) As several patients went through the clinic, the student additionally interviewed the patients as to their perceptions of the process ("going to the gemba", see Chapter 4.) The patient concerns were overlaid on the clinic flowchart; the mood of the patient with diagnosed cancer was expressed in a thermometer form also on the chart. The overall combined process & patient perception flowchart is extremely informative, as a glance at Figure 23-5 below should indicate.

The total chart was used to identify points of stress for patients during their clinic visit, and will be used in the redesign of the clinic operation. (For other useful ways of envisioning information, the reader is referred to the texts by Edward R. Tufte).

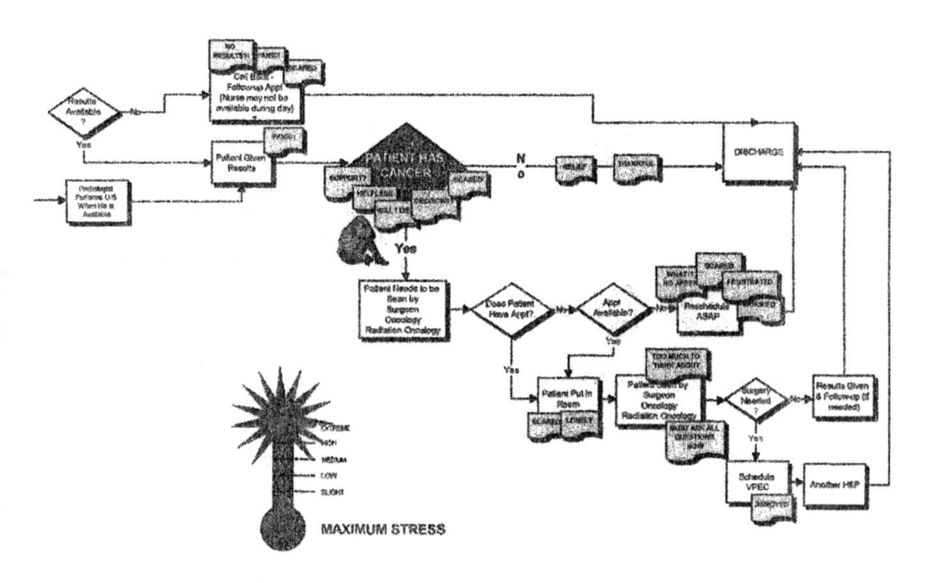

Figure 23-5 Cancer clinic diagnosis/discharge/follow-up section. (Courtesy of http://www.hyperionics.com)

23.5 EKG Analysis Techniques

23.5.1 Background

Author Paul H. King was approached by a physician, who stated: "We have obtained (name deleted) equipment to record telemetered ECGs in live unrestrained mice, and have gotten what seem to be reasonable recordings out of the animals. The data are pretty noisy and others who have the same system tell me that they often need to resort to signal averaging. We are looking at drug effects in wild-type and animals in which cardiac ion channel proteins have been knocked out. This would be a great project for an over-ambitious student, and one bit a while back but never got back to me. Resources would also be available to support collaboration at a more senior level, e.g. a percentage of someone's effort. It will also become an institutional imperative to be able to do this sort of experiment in mice. It even occurs to me that you may have software "lying around" since I think (name deleted) has the same equipment that he is using for rats. Can you point me in the right direction? "

23.5.2 Problem statement

As is normal with the above open-ended statement, development of a problem statement was an evolutionary process. The initial request from the physician consisted of the following (edited):

"... give you a single large file from each experiment, and have a machine derive values from 10-20 averaged ECGs at multiple points in time as well as RR plots as a function of time. I look forward to hearing your verdict on how easy or difficult this may be. " [Data sets were to consist of 2-3 hours of single lead ECGs sampled at 1000 samples per second.]

" My ideal would be to have (technician) do the implant and drug administration parts of the experiments, and to record everything (best in a single large file) and give it to you for an RR time series (every beat), interval measurements at specified times (e.g. 5 min, 10 min, etc, averaged over some number of beats like 5-20), and perhaps a look at particular parts of the record that happened to be interesting from a rhythm point of view (identifiable from the RR plot). ... What are the prospects of getting some system in place in the next month or so, so we could generate data for the ... deadline "

"... is a pediatric cardiology/electrophysiology fellow who is very interested in joining this ECG project. He will be in contact with you about looking at data and acting as a go between for you and (technician) -- and looking at the data with a cardiologist's eye to make sure we are seeing what we want to see and aren't losing data by reducing it too much ..."

" I hope that by the end of the summer we will have a relatively sophisticated add-on to the current system that will allow interval analysis (possibly automated or at least semi-automated), RR analyses, and perhaps RR analysis in the frequency domain. We also need to think a bit about arrhythmia analysis (first cut = how many beats don't fit the sinus template, especially if they are preceded by different RRs), since some of the mice that are coming may be arrhythmia prone..."

From an engineering point of view, the above statements required some serious decision-making about the software platform to be utilized, the speed of the software, and the platform to be used for analysis. The data files generated were huge, the time to analyze them was of concern.

23.5.3 Problem solution

Small sets of data were initially analyzed using Microsoft Excel and visual basic subroutines in order to get a "feeling" for the size of the problem and the techniques needed for analysis per the requesting physician's requests. This was a stopgap measure to get "some results" for analysis of archived data. It was too time consuming for a full analytical procedure on the entire data set.

The following list of alternatives was considered:

- a combination of Microsoft Access and Microsoft Excel and Visual Basic
- a combination of IDL (interactive data language) and Visual C
- a combination of PV-WAVE and C
- a combination of MATLAB and Visual C++ and Excel and Visual Basic.

The following sources were consulted for advice on alternatives:

- others using software on the list (& doing similar work) at Vanderbilt
- the manufacturer of the data collection system
- others in industry (referrals) using the above software packages
- web site information from the above companies
- the documentation provided with the above software packages.

The following criteria were applied to a final determination of software choice:

- completeness of documentation
- ease of use (analysis, display, archiving, ...)

- ability to handle data files up to 13 million data points in length
- user base at this location
- ease of transferal of updating and maintenance tasks to others, such as graduate or undergraduate students
- cost of one or more licenses as necessary
- license particulars
- speed of program in the environment (PC-based)
- prior application and documentation in a similar situation (examples, recommendation from data capture device company, etc.).

A formal procedure, such as using a QFD diagram for this analysis, was not done, it is left as an exercise for the reader as applied to their environment. MATLAB was chosen for the task at hand.

23.6 EKG Analysis Module

23.6.1 Background

Few people consider this, but planning a course from scratch is a design process[8]. Modifying a course fits nicely into a plan-do-study-act type of cycle, as input from constituencies is evaluated (graduates, employers, etc.) How would you design a course?

23.6.2 Problem statement

Given the mandate to do so, design an introductory freshman module (1 credit hour) to allow students potentially interested in your department to sample what they might experience in their remaining three years should they elect your department's major.

23.6.3 One solution

A module titled Electrocardiogram Capture and Analysis was designed for this purpose. Based in part on the above experiences, the specific goals of this course include the introduction of the student to:

- data analysis techniques in electrocardiography,
- medical and engineering nomenclature,
- engineering and engineering applied to medicine,
- technologies involved in cardiology and electrocardiography,
- and societal ramifications of heart-related research.

Specific topics covered via lectures were:

- Cardiac anatomy and normal cardiac rhythm.
- Abnormalities of the heart.
- History of cardiology, from stethoscope to galvanometer to chart form.
- Basics of EKG analysis from the chart.
- Data capture techniques and A/D conversion.
- Basic rhythm analysis using Excel.
- An introduction to analysis using MATLAB (in parallel with a three hour common freshman course teaching MATLAB).
- Electrical pacing, advanced diagnostic procedures.
- Defibrillators (external and implantable).
- Transmitter systems.
- Holter Monitors, databases.
- Visit to a human patient simulator lab.
- Visit to a clinical research facility.
- Basic medical nomenclature.
- And other topics.

Each topic and lecture was aimed at bridging between engineering, science, and medicine, demonstrating how the principles to be stressed later in the curriculum would apply.

23.7 Choosing the Correct Plastic Material

23.7.1 Background

Medical devices are cleaned with many different types of cleaining agents that vary widely in pH. Based on its pH value, a chemical may cause crazing and cracking when placed on various types of plastics. The chemical reaction may also affect the natural tensile strength of the material.

23.7.2 Problem statement

The purpose of the test is to provide rough insight into whether plastic materials subjected to stress are compatible with common cleaning substances. The materials being considered are Valox, Zytel, Cycoloy, and Thermocomp.

23.7.2 Problem solution (9,10)

Protocol:

1. Three ASTM Type I tensile test samples ("dogbones") will be used for each of nine commonly used cleaning substances:

    - Kleen-Aseptic
    - Sporicidin
    - Cidex+
    - Aldiced
    - Virex 256
    - Wescodyn
    - Acetone
    - Bleach
    - Isopropyl alcohol.

    Six samples will be used as controls.
2. Test half the control samples in the tensile test fixture at the commencement of the test.

    - Test each sample to failure
    - Use a speed of 5 mm/min (0.2 in/min) ± 25%.
    - Measure the tensile strength, percent elongation, and modulus of elasticity.

3. The samples, including half the control samples, will be placed in fixtures built by the Louisville facility. The fixtures force each sample to bow, as depicted in Figures 1 and 2 in the GE Plastics publication. A strain of 1% will be used for this test. A base length of 8.19" will be used for the Cycoloy and Valox plastics. A base length of 8.28" will be used for Zytel, and 7.6875" will be used for Thermocomp.
4. A small length of cheesecloth will be saturated with each substance and wrapped around each sample at the center of each bow. Plastic film will be wrapped around the cheesecloth to prevent evaporation of the cleaning substance. The multiple samples used for each cleaning substance will be distributed among the fixtures; the three samples for a given cleaning substance will not all be located on the same fixture. The samples will be exposed in this way to the cleaning substances for seven days.
5. At the end of the exposure period, remove each specimen and wipe clean.
6. Perform the following:
   - Examine each sample for indications of crazing or embrittlement.
   - Bend the bars with the chemically exposed area in tension (at outermost point of the bend).
   - Record any visible effects.
7. Test the samples in the tensile test fixture.
   - Test each sample to failure
   - Use a speed of 5 mm/min (0.2 in/min) ± 25%.
   - Measure the tensile strength, percent elongation, and modulus of elasticity

Results:

Clearly cycoloy would be an inappropriate material for use with the cleaning chemicals, as several of the chemicals fractured the samples outright. By inspection, the Zytel samples appear to have been affected by the chemicals as well. With the Thermocomp and Valox, any differences are less distinct. The following tables indicated test results:

Chemical Applied	Sample Averages	
	Tensile Strength (psi)	Young's Modulus (psi)
Control, non-stressed	8202	148911
Control, stressed	7862	140766
Acetone	N/A (all failed)	N/A (all failed)
Alcide LD	6277	147854
Alcohol	4483 (2 samples)	143564
Bleach	6248	143484
Cidex Plus	3120	127530
Kleen-Aseptic	N/A (all failed)	N/A (all failed)
Sporicidin	2099 (1 sample)	138267 (1 sample)
Virex 256	N/A (all failed)	N/A (all failed)
Wescodyne	6589	148944

Visual notes: acetone samples were blanched and cracked after test. All Kleen-Aseptic, Virex 256, and acetone samples failed. Two sporicidin and one alcohol samples failed.

Table 23-1 Cycoloy Results

Chemical Applied	Sample Averages	
	Tensile Strength (psi)	Young's Modulus (psi)
Control, non-stressed	10795	152478
Control, stressed	9482	111868
2nd control, non-stressed	11059	138446
Acetone	9087	99053
Alcide LD	8039	85013
Alcohol	8565	86903
Bleach	8675	96596
Cidex Plus	8279	87297
Kleen-Aseptic	8156	92696
Sporicidin	8036	78989
Virex 256	8020	77531
Wescodyne	8011	87061

Table 23-2 Zytel Result

Chemical Applied	Sample Averages	
	Tensile Strength (psi)	Young's Modulus (psi)
Control, non-stressed	6032	146531
Control, stressed	6108	131205
Acetone	5975	135291
Alcide LD	6001	132608
Alcohol	6024	131036
Bleach	6025	135290
Cidex Plus	5997	134990
Kleen-Aseptic	5997	131733
Sporicidin	6029	129006
Virex 256	5991	135704
Wescodyne	6002	136874

Visual notes: Large pieces of glass were found embedded in the resin.

Table 23-3 Thermocomp Results

Chemical Applied	Sample Averages	
	Tensile Strength (psi)	Young's Modulus (psi)
Control, non-stressed	7769	116676
Control, stressed	7755	104042
Acetone	7121	107147
Alcide LD	7520	105698
Alcohol	7911	110644
Bleach	7566	120864
Cidex Plus	7663	114774
Kleen-Aseptic	7691	107404
Sporicidin (2 samples)	7564	113090
Virex 256	7520	117873
Wescodyne	7540	108279

Table 23-4 Valox Results

23.8 Choosing the Appropriate Material for Autoclaving

23.8.1 Background

When humidity is required for breathing assistance in infants, incubators contain reservoirs where demineralized water is kept until the humidifier distributes it to the patient area. As part of maintaining the overall system and keeping it free of pathogens, the reservoir must be autoclaved.

23.8.2 Problem statement

Certain materials react well after being subjected to autoclave cycles. Other materials can be show crazing and cracking following repeated autoclave cycles. This can be dependent upon the type of material used, the types of bends in the material made when it was formed, or a combination of both. The purpose of this project was to determine the proper plastic material to survive a minimum of 75 autoclave cycles.

23.8.3 Problem solution

Protocol:

Parts made of injection molded polysulfone and Radel-R will be tested. Two of each part (marked "A" and "B") will be subjected to the test cycles. One of each part (marked "C") will be used as a control and will not be subjected to the test cycles.

1. Check each part for color and structure.
2. Separate the top and bottom parts. Subject them to the following wash cycle:

   - Machine wash cycle: 0.5 hour
   - Machine dry cycle: 0.5 hour
   - Wash Temperature: 49 °C
   - Water: Soft
   - Detergent: Alcojet

3. Place the top and bottom parts together (both parts marked "A" and both parts marked "B"). Subject the parts to 5 autoclave cycles consisting of the following parameters:

   - Conditioning time: ~3.5 minutes
   - Sterilizing time: 20 minutes at 134 °C (273 °F) and 32 PSI
   - Exhaust time: ~21 minutes
   - Total cycle time: ~45 minutes.

4. Remove the parts from the autoclave. Examine each part for discoloration and/or structure changes. Record all observations, listed by the number of autoclave cycles that have been completed.
5. Repeat steps 2 through 4, until a minimum of 75 autoclave cycles have been achieved or significant changes in the color and structure of the parts are observed.

Results:

The polysulfone material showed crazing and small cracks following 25 autoclave cycles. The crazing and cracking increased as the number of autoclave cycles was increased (Figure 23-6). The Radel-R material survived the 75 autoclave cycles with no crazing or cracking.

23.9 Choosing the Correct Cleaning Material

23.9.1 Background

Due to the concern over AIDS issues, many hospitals have begun to use very harsh cleaning agents to clean plastic parts. Because the pH of these materials is very basic, the chemicals react with the plastics, causing crazing and cracking. One example of this type of cleaning agent is Cidex +. Recently, Canada has outlawed the use of Cidex + to clean medical plastics. The alternative is Cidex OPA.

23.9.2 Problem statement

The purpose of this test is to determine the chemical reaction of Cidex OPA to plastic flow sensors made of cycoloy material. Parts will be treated with

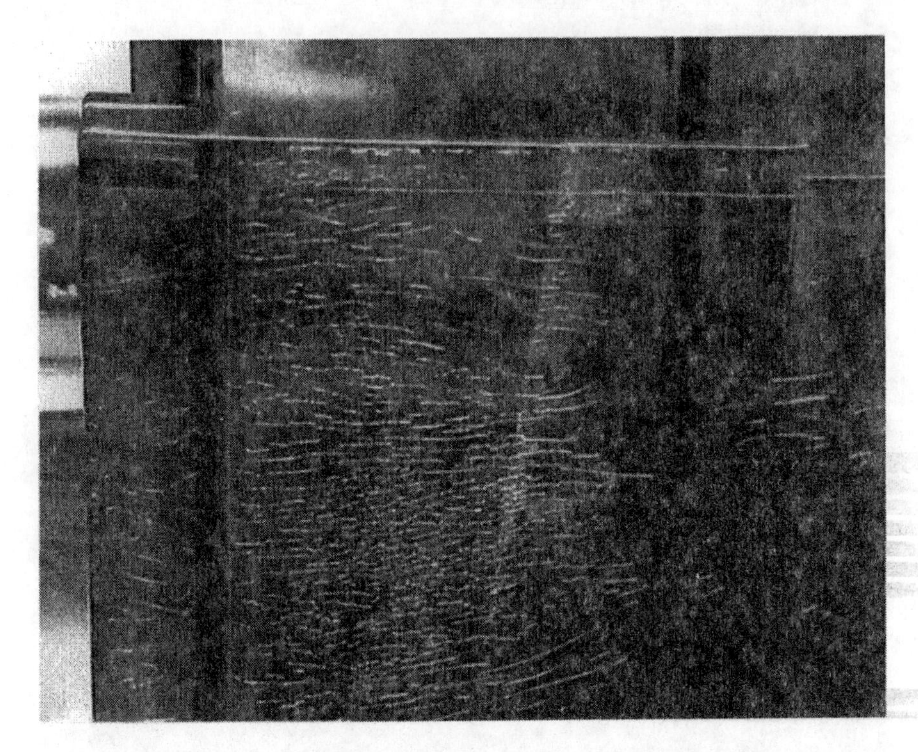

Figure 23-6 Crazing of polysulfone after 40 autoclave cycles

Cidex + as a benchmark. Previous work has indicated cycoloy crazes and cracks when treated with Cidex +. Three sensors will be treated with Cidex OPA, three with Cidex +, and three will receive no treatment as a control.

23.9.3 Problem solution

Protocol:

1. Check each part for color and structure.
2. Place one set of sensors in a container of Cidex OPA, the other in a container of Cidex + for 30 minutes.

3. Remove the traps, rinse them thoroughly, and let them air dry for 60 minutes.
4. Visually inspect the traps for color or structure changes. Compare to the control group. Record any observations, including the number of soak cycles completed.
5. Repeat steps 2 through 4, completing 4 soak and air dry cycles per day.
6. Repeat steps 2 through 5 until the material shows any color and/or structural changes. Record the number of cycles completed.

Results:

Crazing and cracking was noted on the cycoloy material when Cidex + was used. No crazing and cracking was noted when cleaning with Cidex OPA.

Homework Exercises

1. The rectilinear scanner systems in section 23.1 have been replaced by systems using one or more gamma cameras and back projection algorithms. Diagram the two systems and discuss how the gamma camera systems improve image collection efficiency.
2. Section 23.2 discusses testing of anesthetist competency. Discuss the objections you might have if you were the examinee. As the examiner, what ethical questions might come up if an examinee "fails" a test? How would you approach such a question if the examinee were a first year resident? A "seasoned" physician in practice for several years?
3. The apnea detection system in section 23.3 was not continued as the principals involved dispersed due to various conditions. Go to the literature and determine (or estimate) the number of patients lost each year due to episodes of apnea, estimate the device market available if you were to develop an inexpensive monitor of respiration. Given current technology, suggest a design for your device.
4. One of the consequences of the use of certain illegal drugs is apnea. Perform a literature search to determine the causes of this effect, the drugs that cause it, and current suggested ways of prevention of death in drug users due to apnea. Suggest two or more ways to decrease the number of deaths, and discuss the ethics of your choices.

5. The Cancer Clinic charting system detailed in section 23.4 is not unique. Based upon you experience or that of one of your acquaintances, outline (flowchart) a clinic visit and the emotions the visit caused.
6. The EKG analysis technique outlined in section 23.5 could have been presented in a preferences or evaluation chart form (see Chapter 2 selection grids and QFD diagrams.) Take the four proposed problem solution techniques and generate an evaluation chart.
7. The EKG analysis module in Section 23.6 could be extended to a number of other bioelectric signals. Select one and outline the course content for a one-credit hour module for freshmen engineering students.
8. Ethylene oxide has been used for sterilization of medical instruments. Research the several harmful effects of this gas.

References

1. United States Patent Number 3,591,806, July 6, 1971. Inventors James Patton, Jon Erickson, Paul H. King, Aaron B. Brill.
2. "The Design, Construction, and Preliminary Testing of a Mutually Orthogonal Coincident Focal Point Tomographic Brain Scanner", M.S.. thesis of David R. Pickens III, December 1977, Vanderbilt University.
3. Medical Education Technology, Inc, Sarasota Florida and The Eagle Patient Simulator, Palo Alto CA were two U.S. manufacturers of simulators.
4. King, P. H., Blanks, S., Rummel, D., Patterson, D., "Simulator Training in Anesthesiology: An Answer?", *Biomedical Instrumentation and Technology*, July/August 1996 pgs. 341-345.
5. King, P.H., Pierce, D., Higgins, M., Beattie, C. “A Proposed Method for the Measurement of Anesthetist Variability”, Accepted by the *Journal Of Clinical Monitoring and Computing*, June 2000.
6. Smith, B.E., Patel, N.P., King, P.H., Flanagan, J.F. "Automated End-Tidal CO_2 Monitoring in the Postoperative Patient", web site: http://shr.hama-med.ac.jp/iscaic18/AbstractSymposium/Smith-CO2.htm .
7. Design study by Michelle Kandcer, supervised by Dr. Doris Quinn, web site: http://vubme.vuse.vanderbilt.edu/kandcer/ .
8. Waks, S. *Curriculum Design, From an Art Towards a Science*, Tempus Publications, Hamburg, 1995.

9. General Electric, "A Simplified Environmental Stress Cracking, Chemical Resistance Test", from *Design Tips*, GE Plastics publication 10-89TSS, Number 16.
10. ASTM, "Standard Test Method for Tensile Properties of Plastics", ASTM Designation D 638-98.

Chapter 24

Future Design Issues

"When it comes to the future, there are three kinds of people: those who let it happen, those who make it happen, and those who wonder what happened."
John M. Richardson, Jr.

"May you live in interesting times" is a saying meant to be a curse, implying that the recipient of the curse would be overwhelmed in an environment that – in contrast to the current - is interesting. The quotation is variously attributed to ancient Chinese literature (unproven), John Kennedy in 1966 (proven), or early science fiction literature (1950, proven.) These are interesting times in the field of design in general and in the proliferation of topics for design projects in Biomedical and Biological Engineering. This chapter will survey some of these areas in an attempt to give the reader some feeling for the directions that the field of design in biomedical and biological engineering is evolving. This field is interesting and evolving. This chapter is also meant to give the reader a sample of what options are becoming available for future work in this field.

24.1 The NSF Design, Manufacturing, and Industrial Innovation Division

The division of the National Science Foundation that is most responsible for assisting in the development of the process of design in both academia and industry is the division of Design, Manufacturing, and Industrial Innovation. Two of the arms of this group, the SBIR/STTR (Small Business Innovation Research/Small Business Technology Transfer, in the Industrial Innovation Program) and the Engineering Design Program (in the Engineering Decision Systems Program) are of major importance to this section of the text, and will next be discussed.

24.1.1 SBIR/STTR

The SBIR and STTR programs are designed to assist small businesses in the generation of new and innovative products, devices, processes or services in order to facilitate the competitiveness of the industrial sector of the nation. The NSF sets the standards for acceptance of proposals, generally looking for end results that will translate into new jobs or other social benefits. To that end, it guides potential grantees to work in areas it feels is of importance. Thus it generates listings of areas it deems worthy of funding. The listing below (A-T) was posted on the NSF website solicitation for year 2002 proposals (some editing by the authors was done to define or expand terms used.)[1]

A. Genomics (the study of genes and their interaction and influence on biological pathways and physiology)
New capabilities enabling the rapid and massive sequencing of entire genomes of organisms, from microbes to humans, are transforming biological research. Exciting opportunities for commercialization activity have been created, with more yet to be proposed.

B. Proteomics (the study of protein structure, function, and interaction)
The full complement of proteins expressed by complete genomes is now susceptible to analysis, prediction, and modification of structure, function, and interactions, giving rise to new commercial opportunities.

C. Bioinformatics (the science and art of converting data to knowledge)
Computer power and new mathematical methods are required to harness the vast and expanding data sets that are being explosively generated through genomics

and proteomics, creating bioinformatics business opportunities.

D. Biochips

"Biochips" are biologically based microarray and microfluidic devices used for analysis and synthesis. How can they be made at lower cost? How can their applications be expanded?

E. Combinatorial Biotechnology

Proposals are welcome on potential commercial applications of "combinatorial biosynthesis," "combinatorial biocatalysis," and biologically oriented combinatorial chemistry.

F. Computational Biotechnology

Research with commercial objectives is needed for the development and implementation of algorithms and software for:

- the characterization of the relationship of DNA and protein sequence to biological function,
- the design of small molecules with biological activity,
- the analysis of complex dynamic biological systems, and
- multiscale ecological modeling.

G. Environmental Biotechnology (Including Bioremediation)

How can the power of biology be applied to improve and protect the environment?

H. Ecological Engineering and Biocomplexity in the Environment

Research with commercialization potential is sought for the design and management of ecosystems based on ecological principles and incorporating the self-organizing capacity of natural systems. Specific areas include ecosystem rehabilitation, habitat construction or enhancement, and flood prevention or mitigation.

The term "biocomplexity" refers to phenomena that arise as a result of dynamic interactions that occur within living systems, including human beings, and between these systems and the physical environment, both natural and human made. Biocomplexity encompasses ecological engineering as well as other areas. For further discussion, see <www.nsf.gov/home/crssprgm/be>.

I. Agricultural and Food Biotechnology

How can biotechnology be applied to crops and food products? How can it enhance food safety? Biological control of pests is included in this subtopic.

J. Marine Biotechnology and Aquaculture
How can biotechnology be used to enhance the search for valuable products from the sea and/or to improve their production?

K. Industrial Bioproducts
Bioproducts such as industrial enzymes, biopolymers, neutraceuticals, and bioreagents are opening up new opportunities for small businesses.

L. Biosensors
What new biosensors can be developed for commercial applications?

M. Bioprocessing and Bioconversion
Proposals are welcome on new commercial applications for involving bioreactors, bioseparations and purification, and biotechnology for a sustainable environment, for example biomining and bioleaching alternatives to smelting.

N. Biomedical Engineering/Research to Aid Persons with Disabilities
Bioengineering research with commercial objectives is sought to help improve health care and reduce its costs. Proposals are welcome in such areas as:

- deriving information from cells, tissues, organs, and organ systems; extracting useful information from complex biomedical signals to derive new approaches to the design of structures and materials for eventual medical use;
- devising new means for characterizing, restoring, and/or substituting normal functions in humans, such as advanced prosthetics, hearing, speech, vision technologies, and other assistive technologies;
- novel and/or improved medical imaging technologies such as in-vivo molecular and cellular imaging and probes;
- biomedical photonics, such as optical coherence tomography (OCT), and two-photon imaging/microscopy/spectroscopy; and
- home care technologies such as mobility enhancement, manipulation ability, cognitive function, and remote patient monitoring.

O. Tissue Engineering
Tissue-engineering technologies have opened commercial opportunities for developing polymer/cell structures and systems for biomedical applications.

P. Metabolic Engineering
How can the metabolic pathways in organisms be altered in a targeted and purposeful manner to enable or improve the generation of useful products?

Q. Biomaterials
Proposals are sought on developing new materials for bioengineering applications.

R. Pharmaceutical Drug Delivery
What systems, devices, or materials can be developed to enable or improve pharmaceutical dose applications and/or regimens?

S. Biotechnology at the Nanoscale
Research is encouraged on fabrication at the nanoscale involving biomolecules and/or biosystems for potential commercial applications.

T. Newly Emerging Developments in Biotechnology
Proposals are welcome in creative new biotechnology areas as they emerge.

24.1.2 Engineering design program

The following are some relevant issues addressed by the Engineering Design Program at NSF, as published on the web (minor modifications again by the authors):[2]

"***Rapid generation of design alternatives*** -- Designs are chosen from among a set of alternatives. Alternatives are generated by engineers using tools such as computer-aided design (CAD) ... We need tools that can take natural language descriptions and other natural forms of inputs and quickly derive candidate designs.

Easy evaluation of candidate designs -- Evaluation of candidate designs typically requires various forms of analysis, such as finite element analysis (FEA), thermal analysis, hydrodynamic analysis, and so on. Many computer codes exist and new codes are under development for such analyses. But it can be very difficult to interface these codes to work together or even to use CAD representations as the inputs to these analyses. We need methods to facilitate quick, accurate, and complete evaluation of candidate designs.

Rigorous evaluation of design decisions -- A view of engineering design that is providing the basis for many of the significant advances in the field today is that design is a decision-making process. In accordance with this view, design decisions are subject to rigorous analysis using well established principles of decision theory. We need theory and tools for the rigorous evaluation and comparison of design alternatives. This theory could build, for example, on the Von Neumann-Morgenstern axioms of utility theory.

Optimization of designs -- In virtually all cases, a designer is confronted with an infinity of possible design alternatives. Selection of an optimal design can be extraordinarily difficult, and generally impossible. First, it is often not even possible to create a finite taxonomy of design alternatives. Methods are needed to assist designers in creating and categorizing alternatives. Second, the range of alternatives is usually too great even to give consideration to all classes of alternatives. A method for discarding classes of alternatives early in the design process, under substantial uncertainty and risk, is needed. Third, consideration of a class of design alternatives demands that the class be modeled. Better methods for creating system models and methods for reuse of models are needed. Fourth, design intensely involves decision making under uncertainty and risk. Convenient methods of modeling system performance including uncertainty and risk are needed, and these methods must be compatible with the goal of system optimization. Fifth, virtually all products, processes, or systems require huge numbers of variables to describe. Thus, their optimization runs into problems of dimensionality. We need better approaches to the issue of dimensionally in design optimization.

Design information systems --A great deal of data may be generated during the design process. This may include the design itself and documentation of the rationale for the design. We need to find ways of capturing these data and maintaining them in an accessible database. There is also a need for several engineers working together to simultaneously access a design database and to make changes in the database that are instantly accessible by others on the team. At the same time, there is a need for conveying these data to designers at remote locations while providing a high level of security on proprietary designs.

Collaborative design -- More than ever before, engineering design has become a collaborative process that may involve teams and individuals working remotely. Particularly as these teams may be comprised of engineers representing a wide range of different organizations, their objectives may not precisely overlap, and hence the design becomes in the mathematical sense a cooperative game. This raises many issues: How can we manage design teams to assure rational design? How can the results provided by team members be effectively integrated to obtain a desired result? What are the best protocols for the transfer of design data? What forms of communication between team members work well?

Design education -- An emerging view of engineering design holds that design intensely involves decision making under conditions of uncertainty and risk. But current engineering curricula rarely include any principles of decision theory. Value or utility theory, central to all decision making, is largely neglected and almost always treated incorrectly in the engineering community. And probability theory, which comprises the basic mathematics needed for the assessment of uncertainty and risk, is taught in only about half the engineering curricula. We need new pedagogy for design education. We need practical examples, particularly of real design cases. And we need much better approaches to the integration of design education across the engineering curriculum."

Two specific examples of the application of the above list of needs are worth mentioning. The first is the "Open workshop on Decision-based design"[3], which is primarily an interactive web site sponsored for the purpose of exchange of information about the general process of decision-based design. Recognizing that indeed design is a decision-making activity, it seeks exchange of information about that activity, with a parallel interest in the development of definitions and taxonomies of design. It also intends to help develop laws and axioms relating to design, perhaps to parallel the work done by Nam Suh at MIT on axiomatic methods.[4]

The second major development that the NSF has helped sponsor is the publication of "Advanced Engineering Environments: Achieving the Vision, Phase 1 (1999)[5] and Design in the New Millennium: Advanced Engineering Environments: Phase 2, National Academy Press[6] (2000). The messages sent by these publications include the development of design environments, three dimensional imaging and interaction with design computer systems, increased dispersal of design personnel, increased and justifiable use of design software packages, and decreased time-to–market. Computational assistance will become pervasive in the design process.

24.2 The National Institute of Biomedical Imaging and Bioengineering

The National Institute of Biomedical Imaging and Bioengineering (NPBIB) is a newly formed institute (2001) within the National Institutes of Health.[7] The goal of the institute is to support *basic and applied research and research training that improves health by promoting fundamental discoveries, design and development, translation, and assessment of technological capabilities in biomedical imaging and bioengineering. Research projects should be enabled by areas of engineering, the physical sciences, mathematics, and the computational sciences and should result in discoveries that can be translated into applications for specific diseases, disorders, or biological processes. Integrated, multi-disciplinary, and collaborative approaches to addressing biomedical research are encouraged. Proposals can be based on hypothesis-, design-, needs-, development-, or problem-driven research*. Thus, this new institute is fully supportive of design activities, as opposed to hypothesis-driven research as is the case in much of the rest of the NIH.

Some of the current design activities sponsored include:

1. Development of probes for micro imaging the nervous system
2. Development of novel technologies for in vivo imaging
3. Development of new and improved instruments or devices for research
4. Development of new methodologies for biomedical research
5. Development of software to be used in biomedical research
6. Development of rapid, accurate diagnostics for natural and bioengineered microbes and/or toxins (botulism, anthrax, plague, etc.).

Many of these are in conjunction with other branches of the NIH, and are only a brief listings of all activities related to design.

24.3 The National Institute of Science and Technology

The Advanced Technology Program (ATP)[8] at the National Institute of Science and Technology (NIST) is aimed at supporting high-risk, high-payoff proposals from all technology areas. For example, projects covering cutting-edge developments in the areas of tools for DNA diagnostics, photonics, manufacturing, and component-based software have all been supported by the ATP. The Program's focus areas include chemistry and the life sciences, electronics and photonics technology, information technology and applications, and economic assessments. Current information on this and related topics may be found on the NIH Bioengineering Consortium website.[9]

24.4 DARPA – Defense Advanced Research Projects Agency

The DARPA mission is to develop imaginative, innovative and often high-risk research ideas offering a significant technological impact that will go well beyond the normal evolutionary developmental approaches; and, to pursue these ideas from the demonstration of technical feasibility through the development of prototype systems.[10] Some of the more recent solicitations made by this agency include development work in the areas of:

- Bio-Optic Synthetic Systems
- Bio-Magnetic Interfacing Concepts (BioMagnetIC)
- Biological Input/Output Systems (BIOS)
- Brain Machine Interfaces
- Biomolecular Motors (BM)
- Evidence Extraction and Link Discovery (EELD) Program
- BIO-Surveillance System
- Effective, Affordable, Reusable Speech-to-Text (EARS)
- Augmented Cognition
- Speech In Noisy Environments (SPINE)
- Microelectronics
- Micro-electromechanical Systems (MEMS)
- Opto-electronics and/or Photonics Technology.

As may be expected, all of these have defense ramifications as well as potential applications in the general field of human and animal health and welfare.

24.5 Miscellaneous and Other Areas of Future Design Activity

Potential developments in the field of design in Biomedical Engineering encompass many more areas than have been elaborated above. A sampler of topics includes:[11]

- Neural computing, interfacing between the living and the inanimate
- Biotechnology in general, design of organs specifically
- Genetic modification to relieve disease or genetic disorders
- Cloning
- Improved vision correction systems
- Biometrics and biometric technology for site protection
- Improved biomedical optics systems, automated cancer laser surgery
- Improved pharmacogenomics
- Improved mass analysis techniques (microarrays)
- Improved and miniaturized detection systems (biochips)
- Stem cell applications
- Agriculture and food technology interaction with BME
- Advanced medical informatics
- Improved biomaterials
- Improved design software and visualization tools
- Robotic surgery, including nanoscale
- Computational biotechnology.

As long as there is money and interest, there will be design work to be done.

24.6 Conclusions

The future of design in Biomedical Engineering is indeed promising with plenty of challenges and opportunities. Increasing technical sophistication is being accompanied by increasing breadth of research areas, such that the distinction between biomedical engineering and biological engineering is beginning to blur. This blurring of boundaries will give way to enormous numbers of new opportunities now and in the future.

Homework Exercise

1. For any of the items A - T listed in Section 24.1 perform a web search and report out an expanded definition of the terms used. Hypothesize or find an expected benefit from research and development in this field. List several groups performing this activity.
2. Obtain a copy of the "Design in the new millennium" text referred to in Reference 5, read the summary chapter, write a brief review of this chapter.
3. Investigate and report on the current list of NIBIB sponsored projects (see Section 24.2) as reported on the web. Report on one subject of interest to you.
4. Investigate and report on the current list of NIST sponsored projects (see Section 24.3) as reported on the web. Report on one subject of interest to you.
5. Investigate and report on the current list of DARPA sponsored projects (see Section 24.4) as reported on the web. Report on one subject of interest to you.
6. Investigate and report on the current list of miscellaneous projects (see Section 24.5). Report on one subject of interest to you.

References

[1] http://www.eng.nsf.gov/sbirspecs/BT/bt.htm
[2] http://www.eng.nsf.gov/dmii/Message/EDS/ED/ed.htm
[3] http://dbd.eng.buffalo.edu/
[4] *The Principles of Design*, Nam Suh, Oxford Press, New York: 1990.
[5] http://www.nap.edu/catalog/9597.html
[6] http://www.nap.edu/books/0309071259/html/
[7] http://www.nibib.nih.gov/research/investigators.htm#NIBIBfunding
[8] http://www.becon.nih.gov/becon_news.htm#20011220
[9] http://www.becon.nih.gov/becon.htm
[10] http://www.arpa.mil/
[11] Thanks to the class of 2002 at Vanderbilt for the majority of these topics.

Appendix 1

Chi Square Table

υ/γ	0.975	0.950	0.900	0.050	0.100	0.050	0.025
1	0.001	0.004	0.016	0.455	2.706	3.841	5.024
2	0.051	0.103	0.211	1.386	4.605	5.991	7.738
3	0.216	0.352	0.584	2.366	6.251	7.815	9.438
4	0.484	0.711	1.064	3.357	7.779	9.488	11.143
5	0.831	1.145	1.610	4.351	9.236	11.070	12.832
6	1.237	1.635	2.204	5.348	10.645	12.592	14.449
7	1.690	2.167	2.833	6.346	12.017	14.067	16.013
8	2.180	2.733	3.490	7.344	13.362	15.507	17.535
9	2.700	3.325	4.168	8.343	14.684	16.919	19.023
10	3.247	3.940	4.865	9.342	15.987	18.307	20.483
11	3.816	4.575	5.578	10.341	17.275	19.675	21.920
12	4.404	5.226	6.304	11.340	18.549	21.026	23.337
13	5.009	5.892	7.042	12.340	19.812	22.362	24.736
14	5.629	6.571	7.790	13.339	21.064	23.685	26.119
15	6.262	7.261	8.547	14.339	22.307	24.996	27.488
16	6.908	7.962	9.312	15.338	23.542	26.296	28.845
17	7.564	8.672	10.085	16.338	24.769	27.587	30.191

υ/γ	0.975	0.950	0.900	0.050	0.100	0.050	0.025
18	8.231	9.390	10.865	17.338	25.989	28.869	31.526
19	8.907	10.117	11.651	18.338	27.204	30.144	32.852
20	9.591	10.851	12.443	19.337	28.412	31.410	34.170
21	10.283	11.591	13.240	20.337	29.615	32.671	35.479
22	10.982	12.338	14.041	21.337	30.813	33.924	36.781
23	11.688	13.091	14.848	22.337	32.007	35.172	38.076
24	12.401	13.848	15.659	23.337	33.196	36.415	39.364
25	13.120	14.611	16.473	24.337	34.382	37.652	40.646
26	13.844	15.379	17.292	25.336	35.563	38.885	41.923
27	14.573	16.151	18.114	26.336	36.741	40.113	43.194
28	15.308	16.928	18.939	27.336	37.916	41.337	44.461
29	16.047	17.708	19.768	28.336	39.087	42.557	45.722
30	16.791	18.493	20.599	29.336	40.256	43.773	46.979

Appendix 2

Percent Rank Tables

Sample Size = 1

Order Number	2.5	5.0	10.0	50.0	90.0	95.0	97.5
1	2.50	5.00	10.00	50.00	90.00	95.00	97.50

Sample Size = 2

Order Number	2.5	5.0	10.0	50.0	90.0	95.0	97.5
1	1.258	2.532	5.132	29.289	68.377	77.639	84.189
2	15.811	22.361	31.623	71.711	94.868	97.468	98.742

Sample Size = 3

Order Number	2.5	5.0	10.0	50.0	90.0	95.0	97.5
1	0.840	1.695	3.451	20.630	53.584	63.160	70.760
2	9.430	13.535	19.580	50.000	80.420	86.465	90.570
3	29.240	36.840	46.416	79.370	96.549	98.305	99.160

Sample Size = 4

Order Number	2.5	5.0	10.0	50.0	90.0	95.0	97.5
1	0.631	1.274	2.600	15.910	43.766	52.713	60.236
2	6.759	9.761	14.256	38.573	67.954	75.140	80.588
3	19.412	24.860	32.046	61.427	85.744	90.239	93.241
4	39.764	47.287	56.234	84.090	97.400	98.726	99.369

Sample Size = 5

Order Number	2.5	5.0	10.0	50.0	90.0	95.0	97.5
1	0.505	1.021	2.085	12.945	36.904	45.072	52.182
2	5.274	7.644	11.223	31.381	58.389	65.741	71.642
3	14.663	18.926	24.644	50.000	75.336	81.074	85.337
4	28.358	34.259	41.611	68.619	88.777	92.356	94.726
5	47.818	54.928	63.096	87.055	97.915	98.979	99.495

Sample Size = 6

Order Number	2.5	5.0	10.0	50.0	90.0	95.0	97.5
1	0.421	0.851	1.741	19.910	31.871	39.304	45.926
2	4.327	6.285	9.260	26.445	51.032	58.180	64.123
3	11.812	15.316	20.091	42.141	66.681	72.866	77.722
4	22.278	27.134	33.319	57.859	79.909	84.684	88.188
5	35.877	41.820	48.968	73.555	90.740	93.715	95.673
6	54.074	60.696	68.129	89.090	98.259	99.149	99.579

Sample Size = 7

Order Number	2.5	5.0	10.0	50.0	90.0	95.0	97.5
1	0.361	0.730	1.494	9.428	28.031	34.816	40.962
2	3.669	5.338	7.882	22.489	45.256	52.070	57.872
3	9.899	12.876	16.964	36.412	59.618	65.874	70.958
4	18.405	22.532	27.860	50.000	72.140	77.468	81.595
5	29.042	34.126	40.382	63.588	83.036	87.124	90.101
6	42.128	47.930	54.744	77.151	92.118	94.662	96.331
7	59.038	65.184	71.969	90.752	98.506	99.270	99.639

Sample Size = 8

Order Number	2.5	5.0	10.0	50.0	90.0	95.0	97.5
1	0.316	0.639	1.308	8.300	25.011	31.234	36.942
2	3.185	4.639	6.863	20.113	40.625	47.068	52.651
3	8.523	11.111	14.685	32.052	53.822	59.969	65.086
4	15.701	19.290	23.966	44.016	65.538	71.076	75.514
5	24.486	28.924	43.462	55.984	76.034	80.710	84.299
6	34.914	40.031	46.178	67.948	85.315	88.889	91.477
7	47.349	52.932	59.375	79.887	93.137	95.361	96.815
8	63.058	68.766	74.989	91.700	98.692	99.361	99.684

Sample Size = 9

Order Number	2.5	5.0	10.0	50.0	90.0	95.0	97.5
1	0.281	0.568	1.164	7.413	22.574	28.313	33.627
2	2.814	4.102	6.077	17.962	36.836	42.914	48.250
3	7.485	9.775	12.950	28.624	49.008	54.964	60.009
4	13.700	16.875	21.040	39.308	59.942	65.506	70.070
5	21.201	25.137	30.097	50.000	69.903	74.863	78.799
6	29.930	34.494	40.058	60.692	78.960	83.125	86.300
7	39.991	45.036	50.992	71.376	87.050	90.225	92.515
8	51.750	57.086	63.164	82.038	93.923	95.898	97.186
9	66.373	71.687	77.426	92.587	98.836	99.432	99.719

Sample Size = 10

Order Number	2.5	5.0	10.0	50.0	90.0	95.0	97.5
1	0.253	0.512	1.048	6.697	20.567	25.887	30.850
2	2.521	3.677	5.453	16.226	33.685	39.416	44.502
3	6.674	8.726	11.583	25.857	44.960	50.690	55.610
4	12.155	15.003	18.756	35.510	55.173	60.662	65.245
5	18.709	22.244	26.732	45.169	64.578	69.646	73.762
6	26.238	30.354	35.422	54.831	73.268	77.756	81.291
7	34.755	39.338	44.827	64.490	81.244	84.997	87.845
8	44.390	49.310	55.040	74.143	88.417	91.274	93.326
9	55.498	60.584	66.315	83.774	94.547	96.323	97.479
10	69.150	74.113	79.433	93.303	98.952	99.488	99.747

Sample Size = 11

Order Number	2.5	5.0	10.0	50.0	90.0	95.0	97.5
1	0.230	0.465	0.953	6.107	18.887	23.840	28.491
2	2.283	3.332	4.945	14.796	31.024	36.436	41.278
3	6.022	7.882	10.477	23.579	41.516	47.009	41.776
4	10.926	13.508	16.923	32.380	51.076	56.437	60.974
5	16.749	19.958	24.053	41.189	59.947	65.019	69.210
6	23.379	27.125	31.772	50.000	68.228	72.875	76.621
7	30.790	34.981	40.053	58.811	75.947	80.042	83.251
8	39.026	43.563	48.924	67.620	83.077	86.492	89.074
9	48.224	52.991	58.484	76.421	89.523	92.118	93.978
10	58.722	63.564	68.976	85.204	95.055	96.668	97.717
11	71.509	76.160	81.113	93.893	99.047	99.535	99.770

Sample Size = 12

Order Number	2.5	5.0	10.0	50.0	90.0	95.0	97.5
1	0.211	0.427	0.874	5.613	17.460	22.092	26.465
2	2.086	3.046	4.524	13.598	28.750	33.868	38.480
3	5.486	7.187	9.565	21.669	38.552	43.811	48.414
4	9.925	12.285	15.419	29.758	47.527	52.733	57.186
5	15.165	18.102	21.868	37.583	55.900	60.914	65.112
6	21.094	24.530	28.817	45.951	63.772	68.476	72.333
7	27.667	31.524	36.228	54.049	71.183	75.470	78.906
8	34.888	39.086	44.100	62.147	78.132	81.898	84.835
9	42.814	47.267	52.473	70.242	84.581	87.715	90.075
10	51.586	56.189	61.448	78.331	90.435	92.813	94.514
11	61.520	66.132	71.250	86.402	95.476	96.954	97.914
12	73.535	77.908	82.540	94.387	99.126	99.573	99.789

Sample Size = 13

Order Number	2.5	5.0	10.0	50.0	90.0	95.0	97.5
1	0.195	0.394	0.807	5.192	16.232	20.582	24.705
2	1.921	2.805	4.169	12.579	26.784	31.634	36.030
3	5.038	6.605	8.800	20.045	35.978	41.010	45.447
4	9.092	11.267	14.161	27.528	44.426	49.465	53.813
5	13.858	16.566	20.050	35.016	52.343	57.262	61.426
6	19.223	22.396	26.373	52.508	59.824	64.520	68.422
7	25.135	28.705	33.086	50.000	66.914	71.295	74.865
8	31.578	35.480	40.176	57.492	73.627	77.604	80.777
9	38.574	42.738	47.657	64.984	79.950	83.434	86.142
10	46.187	50.535	55.574	72.472	85.839	88.733	90.908
11	54.553	58.990	64.022	79.955	91.200	93.395	94.962
12	63.970	68.366	73.216	87.421	95.831	97.195	98.079
13	75.295	79.418	83.768	94.808	99.193	99.606	99.805

Sample Size = 14

Order Number	2.5	5.0	10.0	50.0	90.0	95.0	97.5
1	0.181	0.366	0.750	4.830	15.166	19.264	23.164
2	1.779	2.600	3.866	11.702	25.067	29.673	33.868
3	4.658	6.110	8.148	18.647	33.721	38.539	42.813
4	8.389	10.405	13.094	25.608	41.698	46.566	50.798
5	12.760	15.272	18.513	32.575	49.197	54.001	58.104
6	17.661	20.607	24.316	39.544	56.311	60.959	64.862
7	23.036	26.358	30.455	46.515	63.087	67.497	71.139
8	28.861	32.503	36.913	53.485	69.545	73.642	76.964
9	35.138	39.041	43.689	60.456	75.684	79.393	82.339
10	41.896	45.999	50.803	67.425	81.487	84.728	87.240
11	49.202	53.434	58.302	74.392	86.906	89.595	91.611
12	57.187	61.461	66.279	81.353	91.852	93.890	95.342
13	66.132	70.327	74.933	88.298	96.134	97.400	98.221
14	76.836	80.736	84.834	95.170	99.250	99.634	99.819

Sample Size = 15

Order Number	2.5	5.0	10.0	50.0	90.0	95.0	97.5
1	0.169	0.341	0.700	4.516	14.230	18.104	21.802
2	1.658	2.423	3.604	10.940	23.557	27.940	31.948
3	4.331	5.685	7.586	17.432	31.279	36.344	40.460
4	7.787	9.666	12.177	23.939	39.279	43.978	48.089
5	11.824	14.166	17.197	30.452	46.397	51.075	55.100
6	16.336	19.086	22.559	36.967	53.171	57.744	61.620
7	21.627	24.373	28.218	43.483	59.647	64.043	67.713
8	26.586	29.999	34.152	50.000	65.848	70.001	73.414
9	32.287	35.957	40.353	56.517	71.782	75.627	78.733
10	38.380	42.256	46.829	63.033	77.441	80.914	83.664
11	44.900	48.925	53.603	69.548	82.803	85.834	88.176
12	51.911	56.022	60.721	76.061	87.823	90.334	92.213
13	59.540	63.656	68.271	82.568	92.414	94.315	95.669
14	68.052	72.060	76.443	89.060	96.396	97.577	98.342
15	78.198	81.896	85.770	95.484	99.300	99.659	99.831

Sample Size = 16

Order Number	2.5	5.0	10.0	50.0	90.0	95.0	97.5
1	0.158	0.320	0.656	4.240	13.404	17.075	20.591
2	1.551	2.268	3.375	10.270	22.217	26.396	30.232
3	4.047	5.315	7.097	16.365	29.956	34.383	38.348
4	7.266	9.025	11.380	22.474	37.122	41.657	45.646
5	11.017	13.211	16.056	28.589	43.892	48.440	52.377
6	15.198	17.777	21.041	34.705	50.351	54.835	58.662
7	19.753	22.669	26.292	40.823	56.544	60.899	64.565
8	24.651	27.860	31.783	46.941	62.496	66.663	70.122
9	29.878	33.337	37.504	53.059	68.217	72.140	75.349
10	35.435	39.101	43.456	59.177	73.708	77.331	80.247
11	41.338	45.165	49.649	65.295	78.959	82.223	84.802
12	47.623	51.560	56.108	71.411	83.944	86.789	88.983
13	54.354	58.343	62.878	77.526	88.620	90.975	92.734
14	61.652	65.617	70.044	83.635	92.903	94.685	95.953
15	69.768	73.604	77.783	89.730	96.625	97.732	98.449
16	79.409	82.925	86.596	95.760	99.344	99.680	99.842

Sample Size = 17

Order Number	2.5	5.0	10.0	50.0	90.0	95.0	97.5
1	0.149	0.301	0.618	3.995	12.667	16.157	19.506
2	1.458	2.132	3.173	9.678	21.021	25.012	28.689
3	3.779	4.990	6.667	15.422	28.370	32.619	36.441
4	6.811	8.465	10.682	21.178	35.187	39.564	43.432
5	10.314	12.377	15.058	26.940	41.639	46.055	49.899
6	14.210	16.636	19.716	32.704	47.807	52.192	55.958
7	18.444	21.191	24.614	38.469	53.735	58.029	61.672
8	22.983	26.011	29.726	44.234	59.449	63.599	67.075
9	27.812	31.083	35.039	50.000	64.961	68.917	72.188
10	32.925	36.401	40.551	55.766	70.274	73.989	77.017
11	38.328	41.971	46.265	61.531	75.386	78.809	81.556
12	44.042	47.808	52.193	67.296	80.284	83.364	85.790
13	50.101	53.945	58.361	73.060	84.942	87.623	89.686
14	56.568	60.436	64.813	78.821	89.318	91.535	93.189
15	63.559	67.381	71.630	84.578	93.333	95.010	96.201
16	71.311	74.988	78.979	90.322	96.827	97.868	98.542
17	80.494	83.843	87.333	96.005	99.382	99.699	99.851

Sample Size = 18

Order Number	2.5	5.0	10.0	50.0	90.0	95.0	97.5
1	0.141	0.285	0.584	3.778	12.008	15.332	18.530
2	1.375	2.011	2.995	9.151	19.947	23.766	27.294
3	3.579	4.702	6.286	14.58‘	26.942	31.026	34.712
4	6.409	7.970	10.064	20.024	33.441	37.668	41.418
5	9.695	11.643	14.177	25.471	39.602	43.888	47.637
6	13.343	15.634	18.549	30.921	45.502	49.783	53.480
7	17.299	19.895	23.139	36.371	51.184	55.405	59.007
8	21.530	24.396	27.922	41.823	56.672	60.784	64.255
9	26.019	29.120	32.885	47.274	61.980	65.940	69.243
10	30.757	34.060	38.020	52.726	67.115	70.880	73.981
11	35.745	39.216	43.328	58.177	72.078	75.604	78.470
12	40.993	44.595	48.618	63.629	76.861	80.105	82.701
13	46.520	50.217	54.498	69.079	81.451	84.336	86.657
14	52.363	56.112	60.398	74.529	85.823	88.357	90.305
15	58.582	62.332	66.559	79.976	89.936	92.030	93.591
16	65.288	68.974	73.058	85.419	93.714	95.298	96.421
17	72.706	76.234	80.053	90.849	97.005	97.989	98.625
18	81.470	84.668	87.992	96.222	99.416	99.715	99.859

Sample Size = 19

Order Number	2.5	5.0	10.0	50.0	90.0	95.0	97.5
1	0.133	0.270	0.553	3.582	11.413	14.587	17.647
2	1.301	1.903	2.835	8.678	18.977	22.637	26.028
3	3.383	4.446	5.946	13.827	25.651	29.580	33.138
4	6.052	7.529	9.514	18.989	31.859	35.943	39.578
5	9.147	10.991	13.394	24.154	37.753	41.912	45.565
6	12.576	14.747	17.513	29.322	43.405	47.580	51.203
7	16.289	18.750	21.832	34.491	48.856	52.997	56.550
8	20.252	22.972	26.327	39.660	54.132	58.194	61.642
9	24.447	27.395	30.983	44.830	59.246	63.188	66.500
10	28.864	32.009	35.793	50.000	64.207	67.991	71.136
11	33.500	36.812	40.754	55.170	69.017	72.605	75.553
12	38.358	41.806	45.868	60.340	73.673	77.028	79.748
13	43.450	47.003	51.144	65.509	78.168	81.250	83.711
14	48.797	54.420	56.595	70.678	82.487	85.253	87.424
15	54.435	58.088	62.247	75.846	86.606	89.009	90.853
16	60.422	64.057	68.141	81.011	90.486	92.471	93.948
17	66.682	70.420	74.349	86.173	94.054	95.554	96.617
18	73.972	77.363	81.023	91.322	97.165	98.097	98.699
19	82.353	85.413	88.587	96.418	99.447	99.730	99.867

Sample Size = 20

Order Number	2.5	5.0	10.0	50.0	90.0	95.0	97.5
1	0.127	0.256	0.525	3.406	10.875	13.911	16.843
2	1.235	1.807	2.691	8.251	18.096	21.611	24.873
3	3.207	4.217	5.642	13.147	24.477	28.262	31.698
4	5.733	7.135	9.021	18.055	30.419	34.366	37.893
5	8.657	10.408	12.693	22.967	36.066	40.103	43.661
6	11.893	13.955	16.587	27.880	41.489	45.558	49.105
7	15.391	17.731	20.666	32.795	46.727	50.782	54.279
8	19.119	21.707	24.906	37.711	51.803	55.803	59.219
9	23.058	25.865	29.293	42.626	56.733	60.642	63.946
10	27.196	30.195	33.817	47.542	61.525	65.307	68.472
11	31.528	34.693	38.475	52.458	66.183	69.805	72.804
12	36.054	39.358	43.267	57.374	70.707	74.135	76.942
13	40.781	44.197	48.197	62.289	75.094	78.293	80.881
14	45.721	49.218	53.273	67.205	79.334	82.269	84.609
15	50.895	54.442	58.511	72.120	83.413	86.045	88.107
16	56.339	59.897	63.934	77.033	87.307	89.592	91.343
17	62.107	65.634	69.581	81.945	90.979	92.865	94.267
18	68.302	71.738	75.523	86.853	94.358	95.783	96.793
19	75.127	78.389	81.904	91.749	97.309	98.193	98.765
20	83.157	86.089	89.125	96.594	99.475	99.744	99.873

Sample Size = 21

Order Number	2.5	5.0	10.0	50.0	90.0	95.0	97.5
1	0.120	0.244	0.500	3.247	10.385	13.295	16.110
2	1.175	1.719	2.562	7.864	17.294	20.673	23.816
3	3.049	4.010	5.367	12.531	23.405	27.055	30.377
4	5.446	6.781	8.577	17.209	29.102	32.921	36.342
5	8.218	9.884	12.062	21.891	34.522	38.441	41.907
6	11.281	13.245	15.755	26.574	39.733	43.698	47.166
7	14.588	16.818	19.619	31.258	44.771	48.739	52.175
8	18.107	20.575	23.632	35.943	49.661	53.594	56.968
9	21.820	24.499	27.779	40.629	54.416	58.280	61.565
10	25.713	28.580	32.051	45.314	59.046	62.810	65.979
11	29.781	32.811	36.443	50.000	63.557	67.189	70.219
12	34.021	37.190	40.954	54.686	67.949	71.420	74.287
13	38.435	41.720	45.584	59.371	72.221	75.501	78.180
14	43.032	46.406	50.339	64.057	76.368	79.425	81.893
15	47.825	51.261	55.229	68.742	80.381	83.182	85.412
16	52.834	56.302	60.267	73.426	84.245	86.755	88.719
17	58.093	61.559	65.478	78.109	87.938	90.116	91.782
18	63.658	67.079	70.898	82.791	91.423	93.219	94.554
19	69.623	72.945	76.595	87.469	94.633	95.990	96.951
20	76.184	79.327	82.706	92.136	97.438	98.281	98.825
21	83.890	86.705	89.615	96.753	99.500	99.756	99.880

Sample Size = 22

Order Number	2.5	5.0	10.0	50.0	90.0	95.0	97.5
1	0.115	0.233	0.478	3.102	9.937	12.731	15.437
2	1.121	1.640	2.444	7.512	16.559	19.812	22.844
3	2.906	3.822	5.117	11.970	22.422	25.947	29.161
4	5.187	6.460	8.175	16.439	27.894	31.591	34.912
5	7.821	9.411	11.490	20.911	33.104	36.909	40.285
6	10.729	12.603	15.002	25.384	38.117	41.980	45.370
7	13.865	15.994	18.674	29.859	42.970	46.849	50.222
8	17.198	19.556	22.483	34.334	47.684	51.546	54.872
9	29.709	23.272	26.416	38.810	52.275	56.087	59.342
10	24.386	27.131	30.463	43.286	56.752	60.484	63.645
11	28.221	31.126	34.619	47.762	61.119	64.746	67.790
12	32.210	35.254	38.881	52.238	65.381	68.874	71.779
13	36.355	39.516	43.248	56.714	69.537	72.869	75.614
14	40.658	43.913	47.725	61.190	73.584	76.728	79.291
15	45.128	48.454	52.316	65.666	77.517	80.444	82.802
16	49.778	53.151	57.030	70.141	81.326	84.006	86.135
17	54.630	58.020	61.883	74.616	84.998	87.397	89.271
18	59.715	63.091	66.896	79.089	88.510	90.589	92.179
19	65.088	68.409	72.106	83.561	91.825	93.540	94.813
20	70.839	74.053	77.578	88.030	94.883	96.178	97.094
21	77.156	80.188	83.441	92.488	97.556	98.360	98.879
22	84.563	87.269	90.063	96.898	99.522	99.767	99.885

Sample Size = 23

Order Number	2.5	5.0	10.0	50.0	90.0	95.0	97.5
1	0.110	0.223	0.457	2.969	9.526	12.212	14.819
2	1.071	1.567	2.337	7.191	15.884	19.020	21.949
3	2.775	3.652	4.890	11.458	21.519	24.925	28.038
4	4.951	6.168	7.808	15.734	26.781	30.364	33.589
5	7.460	8.981	10.971	20.015	31.797	35.493	38.781
6	10.229	12.021	14.318	24.297	36.626	40.390	43.703
7	13.210	15.248	17.816	28.580	41.305	45.098	48.405
8	16.376	18.634	21.442	32.863	45.856	49.644	52.919
9	19.708	22.164	25.182	37.147	50.291	54.046	57.226
10	23.191	25.824	29.027	41.431	54.622	58.315	61.458
11	26.820	29.609	32.971	45.716	58.853	62.461	65.505
12	30.588	33.515	37.012	50.000	62.988	66.485	69.412
13	34.495	37.539	41.147	54.284	67.029	70.391	73.180
14	38.542	41.685	45.378	58.569	70.973	74.176	76.809
15	42.734	45.954	49.709	62.853	74.818	77.836	80.292
16	47.081	50.356	54.144	67.137	78.558	81.366	83.624
17	51.595	54.902	58.695	71.420	82.184	84.752	86.790
18	56.297	59.610	63.374	75.703	85.682	87.979	89.771
19	61.219	64.507	68.203	79.985	89.029	91.019	92.540
20	66.411	69.636	73.219	84.266	92.192	93.832	95.049
21	71.962	75.075	78.481	88.542	95.110	96.348	97.225
22	78.051	80.980	84.116	92.809	97.663	98.433	98.929
23	85.151	87.788	90.474	97.031	99.543	99.777	99.890

Sample Size = 24

Order Number	2.5	5.0	10.0	50.0	90.0	95.0	97.5
1	0.105	0.213	0.438	2.847	9.148	11.735	14.247
2	1.026	1.501	2.238	6.895	15.262	18.289	21.120
3	2.656	3.495	4.682	10.987	20.685	23.980	26.997
4	4.735	5.901	7.473	15.088	25.754	29.227	32.361
5	7.132	8.589	10.497	19.192	30.588	34.181	37.384
6	9.773	11.491	13.694	23.299	35.246	38.914	42.151
7	12.615	14.569	17.033	27.406	39.763	43.469	46.711
8	16.630	17.796	20.493	31.513	44.160	47.873	51.095
9	18.799	21.157	24.058	35.621	48.449	52.142	55.322
10	22.110	24.639	27.721	39.729	52.461	56.289	59.406
11	25.553	28.236	31.476	43.837	56.742	60.321	63.357
12	29.124	31.942	35.317	47.946	60.755	64.244	67.179
13	32.821	35.756	39.245	52.054	64.683	68.058	70.876
14	36.643	39.679	43.258	56.163	68.524	71.764	74.447
15	40.594	43.711	47.359	60.271	72.279	75.361	77.890
16	44.678	47.858	51.551	64.379	75.942	78.843	81.201
17	48.905	52.127	55.840	68.487	79.507	82.204	84.370
18	53.289	56.531	60.237	72.594	82.967	85.431	87.385
19	57.849	60.086	64.754	76.701	86.306	88.509	90.227
20	62.616	65.819	69.412	80.808	89.503	91.411	92.868
21	67.639	70.773	74.246	84.912	92.527	94.099	95.265
22	73.003	76.020	79.315	89.013	95.318	96.505	97.344
23	78.880	81.711	84.738	93.105	97.762	98.499	98.974
24	85.753	88.265	90.852	97.153	99.562	99.787	99.895

Sample Size = 25

Order Number	2.5	5.0	10.0	50.0	90.0	95.0	97.5
1	0.101	0.205	0.421	2.735	8.799	11.293	13.719
2	0.984	1.440	2.148	6.623	14.687	17.612	20.352
3	2.547	3.352	4.491	10.553	19.914	23.104	26.031
4	4.538	5.656	7.166	14.492	24.802	28.172	31.219
5	6.831	8.229	10.062	18.435	29.467	32.961	36.083
6	9.356	11.006	13.123	22.379	33.966	37.541	40.704
7	12.072	13.948	16.317	26.324	38.331	41.952	45.129
8	14.950	17.030	19.624	30.270	42.582	46.221	49.388
9	17.972	20.238	23.032	34.215	46.734	50.364	53.500
10	21.125	23.559	26.529	38.161	50.795	54.393	57.479
11	24.402	26.985	30.111	42.108	54.722	58.316	61.335
12	27.797	30.513	33.774	46.054	58.668	62.138	65.072
13	31.306	34.139	37.514	50.000	62.486	65.861	68.694
14	34.928	37.862	41.332	53.946	66.226	69.487	72.203
15	38.665	41.684	45.228	57.892	69.889	73.015	75.598
16	42.521	45.607	49.205	61.839	73.471	76.441	78.875
17	46.500	49.636	53.266	65.785	76.968	79.762	82.028
18	50.612	53.779	57.418	69.730	80.736	82.970	85.050
19	54.871	58.048	61.669	73.676	83.683	86.052	87.928
20	59.296	62.459	66.034	77.621	86.877	88.994	90.644
21	63.917	67.039	70.533	81.565	89.938	91.771	93.169
22	68.781	71.828	75.198	85.508	92.834	94.344	95.462
23	73.969	76.896	80.086	89.447	95.509	96.648	97.453
24	79.648	82.388	85.313	93.377	97.852	98.560	99.016
25	86.281	88.707	92.201	97.265	99.579	99.795	99.899

Appendix 3

40 Inventive Principles, Engineering Parameters, and Conflict Matrix

40 Inventive Principles

1	Segmentation
2	Extraction
3	Local quality
4	Asymmetry
5	Combining
6	Universality
7	Nesting
8	Counterweight
9	Prior counteraction
10	Prior action
11	Cushion in advance
12	Equipotentiality
13	Inversion
14	Spheroidality
15	Dynamicity

16 Partial or overdone action
17 Moving to a new dimension
18 Mechanical vibration
19 Periodic action
20 Continuity of useful action
21 Rushing through
22 Convert harm into benefit
23 Feedback
24 Mediator
25 Self-service
26 Copying
27 An inexpensive short-life object instead of an expensive durable one
28 Replacement of a mechanical system
29 Use a pneumatic or hydraulic construction
30 Flexible film or thin membranes
31 Use of porous materials
32 Changing the color
33 Homogeneity
34 Rejecting and regenerating parts
35 Transformation of physical and chemical states of an object
36 Phase transition
37 Thermal expansion
38 Use strong oxidizers
39 Inert environment
40 Composite materials

Inventive Principles Ordered by Frequency of Use

35 Transformation of physical and chemical states of an object
10 Prior action
1 Segmentation
28 Replacement of a mechanical system
2 Extraction
15 Dynamicity
19 Periodic action
18 Mechanical vibration

32	Changing the color
13	Inversion
26	Copying
3	Local quality
27	An inexpensive short-life object instead of an expensive durable one
29	Use a pneumatic or hydraulic construction
34	Rejecting and regenerating parts
16	Partial or overdone action
40	Composite materials
24	Mediator
17	Moving to a new dimension
6	Universality
14	Spheroidality
22	Convert harm into benefit
39	Inert environment
4	Asymmetry
30	Flexible film or thin membranes
37	Thermal expansion
36	Phase transition
25	Self-service
11	Cushion in advance
31	Use of porous materials
38	Use strong oxidizers
8	Counterweight
5	Combining
7	Nesting
21	Rushing through
23	Feedback
12	Equipotentiality
33	Homogeneity
9	Prior counteraction
20	Continuity of useful action

Contradiction Table

Feature To Improve / Undesired Result (Conflict)		1 Weight of moving object	2 Weight of non-moving object	3 Length of moving object	4 Length of non-moving object	5 Area of moving object	6 Area of non-moving object	7 Volume of moving object	8 Volume of non-moving object	9 Speed	10 Force	11 Tension, pressure	12 Shape	13 Stability of object
1	Weight of moving object			15, 8, 29, 34		29, 17, 38, 34		29, 2, 40, 28		2, 8, 15, 38	8, 10, 18, 37	10, 36, 37, 40	10, 14, 35, 40	1, 35, 19, 39
2	Weight of non-moving object				10, 1, 29, 35		35, 30, 13, 2		5, 35, 14, 2		8, 10, 19, 35	13, 29, 10, 18	13, 10, 29, 14	26, 39, 1, 40
3	Length of moving object	8, 15, 29, 34				15, 17, 4		7, 17, 4, 35		13, 4, 8	17, 10, 4	1, 8, 35	1, 8, 10, 29	1, 8, 15, 34
4	Length of non-moving object		35, 28, 40, 29				17, 7, 10, 40		35, 8, 2, 14		28, 10	1, 14, 35	13, 14, 15, 7	39, 37, 35
5	Area of moving object	2, 17 29, 4		14, 15, 18, 4				7, 14, 17, 4		29, 30, 4, 34	19, 30, 35, 2	10, 15, 36, 28	5, 34, 29, 4	11, 2, 13, 39
6	Area of non-moving object		30, 2, 14, 18		26, 7, 9, 39						1, 18, 35, 36	10, 15, 36, 37		2, 38
7	Volume of moving object	2, 26, 29, 40		1, 7, 4, 35		1, 7, 4, 17				29, 4, 38, 34	15, 35, 36, 37	6, 35, 36, 37	1, 15, 29, 4	28, 10, 1, 39
8	Volume of non-moving object		35, 10, 19, 14	19, 14	35, 8, 2, 14						2, 18, 37	24, 35	7, 2, 35	34, 28, 35, 40
9	Speed	2, 28, 13, 38		13, 14, 8		29, 30, 34		7, 29, 34			13, 28, 15, 19	6, 18, 38, 40	35, 15, 18, 34	28, 33, 1, 18
10	Force	8, 1, 37, 18	18, 13, 1, 28	17, 19, 6, 36	28, 10	19, 10, 15	1, 18, 36, 37	15, 9, 12, 37	2, 36, 18, 37	13, 28, 15, 12		18, 21, 11	10, 35, 40, 34	35, 10, 21
11	Tension, pressure	10, 36, 37, 40	13, 29, 10, 18	35, 10, 36	35, 1, 14, 16	10, 15, 36, 25	10, 15, 35, 37	6, 35, 10	35, 24	6, 35, 36	36, 35, 21		35, 4, 15, 10	35, 33, 2, 40
12	Shape	8, 10, 29, 40	15, 10, 26, 3	29, 34, 5, 4	13, 14, 10, 7	5, 34, 4, 10		14, 4, 15, 22	7, 2, 35	35, 15, 34, 18	35, 10, 37, 40	34, 15, 10, 14		33, 1, 18, 4
13	Stability of object	21, 35, 2, 39	26, 39, 1, 40	13, 15, 1, 28	37	2, 11, 13	39	28, 10, 19, 39	34, 28, 35, 40	33, 15, 28, 18	10, 35, 21, 16	2, 35, 40	22, 1, 18, 4	
14	Strength	1, 8, 40, 15	40, 26, 27, 1	1, 15, 8, 35	15, 14, 28, 26	3, 34, 40, 29	9, 40, 28	10, 15, 14, 7	9, 14, 17, 15	8, 13, 26, 14	10, 18, 3, 14	10, 3, 18, 40	10, 30, 35, 40	13, 17, 35
15	Durability of moving object	19, 5, 34, 31		2, 19, 9		3, 17, 19		10, 2, 19, 30		3, 35, 5	19, 2, 16	19, 3, 27	14, 26, 28, 25	13, 3, 35
16	Durability of non-moving object		6, 27, 19, 16		1, 10, 35				35, 34, 38					39, 3, 35, 23
17	Temperature	36, 22, 6, 38	22, 35, 32	15, 19, 9	15, 19, 9	3, 35, 39, 18	35, 38	34, 39, 40, 18	35, 6, 4	2, 28, 36, 30	35, 10, 3, 21	35, 39, 19, 2	14, 22, 19, 32	1, 35, 32
18	Brightness	19, 1, 32	2, 35, 32			19, 32, 26								
19	Energy spent by moving object	12, 18, 28, 31		12, 28		15, 19, 25		35, 13, 18		8, 15, 35	16, 26, 21, 2	23, 14, 25	12, 2, 29	19, 13, 17, 24
20	Energy spent by non-moving object		19, 9, 6, 27								36, 37			27, 4, 29, 19

Contradiction Table (Continued)

Feature To Improve \ Undesired Result (Conflict)		14 Strength	15 Durability of moving object	16 Durability of non-moving object	17 Temperature	18 Brightness	19 Energy spent by moving object	20 Energy spent by non-moving object	21 Power	22 Water of energy	23 Water of substance	24 Loss of information	25 Waste of time	26 Amount of substance
1	Weight of moving object	28, 27, 18, 40	5, 34, 31, 35		6, 20, 4, 38	19, 1, 32	35, 12, 34, 31		12, 36, 18, 31	6, 2, 34, 19	5, 35, 3, 31	10, 24, 35	10, 35, 20, 28	3, 26. 18, 31
2	Weight of non-moving object	28, 2, 10, 27		2, 27, 19, 6	28, 19, 32, 22	19, 32, 35		18, 19, 28, 1	15, 19, 18, 22	18, 19, 28, 15	5, 8, 13, 30	10, 15, 35	10, 20, 35, 26	19, 6, 18, 26
3	Length of moving object	8, 35, 29, 34	19		10, 15, 19	32	8, 35, 24		1, 35	7, 2, 35, 39	4, 29, 23, 10	1, 24	15, 2, 29	29, 35
4	Length of non-moving object	15, 14, 28, 26		1, 40, 35	3, 35, 38, 18	3, 25			12, 8	6, 28	10, 28, 24, 35	24, 26	30, 29, 14	
5	Area of moving object	3, 15, 40, 14	6, 3		2, 15, 16	15, 32, 19, 13	19, 32		19, 10, 32, 18	15, 17, 30, 26	10, 35, 2, 39	30, 26	26, 4	29, 30, 6, 13
6	Area of non-moving object	40		2, 10, 19, 30	35, 39, 38				17, 32	17, 7, 30	10, 14, 18, 39	30, 16	10, 35, 4, 18	2, 18, 40, 4
7	Volume of moving object	9, 14, 15, 7	6, 35, 4		34, 39, 10, 18	2, 13, 10	35		35, 6, 13, 18	7, 15, 13, 16	36, 39, 34, 10	2, 22	2, 6, 34, 10	29, 30, 7
8	Volume of non-moving object	9, 14, 17, 15		35, 34, 38	35, 6, 4				30, 6		10, 39, 35, 34		35, 16, 32, 18	35, 3
9	Speed	8, 3, 26, 14	3, 19, 35, 5		28, 30, 36, 2	10, 13, 19	8, 15, 35, 38		19, 35, 38, 2	14, 20, 19, 35	10, 13, 28, 38	13, 26		18, 19, 29, 38
10	Force	35, 10, 14, 27	19, 2		35, 10, 24		19, 17, 10	1, 16, 36, 37	19, 35, 18, 37	14, 15	8, 35, 40, 5		10, 37, 36	14, 29, 18, 36
11	Tension, pressure	9, 18, 3, 40	19, 3, 27		35, 39, 19, 2		14, 24, 10, 37		10, 35, 14	2, 36, 25	10, 36, 3, 37		37, 36, 4	10, 14, 36
12	Shape	30, 14, 10, 40	14, 26, 9, 25		22, 14, 19, 32	13, 15, 32	2, 6, 34, 14		4, 6, 2	14	35, 29, 3, 5		14, 10, 34, 17	36, 22
13	Stability of object	17, 9, 15	13, 27, 10, 35	39, 3, 35, 23	35, 1, 32	32, 3, 27, 15	13, 19	27, 4, 29, 18	32, 35, 27, 31	14, 2, 39, 6	2, 14, 30, 40		35, 27	15, 32, 35
14	Strength		27, 3, 26		30, 10, 40	35, 19	19, 35, 10	35	10, 26, 35, 28	35	35, 28, 31, 40		29, 3, 28, 10	29, 10, 27
15	Durability of moving object	27, 3, 10			19, 35, 39	2, 19, 4, 35	28, 6, 35, 18		19, 10, 35, 38		28, 27, 3, 18	10	20, 10, 28, 18	3, 35, 10, 40
16	Durability of non-moving object				19, 18, 36, 40				16		27, 16, 18, 38	10	28, 20, 10, 16	3, 35, 31
17	Temperature	10, 30, 22, 40	19, 13, 39	19, 18, 36, 40		32, 30, 21, 16	19, 15, 3, 17		2, 14, 17, 25	21, 17, 35, 38	21, 36, 29, 31		35, 28, 21, 18	3, 17, 30, 39
18	Brightness	35, 19	2, 19, 6		32, 35, 19		32, 1, 19	32, 35, 1, 15	32	19, 16, 1, 6	13, 1	1, 6	19, 1, 26, 17	1, 19
19	Energy spent by moving object	5, 19, 9, 35	28, 35, 6, 18		19, 24, 3, 14	2, 15, 19			6, 19, 37, 18	12, 22, 15, 24	35, 24, 18, 5		35, 38, 19, 18	34, 23, 16, 18
20	Energy spent by non-moving object	35				19, 2, 35, 32					28, 27, 18, 31			3, 35, 31

Contradiction Table (Continued)

Feature To Improve	Undesired Result (Conflict)	27 Reliability	28 Accuracy of measurement	29 Accuracy of manufacturing	30 Harmful factors acting on object	31 Harmful side effects	32 Manufacturability	33 Convenience of use	34 Repairability	35 Adaptability	36 Complexity of device	37 Complexity of control	38 Level of automation	39 Productivity
1	Weight of moving object	3, 11, 1, 27	28, 27, 35, 26	28, 35, 26, 18	22, 21, 18, 27	22, 35, 31, 39	27, 28, 1, 36	35, 3, 2, 24	2, 27, 28, 11	29, 5, 15, 8	26, 30, 36, 34	28, 29, 26, 32	26, 35, 18, 19	35, 3, 24, 37
2	Weight of non-moving object	10, 28, 8, 3	18, 26, 28	10, 1, 35, 17	2, 19, 22, 37	35, 22, 1, 39	28, 1, 9	6, 13, 1, 32	2, 27, 28, 11	19, 15, 29	1, 10, 26, 39	25, 28, 17, 15	2, 26, 35	1, 28, 15, 35
3	Length of moving object	10, 14, 29, 40	28, 32, 4	10, 28, 29, 37	1, 15, 17, 24	17, 15	1, 29, 17	15, 29, 35, 4	1, 28, 10	14, 15, 1, 16	1, 19, 26, 24	35, 1, 26, 24	17, 24, 26, 16	14, 4, 28, 29
4	Length of non-moving object	15, 29, 28	32, 28, 3	2, 32, 10	1, 18		15, 17, 27	2, 25	3	1, 35	1, 26	26		30, 14, 7, 26
5	Area of moving object	29, 9	26, 28, 32, 3	2, 32	22, 33, 28, 1	17, 2, 18, 39	13, 1, 26, 24	15, 17, 13, 16	15, 13, 10, 1	15, 30	14, 1, 13	2, 36, 26, 18	14, 30, 28, 23	10, 26, 34, 2
6	Area of non-moving object	32, 35, 40, 4	26, 28, 32, 3	2, 29, 18, 36	27, 2, 39, 35	22, 1, 40	40, 16	16, 4	16	15, 16	1, 18, 36	2, 35, 30, 18	23	10, 15, 17, 7
7	Volume of moving object	14, 1, 40, 11	25, 26, 28	25, 28, 2, 16	22, 21, 27, 35	17, 2, 40, 1	29, 1, 40	15, 13, 30, 12	10	15, 29	26, 1	29, 26, 4	35, 34, 16, 24	10, 6, 2, 34
8	Volume of non-moving object	2, 35, 16		35, 10, 25	34, 39, 19, 27	30, 18, 35, 4	35		1		1, 31	2, 17, 26		35, 37, 10, 2
9	Speed	11, 35, 27, 28	28, 32, 1, 24	10, 28, 32, 25	1, 28, 35, 23	2, 24, 35, 21	35, 13, 8, 1	32, 28, 13, 12	34, 2, 28, 27	15, 10, 26	10, 28, 4, 34	3, 34, 27, 16	10, 18	
10	Force	3, 35, 13, 21	35, 10, 23, 24	28, 29, 37, 36	1, 35, 40, 18	13, 3, 36, 24	15, 37, 18, 1	1, 28, 3, 25	15, 1, 11	15, 17, 18, 20	26, 35, 10, 18	36, 37, 10, 19	2, 35	3, 28, 35, 37
11	Tension, pressure	10, 13, 19, 35	6, 28, 25	3, 35	22, 2, 37	2, 33, 27, 18	1, 35, 16	11	2	35	19, 1, 35	2, 36, 37	35, 24	10, 14, 35, 37
12	Shape	10, 40, 16	28, 32, 1	32, 30, 40	22, 1, 2, 35	35, 1	1, 32, 17, 28	32, 15, 26	2, 13, 1	1, 15, 29	16, 29, 1, 28	15, 13, 39	15, 1, 32	17, 26, 34, 10
13	Stability of object		13	18	35, 24, 30, 18	35, 40, 27, 39	35, 19	32, 35, 30	2, 35, 10, 16	35, 30, 34, 2	2, 35, 22, 26	35, 22, 39, 23	1, 8, 35	23, 35, 40, 3
14	Strength	11, 3	3, 27, 16	3, 27	18, 35, 37, 1	15, 35, 22, 2	11, 3, 10, 32	32, 40, 28, 2	27, 11, 3	15, 3, 32	2, 13, 28	27, 3, 15, 40	15	29, 35, 10, 14
15	Durability of moving object	11, 2, 13	3	3, 27, 16, 40	22, 15, 33, 28	21, 39, 16, 22	27, 1, 4	12, 27	29, 10, 27	1, 35, 13	10, 4, 29, 15	19, 29, 39, 35	6, 10	35, 17, 14, 19
16	Durability of non-moving object	34, 27, 6, 40	10, 26, 24		17, 1, 40, 33	22	35, 10	1	1	2		25, 34, 6, 35	1	10, 20, 16, 38
17	Temperature	19, 35, 3, 10	32, 19, 24	24	22, 33, 35, 2	22, 35, 2, 24	26, 27	26, 27	4, 10, 16	2, 18, 27	2, 17, 16	3, 27, 35, 31	26, 2, 19, 16	15, 28, 35
18	Brightness		11, 15, 32	3, 32	15, 19	35, 19, 32, 39	19, 35, 28, 26	28, 26, 19	15, 17, 13, 16	15, 1, 1, 19	6, 32, 13	32, 15	2, 26, 10	2, 25, 16
19	Energy spent by moving object	19, 21, 11, 27	3, 1, 32		1, 35, 6, 27	2, 35, 6	28, 26, 30	19, 35	1, 15, 17, 28	15, 17, 13, 16	2, 29, 27, 28	35, 38	32, 2	12, 28, 35
20	Energy spent by non-moving object	10, 36, 23			10, 2, 22, 37	19, 22, 18	1, 4					19, 35, 16, 25		1, 6

Contradiction Table (Continued)

No.	Feature To Improve \ Undesired Result (Conflict)	1 Weight of moving object	2 Weight of non-moving object	3 Length of moving object	4 Length of non-moving object	5 Area of moving object	6 Area of non-moving object	7 Volume of moving object	8 Volume of non-moving object	9 Speed	10 Force	11 Tension, pressure	12 Shape	13 Stability of object
21	Power	8, 36, 38, 31	19, 26, 17, 27	1, 10, 35, 37		19, 38	17, 32, 13, 38	35, 6, 38	30, 6, 25	15, 35, 2	26, 2, 36, 35	22, 10, 35	29, 14, 2, 40	35, 32, 15, 31
22	Waste of energy	15, 6, 19, 28	19, 6, 18, 9	7, 2, 6, 13	6, 38, 7	15, 26, 17, 30	17, 7, 30, 18	7, 18, 23	7	16, 35, 38	36, 38			14, 2, 39, 6
23	Waste of substance	35, 6, 23, 40	35, 6, 22, 32	14, 29, 10, 398	10, 28, 24	35, 2, 10, 31	10, 18, 39, 31	1, 29, 30, 36	3, 39, 18, 31	10, 13, 28, 38	14, 15, 18, 40	3, 36, 37, 10	29, 35, 3, 5	2, 14, 30, 40
24	Loss of information	10, 24, 35	10, 35, 5	1, 26	26	30, 26	30, 16		2, 22	26, 32				
25	Waste of time	10, 20, 37, 35	10, 20, 26, 5	15, 2, 29	30, 24, 14, 5	26, 4, 5, 16	10, 35, 17, 4	2, 5, 34, 10	35, 16, 32, 18		10, 37, 36, 5	37, 36, 4	4, 10, 34, 17	35, 3, 22, 5
26	Amount of substance	35, 6, 18, 31	27, 26, 18, 35	29, 14, 35, 18		15, 14, 29	2, 18, 40, 4	15, 20, 29		35, 29, 34, 28	35, 14, 3	10, 36, 14, 3	35, 14	15,. 2, 17, 40
27	Reliability	3, 8, 10, 40	3, 10, 8, 28	15, 9, 14, 4	15, 29, 28, 11	17, 10, 14, 16	32, 35, 40, 4	3, 10, 14, 24	2, 35, 24	21, 35, 11, 28	8, 28, 10, 3	10, 24, 35, 19	35, 1, 16, 11	
28	Accuracy of measurement	32, 35, 26, 28,	28, 35, 25, 26	28, 26, 5, 16	32, 28, 3, 16	26, 28, 32, 3	26, 28, 32, 3	32, 13, 6		28, 13, 32, 24	32, 2	6, 28, 32	6, 28, 32	32, 35, 13
29	Accuracy of manufacturing	28, 32, 13, 18	28, 35, 27, 9	10, 28, 29, 37	2, 32, 10	28, 33, 29, 32	2, 29, 18, 36	32, 28, 2	25, 10, 35	10, 28, 32	28, 19, 34, 36	3, 35	32, 30, 40	30, 18
30	Harmful factors acting on object	22, 21, 27, 39	2, 22, 13, 24	17, 1, 39, 4	1, 18	22, 1, 33, 28	27, 2, 39, 35	22, 23, 37, 35	34, 39, 19, 27	21, 22, 35, 28	13, 35, 39, 18	22, 2, 37	22, 1, 3, 35	35, 24, 30, 18
31	Harmful side effects	19, 22, 15, 39	35, 22, 1, 39	17, 15, 16, 22		17, 2, 18, 39	22, 1, 40	17, 2, 40	30, 18, 35, 4	35, 28, 3, 23	35, 28, 1, 40	2, 33, 27, 18	35, 1	35, 40, 27, 39
32	Manufacturability	28, 29, 15, 16	1, 27, 36, 13	1, 29, 13, 17	15, 17, 27	13, 1, 26, 12	16, 40,	13, 29, 1, 40	35,	35, 13, 8, 1	35, 12	35, 19, 1, 37	1, 28, 13, 27	11, 13, 1
33	Convenience of use	25, 2, 13, 15,	6, 13, 1, 25	1, 17, 13, 12		1, 17, 13, 16	18, 16, 15, 39	1, 16, 35, 15	4, 18, 39, 31	18, 13, 34	28, 13, 35	2, 32, 12	15, 34, 29, 28	32, 35, 30
34	Repairability	2, 27, 35, 11	2, 27, 35, 11	1, 28, 10, 25	3, 18, 31	15, 13, 32	16, 25	25, 2, 35, 11	1	34, 9	1, 11, 10	13	1, 13, 2, 4	2, 35
35	Adaptability	1, 6, 15, 8	19, 15, 29, 16	35, 1, 29, 2	1, 35, 16	35, 30, 29, 7	15, 16	15, 35, 29		35, 10, 14	15, 17, 20	35, 16,	15, 37, 1, 8	35, 30, 14
36	Complexity of device	26, 30, 34, 36	2, 36, 35, 39	1, 19, 26, 24	26	14, 1, 13, 16	6, 36	34, 25, 6	1, 16	34, 10, 28	26, 16	19, 1, 35	29, 13, 28, 15	2, 22, 17, 19
37	Complexity of control	27, 26, 28, 13	6, 13, 28, 1	16, 17, 26, 24	26	2, 13, 15, 17	2, 39, 30, 16	29, 1, 4, 16	2, 18, 26, 31	3, 4, 16, 35	36, 28, 40, 19	35, 36, 37, 32	27, 13, 1, 39	11, 22, 39, 30
38	Level of automation	28, 26, 18, 35	28, 26, 35, 10	14, 13, 17, 28	23	17, 14, 13		35, 13, 16		28, 10	2, 35	13, 35	15, 32, 1, 13	18, 1
39	Productivily	35, 26, 24, 37	28, 27, 15, 3	18, 4, 28, 38	30, 7, 14, 26	10, 26, 34, 31	10, 35, 17, 7	2, 6, 34, 10	35, 37, 10, 2		28, 15, 10, 36	10, 37, 14	14, 10, 34, 40	35, 3, 22, 39

Contradiction Table (Continued)

Feature To Improve	Undesired Result (Conflict)	14 Strength	15 Durability of moving object	16 Durability of non-moving object	17 Temperature	18 Brightness	19 Energy spent by moving object	20 Energy spent by non-moving object	21 Power	22 Waste of enerry	23 Waster of substance	24 Loss of information	25 Waste of time	26 Amount of substance
21	Power	26, 10, 28	19, 35, 10, 38	16	2, 14, 17, 25	16, 6, 19	16, 6, 19, 37			10, 35, 38	28, 27, 18, 38	10, 19	35, 20, 10, 6	4, 34, 19
22	Waste of energy	26			19, 38, 7	1, 13, 32, 15			3, 38		35, 27, 2, 37	19, 10	10, 18, 32, 7	7, 18, 25
23	Waste of information	35, 28, 31, 40	28, 27, 3, 18	27, 16, 18, 38	21, 36, 39, 31	1, 6, 13	35, 18, 24, 5	28, 27, 12, 31	28, 27, 18, 38	35, 27, 2, 31			15, 18, 35, 10	6, 3, 10, 24
24	Loss of information		10	10		19			10, 19	10, 19			24, 26, 28, 32	24, 28, 35
25	Waste of time	29, 3, 28, 18	20, 10, 28, 18	28, 20, 10, 16	35, 29, 21, 18	1, 19, 26, 17	35, 38, 19, 18	1	35, 20, 10, 6	10, 5, 18, 32	35, 18, 10, 39	24, 26, 28, 32		35, 38, 18, 16
26	Amount of substance	14, 35, 34, 10	3, 35, 10, 40	3, 35, 31	3, 17, 39		34, 29, 16, 18	3, 35, 31	35	7, 18, 25	6, 3, 10, 24	24, 28, 35	35, 38, 18, 16	
27	Reliability	11, 28,	2, 35, 3, 25	34, 27, 6, 40	3, 35, 10	11, 32, 13	21, 11, 27, 19	36, 23	21, 11, 26, 31	10, 11, 35	10, 35, 29, 39	10, 28,	10, 30, 4	21, 28, 40, 3
28	Accuracy of measurement	28, 6, 32	28, 6, 32	10, 26, 24	6, 19, 28; 24	6, 1, 32	3, 6, 32		3, 6, 32	26, 32, 27	10, 16, 31, 28		24, 34, 28, 32	2, 6, 32
29	Accuracy of manufacturing	3, 27	3, 27, 40		19, 26	3, 32	32, 2		32, 2	13, 32, 2	35, 31, 10, 24		32, 26, 28, 18	32, 30
30	Harmful side effects	18, 35, 37, 1	22, 15, 33, 28	17, 1, 40, 33	22, 33, 35, 2	1, 19, 32, 13	1, 24, 6, 27	10, 2, 22, 37	19, 22, 31, 2	21, 22, 35, 2	33, 22, 19, 40	22, 10, 2	35, 18, 34	35, 33, 29, 31
31	Harmful side effects	15, 35, 22, 2	15, 22, 33, 31	21, 39, 16, 22	22, 35, 2, 24	19, 24, 39, 32	2, 35, 6	19, 22, 18	2, 35, 18	21, 35, 2, 22	10, 1, 34	10, 21, 29	1, 22	3, 24, 39, 1
32	Manufacturability	1, 3 10, 32	27, 1, 4	35, 16	27, 26, 18	28, 24, 27, 1	28, 26, 27, 1	1, 4	27, 1, 12, 24	19, 35	15, 34, 33	32, 24, 18, 16	35, 28, 34, 4	35, 23, 1, 24
33	Convenience of use	32, 40, 3, 28	29, 3, 8, 25	1, 16, 25	26, 27, 13	13, 17, 1, 24	1, 13, 24		35, 34, 2, 10	2, 19, 13	28, 32, 2, 24	4, 10, 27, 22	4, 28, 10, 34	12, 35
34	Repairability	11, 1 2, 9	11, 29, 28, 27	1	4, 10	15, 1, 13	15, 1, 28, 16		15, 10, 32, 2	15, 1, 32, 19	2, 35, 34, 27		32, 1, 10, 25	2, 28, 10, 25
35	Adaptability	35, 3, 32, 6	13, 1, 35	2, 16	27, 2, 3, 35	6, 22, 26, 1	19, 35, 29, 13		19, 1, 29	18, 15, 1	15, 10, 2, 13		35, 28	3, 35, 15
36	Complexity of device	2, 13, 28	10, 4, 28, 15		2, 17, 13	24, 17, 13	27, 2, 29, 28		20, 19, 30, 34	10, 35, 13, 2	35, 10, 28, 29		6, 29	13, 3, 27, 10
37	Complexity of control	27, 3, 15, 28	19, 29, 39, 25	25, 24, 6, 35	3, 27, 35, 16	2, 24, 26	35, 38	19, 35, 16	19, 1, 16, 10	35, 3, 15, 19	1, 13, 10, 24	35, 33, 27, 22	18, 28, 32, 9	3, 27, 29, 18
38	Level of automation	25, 13	6, 9		26, 2, 19	8, 32, 19	2, 32, 13		28, 2, 27	23, 28	35, 10, 18, 5	35, 33	24, 28, 35, 30	35, 13
39	Productivity	29, 28, 10, 18	35, 10, 2, 18	20, 10, 16, 38	35, 21, 28, 10	26, 17, 19, 1	35, 10, 38, 19	1	35, 20, 10	28, 10, 29, 35	28, 10, 35, 23	13, 15, 23		35, 38

Contradiction Table (Continued)

Feature To Improve / Undesired Result (Conflict)		27 Reliability	28 Accuracy of measurement	29 Accuracy of manufacturing	30 Harmful factors acting on object	31 Harmful side effects	32 Manufacturability	33 Convenience of use	34 Repairability	35 Adaptability	36 Complexity of device	37 Complexity of control	38 Level of automation	39 Productivity
21	Power	19, 24, 26, 31	32, 15, 2	32, 2	19, 22, 31, 2	2, 35, 18	26, 10, 34	26, 35, 10	35, 2, 10, 34	19, 17, 34	20, 19, 30, 34	19, 35, 16	28, 2, 17	28, 35, 34
22	Waste of energy	11, 10, 35	32		21, 22, 35, 2	21, 35, 2, 22		35, 22, 1	2, 19		7, 23	35, 3, 15, 23	2	28, 10, 29, 35
23	Waste of substance	10, 29, 39, 35	16, 34, 31, 28	35, 10, 24, 31	33, 22, 30, 40	10, 1, 34, 29	15, 34, 33	32, 28, 2, 24	2, 35, 34, 27	15, 10, 2	35, 10, 28, 24	35, 18, 10, 13	35, 10, 18	28, 35, 10, 23
24	Loss of information	10, 28, 23			22, 10, 1	10, 21, 22	32	27, 22				35, 33	35	13, 23, 15
25	Waste of time	10, 30, 4	24, 34, 28, 32	24, 26, 28, 18	35, 18, 34	35, 22, 18, 39	35, 28, 34, 4	4, 28, 10, 34	32, 1, 10	35, 28	6, 29	18, 28, 32, 10	24, 28, 35, 30	
26	Amount of substance	18, 3, 28, 40	13, 2, 28	33, 30	35, 33, 29, 31	3, 35, 40, 39	29, 1, 35, 27	35, 29, 25, 10	2, 32, 10, 25	15, 3, 29	3, 13, 27, 10	3, 27, 29, 18	8, 35	13, 29, 3, 27
27	Reliability		32, 3, 11, 23	11, 32, 1	27, 35, 2, 40	35, 2, 40, 26		27, 17, 40	1, 11	13, 35, 8, 24	13, 35, 1	27, 40, 28	11, 13, 27	1, 35, 29, 38
28	Accuracy of measurement	5, 11, 1, 23			28, 24, 22, 26	3, 33, 39, 10	6, 35, 25, 18	1, 13, 17, 34	1, 32, 13, 11	13, 35, 2	27, 35, 10, 34	26, 24, 32, 28	28, 2, 10, 34	10, 34, 28, 32
29	Accuracy of manufacturing	11, 32, 1			26, 28, 10, 36	4, 17, 34, 26		1, 32, 35, 23	25, 10		26, 2, 18		26, 28, 18, 23	10, 18, 32, 39
30	Harmful factors acting on object	27, 24, 2, 40	28, 33, 23, 26	26, 28, 10, 18			24, 35, 2	2, 25, 28, 39	35, 10, 2	35, 11, 22, 31	22, 19, 29, 40	22, 19, 29, 40	33, 3, 34	22, 35, 13, 24
31	Harmful side effects	24, 2, 40, 39	3, 33, 26	4, 17, 34, 26							19, 1, 31	2, 21, 27, 1	2	22, 35, 18, 39
32	Manufacturability		1, 35, 12, 18		24, 2			2, 5, 13, 16	35, 1, 11, 9	2, 13, 15	27, 26, 1	6, 28, 11, 1	8, 28, 1	35, 1, 10, 28
33	Convenience of use	17, 27, 8, 40	25, 13, 2, 34	1, 32, 35, 23	2, 25, 28, 39		2, 5, 12		12, 26, 1, 32	15, 34, 1, 16	32, 26, 12, 17		1, 34, 12, 3	15, 1, 28
34	Repairability	11, 10, 1, 16	10, 2, 13	25, 10	35, 10, 2, 16		1, 35, 11, 10	1, 12, 26, 15		7, 1, 4, 16	35, 1, 13, 11		34, 35, 7, 13	1, 32, 10
35	Adaptability	35, 13, 8, 24	35, 5, 1, 10		35, 11, 32, 31		1, 13, 31	15, 34, 1, 16	1, 16, 7, 4		15, 29, 37, 28	1	27, 34, 35	35, 28, 6, 37
36	Complexity of device	13, 35, 1	2, 26, 10, 34	26, 24, 32	22, 19, 29, 40	19, 1	27, 26, 1, 13	27, 9, 26, 24	1, 13	29, 15, 28, 37		15, 10, 37, 28	15, 1, 24	12, 17, 28
37	Complexity of control	27, 40, 28, 8	26, 24, 32, 28		22, 19, 29, 28	2, 21	5, 28, 11, 29	2, 5	12, 26	1, 15	15, 10, 37, 28		34, 21	35, 18
38	Level of automation	11, 27, 32	28, 26, 10, 34	28, 26, 18, 23	2, 33	2	1, 26, 13	1, 12, 34, 3	1, 35, 13	27, 4, 1, 35	15, 24, 10	34, 27, 25		5, 12, 35, 26
39	Productivity	1, 35, 10, 38	1, 10, 34, 28	18, 10, 32, 1	22, 35, 13, 24	32, 22, 18, 39	35, 28, 2, 24	1, 28, 7, 19	1, 32, 10, 25	1, 35, 28, 37	12, 17, 28, 24	35, 18, 27, 2	5, 12, 35, 26	

The above material is from:
TRIZ: Through the Eyes of an American TRIZ Specialist, A Study of Ideality, Contradictions, Resources, ©1997, Dana W. Clarke, Sr., of Ideation International, by permission of the author.

Appendix 4

Glossary

Accelerated testing

Testing at higher than normal stress levels to increase the failure rate and shorten the time to wearout.

Acceptable quality level (AQL)

The maximum percent defective that, for the purpose of sampling inspection, can be considered satisfactory for a process average.

Acceptance

Sign-off by the purchaser.

Active redundancy

That redundancy wherein all redundant items are operating simultaneously.

Ambient

Used to denote surrounding, encompassing, or local conditions and is usually applied to environments.

Archiving

The process of establishing and maintaining copies of controlled items such that previous items, baselines and configurations can be re-established should there be a loss or corruption.

Assessment

The review and auditing of an organization's Quality Management System to determine that it meets the requirements of the standards, that it is implemented, and that it is effective.

Auditee

An organization to be audited.

Auditor

A person who has the qualifications to perform quality audits.

Baseline

A definition of configuration status declared at a point in the project life cycle.

Burn-in

The operation of items prior to their end application to stabilize their characteristics and identify early failures.

Calibration

The comparison of a measurement system or device of unverified accuracy to a measurement system or device of known and greater accuracy, to detect and correct any variation from required performance specifications of the measurement system or device.

Certification

The process which seeks to confirm that the appropriate minimum best practice requirements are included and that the quality management system is put into effect.

Certification body

An organization which sets itself up as a supplier of product or process certification against established specifications or standards.

Change notice

A document approved by the design activity that describes and authorizes the implementation of an engineering change to the product and its approved configuration documentation.

Checksum

The sum of every byte contained in an input/output record used for assuring the integrity of the programmed entry.

Checklist

An aid for the auditor listing areas and topics to be covered by the auditors.

Client

A person or organization requesting an audit.

Compliance audit

An audit where the auditor must investigate the Quality System, as put into practice, and the organization's results.

Conditioning

The exposure of sample units or specimens to a specific environment for a specified period of time to prepare them for subsequent inspection.

Confidence

The probability that may be attached to conclusions reached as a result of application of statistical techniques.

Confidence interval

The numerical range within which an unknown is estimated to be.

Confidence level

The probability that a given statement is correct.

Confidence limits

The extremes of a confidence interval within which the unknown has a designated probability of being included.

Configuration

A collection of items at specified versions for the fulfillment of a particular purpose.

Controlled document

Documents with a defined distribution such that all registered holders of control documents systematically receive any updates to those documents.

Corrective action

All action taken to improve the overall Quality Management System as a result of identifying deficiencies, inefficiencies, and non-compliances.

Creep

Continuous increase in deformation under constant or decreasing stress.

Critical item

An item within a configuration item which, because of special engineering or logistic considerations, requires an approved specification to establish technical or inventory control.

Cycle

An ON/OFF application of power.

Debugging

A process to detect and remedy inadequacies.

Defect

Any nonconformance of a characteristic with specified requirements.

Degradation

A gradual deterioration in performance.

Delivery

Transfer of a product from the supplier to the purchaser.

Derating

The use of an item in such a way that applied stresses are below rated values.

Design entity

An element of a design that is structurally and functionally distinct from other elements and that is separately named and referenced.

Design review

A formal, documented, comprehensive and systematic examination of a design to evaluate the design requirements and the capability of the design to meet these requirements and to identify problems and propose solutions.

Design view

A subset of design entity attribute information that is specifically suited to the needs of a software project activity.

Deviation

A specific written authorization, granted prior to manufacture of an item, to depart from a particular requirement(s) of an item's current approved configuration documentation for a specific number of units or a specified period of time.

Device

Any functional system.

Discrete variable

A variable which can take only a finite number of values.

Document

Contain information which is subject to change.

Down-time

The total time during which the system is not in condition to perform its intended function.

Early failure period

An interval immediately following final assembly, during which the failure rate of certain items is relatively high.

Entity attribute

A named characteristic or property of a design entity that provides a statement of fact about the entity.

Environment

The aggregate of all conditions which externally influence the performance of an item.

External audit

An audit performed by a customer or his representative at the facility of the supplier to assess the degree of compliance of the quality system with documented requirements.

Extrinsic audit

An audit carried out in a company by a third party organization or a regulatory authority, to assess its activities against specific requirements.

Fail-safe

The stated condition that the equipment will contain self-checking features which will cause a function to cease in case of failure, malfunction, or drifting out of tolerance.

Failure

The state of inability of an item to perform its required function.

Failure analysis

Subsequent to a failure, the logical, systematic examination of any item, its construction, application, and documentation to identify the failure mode and determine the failure mechanism.

Failure mode

The consequence of the mechanism through which the failure occurs.

Failure rate

The probability of failure per unit of time of the items still operating.

Fatigue

A weakening or deterioration of metal or other material, or of a member, occurring under load, specifically under repeated, cyclic or continuous loading.

Fault

The immediate cause of a failure.

Fault iisolation

The process of determining the location of a fault to the extent necessary to effect repair.

Feasibility study

The study of a proposed item or technique to determine the degree to which it is practicable, advisable, and adaptable for the intended

Firmware

The combination of a hardware device and computer instructions or computer data that reside as read-only software on the hardware device.

Form

The shape, size, dimensions, mass, weight, and other visual parameters which uniquely characterize an item.

Grade

An indicator or category or rank relating to features or characteristics that cover different sets of needs for products or services intended for the same functional use.

Inherent failure

A failure basically caused by a physical condition or phenomenon internal to the failed item.

Inherent reliability

Reliability potential present in the design.

Inspection

The examination and testing of supplies and services to determine whether they conform to specified requirements.

Installation

Introduction of the product to the purchaser's organization.

Internal audit

An audit carried out within an organization by its own personnel to assess compliance of the quality system to documented requirements.

Item

Any entity whose development is to be tracked.

Maintainability

The measure of the ability of an item to be retained in or restored to a specified condition when maintenance is performed by personnel having specified skill levels, using prescribed procedures and resources, at each prescribed level of maintenance and repair.

Maintenance

The servicing, repair, and care of material or equipment to sustain or restore acceptable operating conditions.

Major non-compliance

Either the non-implementation, within the quality system of a requirement of ISO 9001, or a breakdown of a key aspect of the system.

Minor non-compliance

A single and occasional instance of a failure to comply with the quality system.

Method

A prescribed way of doing things.

Metric

A value obtained by theoretical or empirical means in order to determine the norm for a particular operation.

Malfunction

Any occurrence of unsatisfactory performance.

Manufacturability

The measure of the design's ability to consistently satisfy product goals, while being profitable.

Mean time between failure (MTBF)

A basic measure of reliability for repairable items.

Mean time to failure (MTTF)

A basic measure of maintainability.

Mean time to repair (MTTR)

The sum of repair times divided by the total number of failures, during a particular interval of time, under stated conditions.

Minimum life

The time of occurrence of the first failure of a device.

Module

A replaceable combination of assemblies, subassemblies, and parts common to one mounting.

Non-compliance

The non-fulfillment of specified requirements.

Objective evidence

Qualitative or quantitative information, records, or statements of fact pertaining to the quality of an item or service or to the existence and the implementation of a quality system element, which is based on observation, measurement, or test, and which can be verified.

Observation

A record of an observed fact which may or may not be regarded as a non-compliance.

Parameter

A quantity to which the operator may assign arbitrary values, as distinguished from a variable, which can assume only those values that the form of the function makes possible.

Parsing

The technique of marking system or subsystem requirements with specified attributes in order to sort the requirements according to one or more of the attributes.

Performance standards

Published instructions and requirements setting forth the procedures, methods, and techniques for measuring the designed performance of equipments or systems in terms of the main number of essential technical measurements required for a specified operational capacity.

Phase

A defined segment of work.

Population

The total collection of units being considered.

Precision

The degree to which repeated observations of a class of measurements conform to themselves.

Predicted

That which is expected at some future time, postulated on analysis of past experience and tests.

Preventive maintenance

All actions performed in an attempt to retain an item in specified condition by providing systematic inspection, detection, and prevention of incipient failures.

Probability

A measure of the likelihood of any particular event occurring.

Probability distribution

A mathematical model which represents the probabilities for all of the possible values a given discrete random variable may take.

Procedures

Documents that explain the responsibilities and authorities related to particular tasks, indicate the methods and tools to be used, and may include copies of, or reference to, software facilities or paper forms.

Product

Operating system or application software including associated documentation, specifications, user guides, etc.

Program

The program of events during an audit.

Prototype

A model suitable for use in complete evaluation of form, design, and performance.

Purchaser

The recipient of products or services delivered by the supplier.

Qualification

The entire process by which products are obtained from manufacturers or distributors, examined and tested, and then identified on a qualified products list.

Quality

The totality of features or characteristics of a product or service that bear on its ability to satisfy stated or implied needs.

Quality assurance

All those planned and systematic actions necessary to provide adequate confidence that a product or service will satisfy given requirements for quality.

Quality audit

A systematic and independent examination to determine whether quality activities and related results comply with planned arrangements and whether these arrangements are implemented effectively and are suitable to achieve objectives.

Quality control

The operational techniques and activities that are used to fulfill requirements for quality.

Quality management

That aspect of the overall management function that determines and implements quality policy.

A technique covering Quality Assurance and Quality Control aimed at ensuring defect free products.

Quality policy

The overall intention and direction of an organization regarding quality as formally expressed by top management.

Management's declared targets and approach to the achievement of quality.

Quality system

The organizational structure, responsibilities, procedures, processes, and resources for implementing quality management.

Record

Provides objective evidence that the Quality System has been effectively implemented.

A piece of evidence that is *not* subject to change.

Redundancy

Duplication, or the use of more than one means of performing a function in order to prevent an overall failure in the event that all but one of the means fails.

Regression analysis

The fitting of a curve or equation to data in order to define the functional relationship between two or more correlated variables.

Reliability

The probability that a device will perform a required function, under specified conditions, for a specified period of time.

Reliability goal

The desired reliability for the device.

Reliability growth

The improvement a reliability parameter caused by the successful correction of deficiencies in item design or manufacture.

Repair

All actions performed as a result of failure, to restore an item to a specified condition.

Review

An evaluation of software elements or project status to ascertain discrepancies from planned results and to recommend improvement.

Review meeting

A meeting at which a work product or a set of work products are presented to project personnel, managers, users, customers, or other interested parties for comment or approval.

Revision

Any change to an original document which requires the revision level to be advanced.

Risk

The probability of making an incorrect decision.

Safety factor

The margin of safety designed into the application of an item to insure that it will function properly.

Schedule

The dates on which the audit is planned to happen.

Screening

A process of inspecting items to remove those that are unsatisfactory or those likely to exhibit early failure.

Service level agreement

Defines the service to be provided and the parameters within which the service provider is contracted to service.

Shelf life

The length of time an item can be stored under specified conditions and still meet specified requirements.

Simulation

A set of test conditions designed to duplicate field operating and usage environments as closely as possible.

Single point failure

The failure of an item which would result in failure of the system and is not compensated for by redundancy or alternative operational procedures.

Software

A combination of associated computer instructions and computer data definitions required to enable the computer hardware to perform computational or control functions.

Software design description

A representation of a software system created to facilitate analysis, planning, implementation, and decision making.

A blueprint or model of the software system.

Source code

The code in which a software program is prepared.

Specification

A document which describes the essential technical requirements for items, material, or services.

Standards

Documents that state very specific requirements in terms of appearance, formal and exact methods to be followed in all relevant cases.

Standard deviation

A statistical measure of dispersion in a distribution.

Standby redundancy

That redundancy wherein the alternative means of performing the function is not operating until it is activated upon failure of the primary means of performing the function.

Sub-contractor

The organization which provides products or services to the supplier.

Supplier

The organization responsible for replication and issue of product.

The organization to which the requirements of the relevant parts of an ISO 9000 standard apply.

System

A group of equipments, including any required operator functions, which are integrated to perform a related operation.

System compatibility

The ability of the equipments within a system to work together to perform the intended mission of the system.

Testing

The process of executing hardware or software to find errors.

A procedure or action taken to determine, under real or simulated conditions, the capabilities, limitations, characteristics, effectiveness, reliability, and suitability of a material, device, or method.

Tolerance

The total permissible deviation of a measurement from a designated value.

Tool

The mechanization of the method or procedure.

Total quality

A business philosophy involving everyone for continuously improving an organization's performance.

Traceability

The ability to track requirements from the original specification to code and test.

Trade-off

The lessening of some desirable factor(s) in exchange for an increase in one or more other factors to maximize a system's effectiveness.

Useful life period

The period of equipment life following the infant mortality period, during which the equipment failure rate remains constant.

Validation

The process of evaluating a product to ensure compliance with specified and implied requirements.

Variable

A quantity that may assume a number of values.

Variance

A statistical measure of the dispersion in a distribution.

Variant

An instance of an item created to satisfy a particular requirement.

Verification

The process of evaluating the products of a given phase to ensure correctness and consistency with respect to the products and standards provided as input to that phase.

Version

An instance of an item or variant created at a particular time.

Wearout

The process which results in an increase in the failure rate or probability of failure with increasing number of life units.

Wearout failure period

The period of equipment life following the normal failure period, during which the equipment failure rate increases above the normal rate.

Work instructions

Documents that describe how to perform specific tasks and are generally only required for complex tasks which cannot be adequately described by a single sentence or paragraph with a procedure.

Worst case analysis

A type of circuit analysis that determines the worst possible effect on the output parameters by changes in the values of circuit elements. The circuit elements are set at the values within their anticipated ranges which produce the maximum detrimental output changes.

Index